# CARING FOR THE DYING PATIENT AND THE FAMILY

**Second edition**

# CARING FOR THE DYING PATIENT AND THE FAMILY

**Second edition**

Edited by Joy Robbins

**Harper & Row, Publishers**
London

Philadelphia
New York
St. Louis
Sydney

San Francisco
London
Singapore
Tokyo

Harper & Row Ltd.
Middlesex House
34–42 Cleveland Street
London
W1P 5FB



Care of the dying patient and family.—
2nd ed.
1. Terminally ill patients. Care
I. Robbins, Joy
362.1′75

ISBN 0–06–318433–8

Typeset by J&L Composition Ltd, Filey, North Yorkshire
Printed and bound by The Alden Press, Oxford

# Contents

# Preface

This second edition has revised and expanded the content of the previous book. Much remains as valid as it was five years ago, but more recent trends have been emphasized. There is further information on the culture and beliefs of the main religious groups in the UK, especially those of ethnic minorities. A new chapter is included on care of the dying patient with AIDS. The important role of the physiotherapist is recognized by devoting a separate chapter to the subject. The chapter on creative activities includes the developing use of poetry-writing. A number of care studies have been incorporated, for example, of the dying child as a means of drawing together the many facets of care discussed. As in the previous edition, the essential place of the patient's family is a continuing thread, rightly appearing in every chapter.

It is hoped that this new edition will be useful to all trained nurses, particularly to those who aim to specialize in the field of terminal care, and who therefore need to teach and to guide student nurses and various members of staff. They will find references on every topic presented in the book, enabling the widening of knowledge and expertise by further reading. This indicates that no one book can give equal emphasis to all aspects of care, or do perfect justice to any. It is hoped that colleges of nursing will wish to include the book in the library for student nurses, and that it will be of interest to members of other professions. The philosophy of terminal care as a team endeavour continues to be the main thrust of the book. Readers will therefore find that many important principles of care are reiterated in more than one chapter with, of course, the emphasis varying according to the role of the contributor.

# Acknowledgements

I am greatly indebted in the preparation of this second edition to Helen Collyer who gave me considerable help and support. Thanks are also due to Sister Joan, Matron of St Joseph's Hospice, Doctor James Hanratty, Medical Director of St Joseph's Hospice and Jean Pegg, Senior Tutor, for their encouragement and advice. A number of people assisted with secretarial work, especially Joan Fitzgerald. I also wish to acknowledge the help and advice of Griselda Campbell, Editor, Harper & Row, publishers. In expressing thanks to these and others not mentioned, I end last and not least with the contributors who expended time and effort in producing the final project. This statement of acknowledgements can suitably end as in the first edition: one is mindful of uncounted numbers of dying patients and their families in whom those who wrote this book found their inspiration.

**Note:** All Royalties from sale of this book will go to St Joseph's Hospice.

# List of Contributors

Sister Marcella Cassells, RGN
Ward Sister, St Joseph's Hospice, London

John W. Collins, MB ChB DRCOG MRCGP
General Practitioner, Wapping, London. Honorary Lecturer in Department of General Practice and Primary Care, St Bartholomew's and The London Hospital Medical College

Helen Collyer, MBE RGN SCM RNT
Bereavement Counsellor, St Christopher's Hospice

Harriet Copperman, RGN SCM NDNCert
Nursing Director, Home Care Service, North London Hospice Group

Mother Frances Dominica, RGN RSCN FRCN
Director, Helen House, Oxford

Sister Catherine Egan, RGN
Ward Sister, St Joseph's Hospice, London

Jane Eisenhaur, BA Hons
Research Associate, St Joseph's Hospice, London

Christine Fox, RGN
Staff Nurse, St Joseph's Hospice, London

Sister Paula Gleeson, RGN
St Vincent's Hospital, Dublin (formerly Matron, St Joseph's Hospice)

James Hanratty, OBE MB ChB MRCGP
Medical Director, St Joseph's Hospice, London

Marion Judd, MNZSP SPR
Community Physiotherapist, Islington, London

Margaret Linton, RGN SCM
Midwifery Tutor, City and Hackney Health District, London

Elizabeth Loughlin, RGN OND
Sister, Home Support Team, St Mary's Hospital, Paddington, London

Reverend Leonard A. Lunn
Chaplain, St Christopher's Hospice, London

Sister Helena Marie McGilly, RGN SCM DNCert
Ward Sister, St Andrew's Hospice, Airdre, Scotland

Sister Finbarr Malone, RGN
Administrator, St Margaret's Hospice, Clydebank, Scotland

Reverend David Morrell
Chaplain, Rowcroft, Torbay and South Devon Hospice

Beryl Munns, MSc BA RGN SCM QN HVCert
Nurse Researcher (formerly St Joseph's Hospice)

Sister Anthonia O'Connor, RGN
Linden Convalescent Home, Dublin

Father Tom O'Connor
Resident Chaplain, St Joseph's Hospice, London

Jennie Pardoe, MA CQSW
Director, Care and Counselling, St Mary Magdalene's Church, Holloway Road, London

Joy Robbins, BA RGN SCM RNT
Lecturer, North Herts. Hospice Care Association (formerly Senior Tutor, St Joseph's Hospice, London)

Bernadette Ross, RGN
Deputy Ward Sister, St Joseph's Hospice, London

Barbara Saunders, RGN RCNT
Director, Home Care Service, St Christopher's Hospice, London

Sister Mary Wynne
Sister-in-Charge, Recreational and Day Centre, St Joseph's Hospice, London

**Note:** The title Sister denotes members of the Sisters of Charity.

# 1. Attitudes to Death and Dying

In his monumental study of attitudes to death, spanning a thousand years, Philippe Aries (1981) reminds us that changes in attitudes to this basic human condition either take place very slowly or else occur between long periods of immobility. He took as the beginning of his study the early Middle Ages but makes the point that many of the phenomena occurring then were part of a chain of traditions going back to early antiquity and indeed to the dawn of history. In attempting to understand attitudes at the end of the twentieth century, the whole pattern of present-day society, its beliefs, way of life and all that influences it must be taken into account. This situation is no different from that of preceding centuries, and explains why in some respects attitudes become so startlingly different as society itself changes–sometimes rapidly and at other times over a long period.

## AGE AT WHICH PEOPLE DIE

Although there are no systematic data available, it is known that about 200 years ago most people died at what would now be regarded as the prime of life, or in infancy when the death rates were particularly high. By 1840 the population in most European countries had a life expectancy of 40-plus years; by 1930 this was 60-plus years and by 1950 it had risen to 70-plus years. In 1989 men could expect to live to about 71 years and women to 77 years.

The dramatic change in this century (the infant mortality rate has fallen remarkably) arose mainly because of overall improvement in living standards – better housing, sanitation and agricultural methods resulting in more food being available. The rapid advances in twentieth-century medicine further reduced the mortality rate. Thus an environment of 'controlled mortality' now prevails, and this has produced a very different life-style from that in previous centuries. Family size is smaller, by choice, and great emotional and financial resources are invested in the children because they, like their parents, are expected to have a long life. More time is devoted to formal education and much energy and money is devoted to research and therapy aimed at curing disease and further extending life. The remoteness of death diminishes the orientation towards religious explanations of the ultimate end.

The technological revolution in the West has made available at all levels of social class an array of consumer durables undreamt of by a generation only a few decades away. This is linked to economic recovery since the Second World War. In Britain 63 per cent of homes are now owner-occupied, and the quality of homes is better. Of households, 97 per cent have a bath or shower, 69 per cent have central heating and 98 per cent have a television set. This is not to hide the fact that many people are relatively poor, but compared to poverty between the two world wars, and thus within living memory, even in the poorest section of today's society life is definitely more affluent. Consumerism is visible on all sides, and it produces its own pressures in persuading people to aspire to ever-higher standards of living. In the midst of so much plenty and comparative ease, death no longer hovers over the horizon due to lack of basic needs – food, shelter and water. When television and newspaper pictures force Western audiences to witness scenes of famine-ridden people in far-off lands, a feeling of shocked unbelief prevails that human beings can actually die of starvation.

## CAUSES AND LOCATION OF DEATH

In Western society the main causes of death are degenerative diseases, particularly of the cardiovascular system, malignant diseases and accidents. This last category leads to the fact that in our present century, unnatural forms of death have increased dramatically, including homicide, self-destruction and road-traffic accidents.

Regrettably, human beings have always killed each other, but it is the sheer size of the phenomenon that is startling. Apart from the two world wars, the Nazi gas chambers (killing 6 million Jews and other 'undesirables'), the explosion of the atom bombs at Hiroshima, and international terrorism are global reminders of the contemporary face of death. The tensions of modern life have contributed to the marked rise in suicides in developing countries. Yet Western society now finds public execution revolting and, indeed, in the main has rejected imposition of the death penalty for serious crime. Such are the complex issues present in the development of cultural attitudes.

Whereas in the past most people died at home, a shift has occurred in this century, removing death from the home into an institution. About 60 per cent of deaths in this country occur in general hospitals. This tends to isolate further the dying person from the rest of society, and the fact of death as a natural part of everyday life. More people grow up from childhood to maturity without witnessing the natural death of a close relative, although paradoxically much entertainment for adults and children concerns killings.

Apart from entertainment, violence is perceived to be an increasing part of modern society, including violent death. Not only is this present in various armed conflicts around the world but also in acts of terrorism on our own doorsteps, civil riots and deaths caused by drunken drivers. In fact, since aggression is an innate human instinct, violence has never been completely absent from any society. Today, the ease of travel and communications make it instantly present to large numbers of people.

## COMMUNICATING THE FACTS OF DEATH AND DYING

In trying to assess attitudes in communications about the subject, it would seem that today there are two distinct levels – the public and the private. With the high profile of journalism, and almost universal literacy, people can read daily accounts of sudden death and accounts of well-known people who have died as a result of natural causes. Television and radio not only report the more horrifying aspects of death and dying but increasingly offer serious programmes discussing death, dying and bereavement as natural events and with first-hand experiences sensitively presented. There have been, for instance, notable programmes on stillbirth and the more enlightened attitudes towards bereaved parents in maternity hospitals. That such programmes are well-received and arouse considerable interest is a positive step towards promoting healthy attitudes among the public.

At the private level, a different picture emerges. Society does not encourage individuals to talk openly about death in a personal way. Sarah Boston (1987) describes her experiences when interviewing people in connection with a television series, *Merely Mortal*. Those with a professional interest, e.g. counsellors, undertakers, stonemasons (mainly men), could only discuss death with ease from a professional standpoint; the subject was quickly changed if there was any direct move to a discussion of attitudes towards their own deaths.

This inhibition was less pronounced among the women interviewed, but in general there was a reticence to talk about death. This had an element of fear, and to talk about one's own death was considered morbid. It is interesting that in choosing a title for the programme it was decided that the word 'death' would turn the viewing public off:

> Our British embarrassment, our view that death is a private matter and our silence are peculiar to our culture and century. Although other societies have used a variety of words, secular and sacred to talk of death, they have all talked. We have not in the twentieth century been able to avoid the subject completely but what we have done is to develop a new and evasive language.
>
> (Boston, 1987, p. 14)

## GRIEF AND MOURNING

Grief and mourning are not new, but attitudes change with societies. People need to grieve in their own way, and to be reassured that the common physical reactions so comprehensively described by Colin Murray Parkes (1986) are normal and will pass, however painful. Most people's grief does not need to be treated as a psychiatric disorder (although it may lead to this) but needs to be recognized and the bereaved person supported. Unfortunately, overt manifestations of grief such as weeping are often felt to be embarrassing and should be done in private. This can increase the isolation and loneliness that adds to the pain. One positive modern advance is that bereaved people themselves have come to realize that they can help each other to work through their grief, and self-help groups have increased with the assistance of such organizations as CRUSE and the Society of Compassionate Friends (for parents whose child has died).

One problem for bereaved people in Western society is that there are no parameters set for the mourning period as in other cultures, and other centuries in our own society. Special mourning clothes are rare so that there is no outward sign that the person is in mourning. After the funeral, there is no recognizable time set aside, and it may be assumed that the bereaved person should now be over their grief and behave as though nothing has happened. In fact, people who are employed may be allowed a week's compassionate leave, which is certainly setting a time, but it bears no relation to the length and extent of their deep grief. Another factor missing in urban society is the sense of a close community, even in the road in which one lives. Knowing the next-door neighbour sufficiently to pass the time of day, and hardly knowing the names of others in the road, is not uncommon. A dying person is more likely to end his or her days away from home, to go straight to the undertaker's chapel of rest and thence to the funeral and cemetery. Funeral cars travel fairly quickly through the streets with scarcely a passing glance from passers-by. The one surviving ritual of mourning that is almost universally observed is the refreshments after the funeral, usually taken in the home of one of the family members. This still achieves, to some degree, the comfort for the mourners as described in the autobiographical account of country life at the end of the last century, *Lark Rise to Candleford* (Thompson, 1973, p. 489).

> The return of the mourners after the final parting and their immediate outbursts of grief. Then, as they grew calmer the gentle persuasion of those less afflicted that the widow or widower or the bereaved parents, for the sake of the living still left to them, should take a little nourishment. Then their gradual revival as they ate and drank. Tears would still be wiped away furtively but a few sad smiles would break through until, at the table, a sober cheerfulness would prevail. They had, as they told themselves and others told them, to go on living, and what greater restorative have we poor mortals than a good meal in the company of loving friends?

## ATTITUDES OF DYING PEOPLE

When a person is actually dying many thoughts and emotions may occupy the mind. The nature of those is well recognized and documented; it should be realized that every human being will react differently and emotions will often be mingled and change from one extreme to the other quite frequently if dying is gradual. Elizabeth Kubler-Ross (1970 and 1982) has by her research provided a major contribution in this field.

The following emotions will be witnessed in dying patients but not necessarily in any particular order or all in one person.

## Anxiety and fear

The instinctive fear of approaching dissolution may be observed if the patient suspects that his or her illness is a fatal one, and has not been able to come to terms with it. The facial expression will be anxious and restlessness and tension will be apparent. On the other hand, patients may conceal their fears, perhaps because they cannot face them, or because they find that no opportunity is given to discuss them with a sympathetic listener. Some of the sources of the fears may be tangible, such as possible effects of their disease. For instance, a patient with malignant growth in the thorax may fear that he or she will suffocate. The patient who is aware of increasing girth and discomfort from an abdominal mass may have a vivid picture of bursting open. A husband or wife may be very anxious about the welfare – financial and otherwise – of the spouse and any children who will be left alone after the death. Patients may be frightened of being left alone, or of dying alone whilst asleep.

## Depression and sadness

These are very understandable reactions in a patient who has had a long illness with possible painful and protracted treatment, particularly for cancer. In the terminal stages of his or her illness, and with increasing sensations of weakness, he or she may feel that all the endurance of such treatment was futile. Anger and resentment – 'Why me?' – may merge with depression, and if a sense of withdrawal by relatives and staff unable to cope with their own painful emotion is added, the patient may well find the situation intolerable. Inadequate relief of symptoms is itself an important cause of misery and depression. These facts should lead nurses and doctors to reflect seriously on their responsibilities and practice in the care of dying patients.

## Denial and acceptance

Considerable research has taken place into the insight of dying patients about their true condition and prognosis, and those with experience will testify how difficult it is in many cases to be sure of what the patient understands and believes. It is generally accepted among those working closely with dying patients that the patient's right to indicate whether he or she wishes to discuss his or her illness in depth or not must be respected. A number of research projects, such as those undertaken by Elizabeth Kubler-Ross (1970 and 1982), show that many patients do realize that they are dying, through their own intuition. Sometimes a patient may have requested a frank discussion and have apparently understood that his or her life-span is expected to be a short one. Other emotions may then intervene, such as hope that the doctor may be mistaken – the patient practising a denial of the information given, as a defence mechanism. Younger patients may go through a distressing phase of struggling against the inevitable outcome, with bitterness and resentment.

Fortunately, most dying patients become peaceful and calm during their last few hours, many during the final weeks, providing that sufficient help has been given in total care, that is, physical, mental, social and spiritual.

# THE PATIENT AND THE FAMILY

While there is still some uncertainty whether a person's illness, although grave, is a mortal one, the patient or more likely the family may search frantically for a cure, seeking further opinions from more than one doctor or trying unorthodox forms of healing. Those with a religious faith will pray earnestly for a cure, and may take the patient to a shrine such as Lourdes. The professional team should respect these actions, and when there is final realization and acceptance of approaching death, the family is often comforted by the thought that they have done all they could for their loved one in an effort to preserve his or her life.

Some people may struggle against their inevitable progress towards death until the very end, and it will be distressing for those caring for such patients to witness their fear and lack of peace. John Hinton in his book *Dying* (1972) suggests that the person in this condition may need the hope and refusal to surrender, rather than the desolation of no hope at all.

In contrast, a peaceful acceptance of death is common among the elderly, who may find particular comfort in the continuity of their family life in their children and grandchildren. For those who have made careful preparation for death in the matter of their personal affairs, this in itself can give an emotional satisfaction and relaxation.

The relevance of religious belief to dying people is, of course, important. A research study into a group of dying patients (Hinton, 1972) revealed that those who had a firm religious faith were the most free from anxiety. Those who maintained that they had no religious beliefs also appeared calm during their last illness. The group who showed most anxiety were those who were uncertain and wavering in their belief in and practice of a religious faith.

One attitude of close relatives that, though understandable, will cause sadness to the dying person is an emotional withdrawal at the very time when he or she most needs companionship and understanding from those he or she loves. This situation may be due to embarrassment as to how to behave or what to say, or to an increasing sense of grief at the impending separation, which the relative feels unable to share with the dying person.

Close relatives often exhibit some or all of the emotional stages through which the dying person is passing. The sense of loss begins before the actual death and anticipatory grief will be experienced as part of bereavement.

## ATTITUDES OF THE NURSE

Since attitudes are related to behaviour, it is important that the nurse who will care for dying patients and their families recognizes the effect of his or her personal thoughts and feelings about death – his or her own and other people's. Nurses, like doctors, are sometimes placed on a pedestal and expected to show supernatural qualities of strength and equability in any situation. They may themselves suppress their own fears and anxieties by erecting barriers in their professional work, allowing only a superficial interaction with their patients – a 'them' and 'us' relationship. Acknowledging a common humanity, which includes at times feelings of inadequacy and anxiety, and talking over problems with colleagues, is a sign of growth not weakness.

The student nurse is usually young and, like his or her contemporaries, has quite probably never met death and dying at first hand before. Unlike his or her friends entering other professional trainings or various forms of employment, he or she must face the sure prospect of intimate contact with dying people, of witnessing the anguish of families facing the loss of a loved one, and of providing the physical care to the dead body before this is relinquished to the funeral director. It is understandable if the anticipation of these responsibilities may cause some apprehension. Most nurses remember clearly when they first looked upon the face of a dead person and found with relief that the sight was peaceful and not frightening.

Attitudes of respect in handling the body and carrying out Last Offices are well-established at an early stage of training and passed on to junior colleagues by precept and example. Few nurses appear to have lasting difficulties in this sphere, although this refers to death from natural causes, at home or in hospital. The sight and handling of mutilated bodies in war or from major accidents will inevitably be unpleasant and emotionally difficult to manage.

It is in the area of communication with dying patients and grieving relatives that difficulties often occur for the nurse in trying to acquire attitudes that will be of maximum help. It is encouraging to remember that actions speak louder than words, and the nurse who demonstrates gentle, effective physical care for the patient, given in an unhurried manner, or simple courtesy and concern for a tired and anxious relative is communicating a positive and caring attitude. To be prepared to listen with whole-hearted attention and to respond to the best of one's ability, offering to bring a more experienced colleague to continue the dialogue if appropriate, is to give a valuable service. The ability to convey a warm, positive attitude is an important attribute and helps to surround the patient with a natural, pleasant atmosphere without false brightness and over-optimism.

Possession of a religious faith, or a stable philosophy about the fundamental issues of life and death, helps to provide an inner strength for the nurse which in turn aids his or her in caring for patients and families in distress.

Nurses themselves may have suffered a bereavement and thus have insight into the feelings of a grieving family. Even if they have never lost a close member of their own family, many forms of loss, e.g. loss of self-esteem or a valued possession, or a broken engagement, mirror in some degree the pain of actual bereavement. Reflecting on such experiences can assist in developing helpful attitudes to bereaved relatives, when shared with experienced colleagues.

Death itself is a mystery and one has no personal point of reference, i.e. personal experience. Unfortunately, lack of understanding and avoidance of facing the problem has meant that for many years the fears and loneliness associated with dying have not been openly considered and helped sufficiently by those professional groups, including nurses, who are in the best position to do so. This situation is gradually changing for the better, and continuing education in these matters for all concerned is spreading. By learning from observing more experienced colleagues, by reading from the considerable literature now available, and by overcoming any tendency to avoid dying patients because of painful and inadequate feelings in ourselves, we can demonstrate a more confident attitude to the dying patient in our efforts to make his or her dying comfortable in body, mind and spirit.

## IS THERE LIFE AFTER DEATH?

In previous centuries this question would not have been publicly raised. Archaeologists have provided irrefutable evidence from antiquity that the dead were provided with articles of everyday living to sustain them on their journey to the next life. Written and oral traditions from every part of the world reinforce this fundamental belief although the perceived nature of the after-life varies greatly. European history, with its Christian roots as a major influence, has consistently shown a belief in the due-course resurrection of the body and the immortality of the soul. Death is thus seen as only a gateway to eternal life.

The awesome advances in scientific knowledge and the decline in universal religious practice and belief in the twentieth century have produced a major change from the past in formulating attitudes to the leading question, is there life after death? In dealing with such a complex issue, it is only possible here to summarize the situation that can be found in the UK. There appear to be three types of attitudes:

(1) A firm belief in an after-life among those who practise a particular religious faith with a full acceptance of all its tenets. The exact nature of this after-life is recognized by many to be unclear.
(2) An open mind on the subject, not ruling out the possibility but with no definite conviction. Some people in this group may be nominally Christian and in facing their own death when the time comes may seek help in sorting out their attitudes. Others remain agnostic till the end.
(3) Those who are quite clear that for them death is the absolute end of human existence, except for the memories that people leave behind of themselves.

Because these different standpoints may change throughout a person's life, including the last days, there is no exactitude about proportions of people holding a certain attitude at any one time. There is increasing interest in connection with this matter in what is known as *near-death experience*.

Records show that more people than ever are returning from the threshold of death due to the advances in medical technology. Examples are resuscitation of a patient in cardiac arrest, and emergency treatment of one becoming rapidly moribund through a massive haemorrhage. During these moments of suspended animation, extraordinary experiences have been recounted by certain people following the type of crisis described. Thousands of people have been interviewed by a number of doctors and the results published. There is a recurring pattern of events including the following.

All patients felt that they were losing consciousness and this indeed seemed to be the case according to onlookers. A common sensation was that the patients felt themselves entering a black void or tunnel, through which they floated towards a brilliant light that did not hurt their eyes. After a momentary fear reported by some, the experience was very peaceful and happy; many said that they did not want it to end. Some described entering a pastoral scene of great beauty, and seeing deceased relatives or figures that had a religious connotation. All described their situation as if it had happened outside their physical body. A frequent description was that 'they' – a conscious non-material identity – floated above their physical body, which they could see on the bed or operating table below them, and were later able to describe minute details of resuscitation procedures that were confirmed by their attendants as completely accurate.

In 1982 an American cardiologist and professor of medicine published results of a five-year research study conducted under rigorous scientific methods. Having been extremely sceptical at the onset of his research he finally concluded that no complete explanation is possible on a purely-physical plane: 'It is here, at the point of near-death that scientific facts and theories interface with religious doctrines and speculations' (Sabom, 1982, p. 186). Doctor Peter Fenwick, clinical neurophysiologist at St Thomas's Hospital, London, is currently studying the phenomena from the viewpoint of the science of human consciousness. He believes that although various theories may be proved correct in explaining some of the experiences attested, there still remain questions to be answered as to why they happen to certain people, and as to the significance of the whole mystery. He suggests that one scientific answer may be that in every person's brain there is a special encoded function that prepares one for death – either to oblivion or to a new life, according to one's beliefs. If the trigger is pulled prematurely, the person returns to the state called consciousness to resume living again. It is evident that there is still much to learn about consciousness, and science has, as yet, still no satisfactory explanation. A final interesting fact is that those who have undergone a near-death experience find that their attitudes to life and death are altered in a profound way.

## REFERENCES AND FURTHER READING

Aries, P. (1981) *The House of our Death*, Allen Lane, London.
Boston, S. and Trezise, R. (1987) *Merely Mortal*, Methuen, London, in association with Channel 4 Television Company Ltd.
Central Office of Information (1988) *Britain Today*, HMSO, London.
Hinton, J. (1972) *Dying*, Pelican, Harmondsworth.
Kubler-Ross, E. (1970) *On Death and Dying*, Tavistock, London.
Kubler-Ross, E. (1975) *Death, the Final Stage of Growth*, Prentice-Hall, Inc. Englewood Cliffs, N.J.
Kubler-Ross, E. (1982) *Living with Death and Dying*, Macmillan, London.
Office of Health Economics (1984) *Compendium of Health Statistics*, HMSO, London.
Parkes, C. Murray (1986) *Bereavement*, Penguin, Harmondsworth.
Sabom, M. B. (1982) *Recollections of Death*, Harper & Row, New York.
Thompson, F. (1973) *Lark Rise to Candleford*, Penguin, Harmondsworth.

## ACKNOWLEDGEMENT

I would like to express my thanks to Doctor Peter Fenwick for help with the section on near-death experience.

# 2. Communications with Patient and Family

'Communication is so important with people like us; if you can get through to someone it automatically lifts the fear.' This view was expressed by Mrs Jones shortly before she died. She had been ill for a long time, was aware of her prognosis and had experienced pain and fear. Her understanding of the concept of communication was comprehensive, in that she saw it as part of all human interaction, and as including not only words, but tone, gesture, touch, sound and the use of many symbols. Mrs Jones realized too that if communication was to be meaningful then those at both ends of the communication channel needed to be able to understand each other and to be competent and willing in their interaction.

Since there are so many elements involved it is not surprising that effective communication is difficult to achieve. Misunderstanding is a common experience in everyday life. This situation cannot be afforded in nursing, when the welfare of patients is at stake, and no field is more important in this respect than that of the care of dying patients. Here good care depends to a great extent on really efficient communication between nurse, patient and the family, and within the whole health-care team. Yet it is just in this area of care that communication difficulties or barriers arise to make achievement that much harder.

This chapter discusses these extra barriers, whilst recommending a general study of human interaction, on which subject several books have been written. It then examines some of the messages that are communicated to patients and their families and the means by which they are conveyed.

# BARRIERS ON THE NURSE'S SIDE

Several barriers can arise on the nurse's side. They stem from attitudes and values that are not entirely negative in themselves but suited more to one situation than another, and which may hinder communication in the care of the dying. The nurse acquires these attitudes during his or her socialization as a member of society and during his or her professional training and experience.

## Society's barriers

In the twentieth century members of Western societies are not well prepared to consider death and dying, except in an impersonal way as presented by the media. In previous eras the frequency of death in early life meant that dying was not divorced from everyday family awareness, and religious teaching often centred round this theme. Therefore, people learned to accept the end of life as well as the beginning.

Today people are healthier and live longer; greater population mobility splits the extended family so that there is less contact with the older family members. It is, therefore, possible to reach adulthood having had little association with death or bereavement. The result is that the very natural fear of death becomes enlarged and unacceptable. People become embarrassed in the presence of the terminally-ill patient and his or her family. A barrier of defence is set up and the coping method chosen is one of avoidance whenever decently possible.

## The barrier of the value given to cure

Over the past years there have been many wonderful advances in medicine and so it is often possible to think in terms of cure. Other discoveries mean that the ultimate – prevention – may now be achieved. Consequently there is great emphasis on prevention and cure. Indeed, research has found that many persons enter the health-care professions motivated by the goal of cure. When this is no longer possible, there is frequently then a deep sense of failure.

It is unrealistic, however, to think in terms of cure for large numbers of patients who are chronically sick, or in the terminal stages of disease. The problem is that with the sense of failure there is often the feeling that no clear or worthwhile goal is left. This seems somewhat strange in nursing, which is a caring rather than curing profession, but this attitude contributes to the embarrassment some nurses feel with dying patients, which they meet by cutting down the time spent in patient contact.

The answer to this situation is the recognition that new and more appropriate goals may be adopted, which can bring great comfort to patients and their families, and these will be discussed later in this chapter. When these goals are met, the aimless feeling need no longer cloud the view of those working with patients for whom cure is no longer possible.

## The barrier of stereotype

The system of viewing patients within diagnostic categories has developed over the years. It is useful in that specialization brings greater skills to care and this labelling provides a form of shorthand for indicating the types of observations, precautions and treatment needed. It provides little understanding, however, of persons as individuals. The effect may be negative in that when another form of label is applied – that of 'dying' – all the inhibitions surrounding the subject become attached to the patient.

It is often necessary to recognize, of course, that a terminal stage of illness has been reached, but this knowledge should not diminish the view of the patient as an individual. John, policeman, husband, father of four, supporter of widowed mother, athlete, reader of thrillers need not become John, dying, needs to be kept comfortable. Whilst John remains within himself much the same, or perhaps a little enlarged because his situation has given him the opportunity to explore his feelings or develop an interest that he has not had time for before, professionals can see him as diminished. If communications are based on the narrower view then the goals of care lack imagination. This situation calls for correction of view based on sensitive personal communications with John and his family.

## The barrier of activity

There are many reasons for an emphasis on physical activity. Nursing uses a variety of practical skills and the importance given to rules of procedure is necessary to ensure safe practice. Staff shortage over the years has meant that nurses have considered it necessary to give priority to essential practical tasks such as making beds. It is not surprising therefore that nursing has often been task oriented and that nurses tend to feel guilty when 'just' quietly sitting, talking to a patient.

Today, through the nursing process, we are beginning to use in a systematic way the knowledge that has been intuitively felt for years, namely that good nursing care can only result from an understanding of the patient as a whole person in a social situation. This knowledge must be obtained through good communication with the patient, his or her family and with other professional people who now share his or her support or who have been involved with him or her in the past.

Sometimes it is necessary to be still, to listen, and to share with the patient, at other times a quality of listening and responsiveness whilst undertaking the practical task will be sufficient. However achieved, meaningful communication is vitally important in the care of dying patients where there is a battle with fear, anxiety and physical symptoms such as pain and nausea. These cannot always be separated from each other. The sharing of fear may of itself reduce tension and relieve pain or point the way to some new beneficial approach. Therefore the value placed on practical activity should not be allowed to bar communication, which could meet the need more efficiently than a multiplicity of tasks.

## The barrier of the value of secrecy

This value can create a great barrier between nurse and patient, for nurses are often placed in a very difficult position when they are aware that the patient has not been told of his or her prognosis. They tend to cope with a bright and rather brusque manner, and with avoidance behaviour, to discourage awkward questions they feel they should not answer.

However, this type of reaction does convey something to patients. Mrs Smith returned from the theatre where it had been discovered that she had an inoperable carcinoma. Long before her doctor told her about this, she has correctly assessed the behaviour of the staff and knew of her situation. This meant that at that time of weakness she was presented with a fearsome knowledge without the reassurance, comfort and support that should go with it. Many patients may be in this position; a recent survey of 482 patients admitted to a hospice in a terminal condition found that over 20 per cent knew or were suspicious of their situation despite having been given no clear information on the subject. This is not to suggest that this was all due to the behaviour of professionals, but silence of staff and family played a part.

To be told the truth is, however, a traumatic experience for nearly everyone, calling for inner resources that, according to the patient's condition, may be available more at one time than another. It is therefore right that caution should be exercised as to when to tell and how much to tell and what way to tell it. A policy of many is not to force unwelcome news upon an unsuspecting and unready patient but to be very sensitive to his or her cues indicating desire for knowledge, so that his or her requirements may be met at the right time and in the right depth. Enquiring patients have a right to know. They may then be able to manage their remaining days as they wish, perhaps seeking to achieve some special goal, making arrangements for dependants or exploring spiritual issues.

The decision 'to tell' is an important one and needs to be based on sound information provided by the care team. The nurse, particularly a junior one, is often important here, for he or she has the greatest contact with the patient. Whilst he or she is caring for the patient, the patient often communicates his or her fears and poses slanted questions. These can be relayed to senior team members. The patient may ask direct questions and it can be quite natural to reflect the question back – for example, 'You seem to be concerned about . . . would you like to talk about it with someone who has more details, sister or doctor?' The request can then be passed on promptly.

The secrecy barrier means that nurse–patient communications are often surrounded by fear on both sides and become unnatural. If the nurse is prepared to meet questions rather than avoid them he or she will be less likely to convey his or her awkwardness and fear to the patient. If his or her sensitivity to the patient's cues for knowledge has enabled him or her to play a part in the patient receiving the right information, he or she may well be rewarded by seeing a release from tension on the patient's part and a greater trust in relationships. He or she will then no longer be afraid to give him- or herself to patients in meaningful communication.

## The barrier of hierarchy

Nurses have always been very conscious of hierarchies, both in the institution and within each nursing team. Channels of command help to provide an orderly setting for care but can be restrictive in that the junior members of staff, who often see most of the patient, have little influence in the decisions that are made on behalf of the patient.

This situation is not helpful in the area of terminal care where a very broad spectrum of factors is involved; those that are physical, psychosocial and spiritual. The team has to be multidisciplinary and include all the members of each discipline. Each nurse needs to value his or her potential to contribute to team knowledge and decision-making, and must be prepared to express his or her own objective professional opinion as well as to communicate the patient's feelings and wishes.

Good communications within the team, based on mutual respect, will enhance the effectiveness of care, and the resulting atmosphere of unity will be sensed by patients, who will then be encouraged to enter into trusting relationships.

## Towards breaking nurse barriers

It would be foolish to assume that long-held attitudes and fears may be instantly removed in pursuit of better nurse–patient communications, but the following suggestions may help to initiate the process.

(1) *Be gentle and patient with yourself* Those who have had long experience in the field of terminal care recognize that it takes many months, perhaps up to two years, for staff to feel comfortable and confident working with dying patients. It may become less difficult very gradually, or there may be more of a sudden breakthrough that relates to some specific experience or achievement with a patient.
(2) *Seek to understand your feelings* Sharing them with other members of the team helps, as does not being afraid to express the emotions that will arise. Are any of the barriers just discussed yours? It is difficult to come to terms with the situation of patients before one has honestly examined one's own feelings about personal mortality.
(3) *Seek to learn* as much as possible about the processes of dying. Understanding them brings the knowledge of how best to cope with patients' problems whether they be physical or emotional. Success helps to bring confidence. Many books have been written on the subject and amongst the most inspiring are the accounts of people who are facing dying. Through them we realize something of the feelings involved and, most important, that this experience can have positive as well as negative aspects. This encourages the search for extra goals that centre around quality of life.

(4) *Plan goals* Communication is rather circular in effect. We share some time with patients and begin to understand them as individuals. This knowledge helps us to look for positive goals, based on their values, and we are then able to communicate on a deeper level. Some goals are more positive than others. For example 'tender loving care' (TLC) has often been used by the health-care professions to denote the attention needed by the chronically-sick or terminally-ill patient. It suggests gentleness and compassion without which there would not be the insight to use skills. It also suggests endeavour to keep the patient as comfortable and free from unpleasant complications as possible. It does not necessarily emphasize the achievement of other and extra goals that may greatly add to the patient's quality of life.

Mrs Peters, a young patient, was struggling to finish knitting a scarf and was finding it difficult to cope with the thick wool and large needles. She could not manage to 'cast off'. A passing nurse spent a few minutes doing this for her while she explained the method. Mrs Peters' face lit up with pleasure and she said, 'I have never in all my life had a finished piece of knitting'. She went on with great enthusiasm to make another scarf and this time completed it herself. This may seem a relatively-small achievement but it added an extra quality to her last days.

Sensitive communication with patients helps the nurse, as part of a team, to provide the right environment for individuals to meet their own needs, whether they result from activity or from quiet thought. When, in a caring environment, patients are seen to renew relationships or turn from fear and bitterness to peaceful trust, the reward to the nurse is great. It heightens the awareness of the potential of communicaton in all its forms and sustains the nurse through the many difficulties he or she experiences.

## BARRIERS ON THE PATIENT'S SIDE

Patients often experience factors that make effective communication more difficult for them. These may relate to the patients' expectations of their role in the ward situation, to physical and emotional states, as well as to the environment provided for them.

### 'Taking the sick role'

'Taking the sick role' is a phrase used to describe a set of attitudes and behaviour adopted by people when they become ill, particularly when they are admitted to an institution such as a hospital. It is helpful to patients in that they are expected to opt out of the responsibilities of life and take a passive resting role, leaving large and small decisions to others. It is easy to encourage this legitimate behaviour because it assists the running of wards and is also necessary for safety. Essentially, patients relinquish their autonomy for their own welfare and that of others.

When patients are in a terminal stage of illness the situaton is somewhat different. They are not giving up in the short term for a long-term gain; the present is the only time that they have for making wide-ranging decisions for their own lives and that of others. Their state also demands that every effort be made to bring their own values of quality into their daily lives. In order for this to be achieved, patients must feel invited to communicate their thoughts and wishes. If, however, the 'sick-role' expectations are carried over from previous experiences, they will be inhibited.

Through their interest and concern for each patient as a unique individual, nurses can help patients feel free to express their feelings, so that their needs may be met, in that they may be supported in their own decision-making.

## Physical condition

However much patients may wish to communicate with those around, their ability may be limited by their physical condition. They may have a tumour of the larynx, for example. Many patients in a terminal stage of disease are elderly, as are relatives, and so they may suffer from diminished sight or hearing. Loss of any sense makes it harder in a general way to send or receive messages, since the senses depend upon each other to produce total pictures.

Meaningful communication also requires clear perception and this may be clouded where there is cerebral disturbance or the presence of various combinations of drugs. Extreme fatigue, so often experienced by dying people, lowers perception levels and limits the time available for communications. When the day is punctuated with sleep episodes it is easy to lose track of events, everything becoming somewhat blurred. In times of exhaustion patients and their hard-pressed relatives need to be freed from the compulsion towards verbal communication and reassured that a comforting, quiet presence may convey the message of love as effectively.

It is not safe to assume levels of consciousness. Long after the patient has lost the ability to communicate he or she may be receptive to touch and hearing. Mary had appeared to be unconscious for several hours and had not in the past given any indication that she was aware of her condition. A visitor stood by her bed and said to a nurse, 'Poor thing, she hasn't long to go now, has she?' Immediately a stream of tears was seen to trickle from under Mary's closed eyelids. She died shortly after. It is so important that nurses are aware of this situation and that they convey this awareness to relatives. This knowledge can then be used to good rather than bad effect when the family are able to communicate comforting words.

There is much that nurses can do when the patient's condition makes communications difficult. They may first of all encourage with real interest and patience, employing all the senses. Then there are a variety of aids ranging from the simple picture chart to the electronic. Last, when the patient appears unconscious, gentle touch and simple cheerful words may be able to continue to bring comfort and support.

## Emotional states

The days or weeks of terminal care are often ones of stress for the patient and his or her family when each is trying to come to terms with the situation. The family may be exhausted after trying to cope at home; a wife, for example, having to shoulder the care of her husband and his business responsibilities on top of her usual commitments. Even when the patient is in hospital the continual visiting is physically and emotionally tiring and disruptive of the daily routine.

In such times of stress, various defence mechanisms and reactions emerge and these affect communication. Relatives may feel numb and appear to lack any emotion, they may become depressed, or they may become angry and direct their anger on to some aspect of care. Thus a presenting problem, generating much feeling, may be not enough sugar in a patient's cup of tea, but the real problem a deep anguish and sense of guilt about not being able to cope any longer with the loved one at home. Families are in a state of anticipated bereavement; they may be extra sensitive, or the anxiety that they suffer may prevent them from absorbing information. It is sometimes necessary to repeat explanations several times.

Patients who are becoming aware of their prognosis experience various emotional states that have been defined as denial, anger, bargaining, depression and acceptance. Feelings may vary with the appearance and disappearance of symptoms; so that successful control of symptoms can lead to denial once more of the true situation. There is, therefore, often no firm basis for a communication approach, and it is necessary to be constantly observant and perceptive.

A further complexity arises from the need to understand how best to offer help. Differences in personality and background provide diverse means of expression requiring different responses; thus, the same degree of resentment might be felt by a little old lady and a young man but each would be likely to express it in a different way. One might prefer a silent empathy, the other encouragement to talk. Many people respond to gentle touch but not all. Sensitivity is needed to discern what is required.

It is not easy to cope in all circumstances and surely learning how to do so is a life-long task. When there are problems it does help if the various manifestations of feeling can be steadfastly and uncritically accepted by the nurse, who can offer a listening presence. The shared wisdom of the team can also be applied to meeting a need, and this will provide support to all concerned.

## The social environment

It is not very often that the patient's needs for communication in human interaction can be entirely met by staff and personal visitors. Patients derive much comfort from each other and from each other's visitors. Here they depend upon the perception and willingness of nurses to place them near to compatible persons.

This is often far from easy in a hospital ward, where there may be frequent admissions and discharges of those not terminally ill, or in a special unit, where deaths occur when relationships have been made and there is always the possibility of being placed with someone who is unable to communicate. The effects can be far-reaching, for example an aphasic patient may become extremely depressed if he or she is placed for long periods next to one who is unconscious. He or she could benefit from watching others who are more active, communicating with them in non-verbal ways. Similarly one who needs to talk should not constantly accompany one who lacks this ability. Compatibility with others may also have much to do with personality and life experience as well as physical ability to communicate.

It would be unrealistic to think that communication systems may be tailored closely to the needs of each patient all the time. Frequent movement may have to be balanced against the needs for stability. However, there can be a continual awareness of social-contact needs, and a review whenever there is change, with the goal of placing compatible persons together for at least part of each day.

## MESSAGES WE SEEK TO COMMUNICATE TO PATIENTS AND THEIR FAMILIES

If we had to choose one word to describe the overall content of messages to patients and their families, this could well be safety or security. We want them to know that even if cure is not possible they may feel safe in hands that are skilled to meet the needs of the present circumstances. We want them to understand that all our skills will be applied to the detection and treatment of symptoms and that through every emotional upheaval patients and their families will be accepted and supported as unique and valuable individuals. These safety messages must be clear and addressed to general and specific situations.

In general it is not easy to send clear messages even though attitudinal barriers have been overcome. There are many components of communication and clarity demands that they be in accord with one another. For example, a nurse might greet a patient, 'Good morning, Mrs Brown. How are you today?' This enquiry may be perceived in different ways by Mrs Brown depending on how she is feeling and also on how the components of the message relate to each other. There are at least five important aspects of this communication apart from the words that are spoken; tone of voice, eye contact, proximity to Mrs Brown, bodily movement of the speaker and use of pause for reply.

Mrs Brown will be helped to confide her worries if she senses genuine concern behind the question and feels the nurse wants to give of his or her time. The nurse will best convey this attitude if there is interest in his or her tone of voice, if he or she engages in eye contact, stands close enough to the bed to encourage conversation, stills his or her bodily movements that would indicate he or she might be in a hurry, and pauses to allow Mrs Brown time to reply. It would perhaps be even more helpful if the nurse is able to sit either on or by the bed so that he or she is on the same level as the patient.

Patients who are aware that their conditions are deteriorating are likely to have a number of specific fears, which are shared by the family on their behalf – ‘Perhaps I am going to die – what will dying be like? Will I be able to bear pain and sickness? What if I should choke or end up being unable to swallow? Will there be help when I need it – suppose I should be helpless and there were to be a fire?’

Other fears relate to loss of role and acceptability. ‘How will the family manage if I die? Suppose I have to depend on others for absolutely everything and lose all my dignity, how could I bear that? Will I become incontinent or smell or look horrible so that people will not want to be near me? Will I be on my own when I die? What has been the point of my life? These are some of the concerns expressed by people who are dying, to which safety messages are addressed in a variety of different ways.

## Communicating security through the environment

Even when one is in full health it can be frightening to meet with a strange environment. Patients who enter an institution for terminal care may have been fighting off admission for some time even though they are acutely uncomfortable. To consent to be admitted is to agree openly that things are not improving; it is to relinquish what may be seen as the last vestige of normality and to consider more fully that perhaps life is coming to an end. For the relatives, it may mean accepting that they no longer are fully able to cope, which often carries an undeserved feeling of guilt. The time of admission therefore is one of extreme sensitivity and first impressions are very important. The components of the security messages here are an attractive physical environment and a warm welcome.

A pleasing environment has much to say. A clean, bright, building conveys the sense of good management, order and care through which the hidden areas such as the kitchens will be safe. Bright curtains and furnishings are cheering, and carefully tended flowers and plants are reminders of hope, love and the natural world outside. They may speak to some of a Creator who cares for details. Carefully chosen pictures convey the feeling that here is a place that is aware of more than physical need. Last but not least, a smiling staff who look neat and attractive transmit the message of high morale and a happy atmosphere.

Security is also derived from a sense of belonging, of being drawn into the life of the ward. Patients are introduced to each other and told or shown the ward arrangements and details of the daily routine. They are greeted by name, and concern is shown for their belongings and for their individuality and personal tastes. The family will feel more secure if they know of expectations regarding visiting, where the visitors' lavatories are situated, where they may rest or have a snack or buy extras for the patient. Whenever possible, patients and their families are offered a tray of tea.

Attention to these small details has great value, not only because each is important in its own right, but because together they closely follow the pattern of Western social custom that denotes hospitality and acceptance in a variety of situations.

## Communicating security through availability and awareness

One of the greatest supports to the patient and his or her family is the knowledge that someone is available to help when needed. The problem is that in a busy ward it is difficult to be available to everyone all the time. To some extent, ward staffing-levels rely on the fact that only a few needs will be presented at any one time. When this is not the case, nurses have to make good use of the factors that communicate interest and willingness to give attention as soon as possible.

Some relatives stood by the bedside of an elderly lady who had been knocked down by a car. It was thought that she might not live and because of her bad condition she had been placed near to the sister's desk. The sister was busy writing and did not look up or greet them. They wanted to speak to her but even though they approached the desk she still did not raise her eyes to show she was available. After an hour they sadly left, not liking to disturb a professional person who seemed to be intent on some important task. They could not help feeling that they mattered so little; they also worried that staff might be too busy to cope if something suddenly went wrong with their mother. This sister might well have had a hectic day and have been under pressure to catch up on her administrative work, but a glance and smile would have been sufficient to indicate that she was aware of the family and would give her full attention when she could.

Whether we are passing visitors in the corridor or a patient who does not need us at present, it is so important to indicate that we are aware of their presence. To show awareness means to acknowledge the person, to communicate that they matter; it transmits empathy in a traumatic situation and gives patients and relatives good reason to feel that their needs will be readily observed. To express this awareness is, of course, no substitute for giving our whole attention to the patient when required, but when we are very pressurized it does enable people to wait for a short time secure in the knowledge that we both know and care about them.

Nurses are often afraid of the situation where an insecure patient makes constant demands on their attention and react with feigned unawareness and avoidance behaviour. This tends to make matters worse. We need to use the time spent on bedside nursing to offer our whole attention to patients so that through conversation and use of silence they may be encouraged to express their fears. They may well be helped towards calmness if they are sure of their means of communication, for example a bell placed at hand and secured so that it cannot slip. We may be able to enlist the help of volunteer helpers to sit with frightened patients, or organize visits from the family so that they are a little spread out. Our willingness to accept the patient's feelings indicates our ready involvement in the total situation, and if this is offered steadily and uncritically through all the manifestations of fear, anger and grief, then it communicates to the patient that as a unique person he or she is secure.

As the patient's life draws to a close our previous meaningful communication with him or her and his or her family may help us to perceive what he or she would like best. Many people are comforted by the presence of someone else, not necessarily a nurse, at this lonely time. This will bring security not only to the individual concerned but to other patients who will be watching. Another form of availability is to be prepared to support patients according to their own cultural values and beliefs, so whatever our own ideas we must be ready, for example, to read a prayer or a passage from appropriate scriptures, or to find someone who will better be able to help. It is not easy to act in this way, especially at first, as our natural inhibitions and professional training have often taught us to deny such situations. It is, however, what true availability demands.

## Communicating security through practical skills

Skilled nursing has great potential for communicating security at all levels. For example, the hot, sticky patient who has tossed around in bed is expertly washed and handled with gentle assurance. Lying in bed, cooler, and in a new position, she feels physically comforted and secure.

But this is not where her comfort ends; the gentleness of the nurse and the personal interest he or she has taken have eased her general fears, particularly if she has been able to confide a little. The care the nurse has taken to preserve her privacy and to involve her in every possible decision – 'What nightdress would you like today – how many pillows?' – has boosted her dignity and made her feel a little more like a real person. Last, the attention the nurse has given to replacing her things on the locker as she will require them has indicated that her needs are anticipated. She then has reason to believe that should she become helpless and inarticulate she will be in safe hands. What a lot of security is obtained from the 'ordinary' task.

## Communicating security through systematic observation and enquiry

Perhaps one of the greatest boosts to a patient's sagging morale is to experience relief from some long-standing symptom such as pain. It can bring the feeling that despite everything life is still worth living. This type of relief often results from the close observation and attention to detail of each member of the care team, who will enquire regularly about the patient's state.

Of itself this enquiry will bring the patient a sense of safety, especially if it is made clear that small details are important. Patients so often feel they should not bother busy staff with items they see as trivial. The nurse may also use a planned nursing-process-type assessment to give breadth as well as depth to his or her enquiry, and his or her systematic approach will be another source of confidence for the patient. His or her findings will assist other members of the team in their own forms of enquiry.

When the combined approach of the team brings symptom control in one area, then the patient is encouraged to trust for the future despite his or her fears and to feel secure in safe hands.

## Communicating security through offering 'the extra'

We all have expectations of a variety of situations in life, and these are based on our attitudes and the values we have absorbed from society. We therefore accept certain standards of behaviour as normal and are aggrieved when they are not met with, rather than appreciative when they are. When something happens that is above our expectations, this then has an impact.

This something extra may be the means through which a breakthrough in trusting relationships is achieved. For example, patients arriving at some units are met and welcomed by a very senior member of staff. This really emphasizes to the patient his or her importance as an individual and the concern that is felt for him or her. Much depends upon the possibilities within each institutional setting; many such extras cannot be planned in advance but are imaginative personal responses to the needs of the time.

Thus one nurse may go to great lengths to find something special for his or her patient to eat, the ward staff may combine to plan a celebration of a patient's birthday or relax their own ideas of ward arrangement to meet the differing expectations of someone from a different cultural background. Another member of staff may show interest and respect for the patient in taking time to learn from him or her or to facilitate his or her participation in a hobby. An exhausted relative whose numb feelings make him or her feel guilty and callous may be surprised to meet with real sympathy and understanding.

The point is that the patient's expectations rather than the nurse's ideals are exceeded, and a perceptive nurse may find many occasions in which he or she can bring surprise and pleasure to the patient. When circumstances make it very hard to trust, it is these kinds of 'extras' that help lift the fear.

Meaningful communication with the patient, the family and with other members of the health-care team is the basis of effective terminal care. Many hazards can be encountered, not least the attitudes and expectations of all concerned. These need to be honestly identified. Once this has been accomplished, safety messages may be sent. If they are to be clearly received, their components must be skilfully blended to form a united picture. This choosing and blending process has potential for great reward – the comforting of body and mind of the patient and his or her family, and perhaps some achievement of a goal that is special to him or her. This presents an exciting challenge that must be met with both the science and art of nursing.

## FURTHER READING

Koff, H. (1980) *Hospice – A Caring Community*, Winthorp, London.
Kubler-Ross, E. (1985) *On Death and Dying*, Tavistock, London.

Parkes, C. Murray (1986) *Bereavement*, Pelican, Harmondsworth.
Saunders, C. M., Summers, D. and Teller, N. (1981) *Hospice: The Living Idea*, Edward Arnold, London.
West, T. S. and Kirkham, R. R. (1981) 'The Family', in C. M. Saunders *et al.* (eds) *Hospice: The Living Idea*, Edward Arnold, London.

# 3. Nursing Assessment

The principles of the nursing process are relevant in the total care of the dying patient and the family whether the nurse is working in the patient's home or in a residential institution. The stages of the nursing process are now well known to nurses, i.e.:

(1) Assessment of the patient's condition and identifying nursing problems.
(2) Planning the nursing care as a result of the initial assessment.
(3) Implementing the care plan.
(4) Evaluating the effectiveness of the care and modifying the care plan as often as is necessary.

These principles can also be applied to the care of the family.

A necessary tool in the nursing process is the keeping of accurate and relevant records so that all involved in the care will find them useful in maintaining a high quality of communications between staff, thus enhancing the care provided. It must be realized that the time-span between the patient first coming under the responsibility of the nurse and his or her death may be very short, even less than 24 hours. Also, the patient's condition may change rapidly and frequently, and so some aspects of the care plan may, as a result, have to be altered several times during the day, for instance, evaluating the efficacy of methods of pain control. Therefore, elaborate and time-consuming record-keeping is out of place. Simplicity should be the keynote. The trained nurse will, of course, be responsible for supervising record-keeping and the modification of the care plan, as well as its implementation. Student nurses and nursing auxiliaries will all play a part in verbal reporting on the changing needs of the patient and family. Written records will be kept by student nurses as part of their learning process, and nursing auxiliaries may take some part – at the discretion of the trained nurse and according to the nursing authority's policy.

# ASSESSMENT OF THE DYING PATIENT

It is important to remember that the patient may have one or more problems not directly related to the main diagnosis and causing considerable discomfort and worry. For instance, the patient with advanced breast cancer may also have such problems as toothache, painful corns or joint pains due to arthritis. Just as the doctor should carry out a thorough physical examination and take a careful medical history, so must the nurse make a complete assessment of the patient in order to ascertain the nursing needs.

## First meeting with the patient

It is a truism that first impressions are crucial in any situation where two people are hoping to build up a relationship. Unless the dying patient is deeply unconscious, he or she is also making observations about the nurse at their first meeting. Thus the assessment stage is mutual although, of course, from different standpoints.

The nurse's aim is to gather essential information by observation, examination and discussion with the patient in order to plan the best possible nursing. The dying patient's aim, whether formulated or not, is to judge from observing the nurse whether he or she is interested in him or her, compassionate, and whether the nurse inspires confidence in his or her ability to relieve distressing symptoms, which may include fear and loneliness with a longing to find a sympathetic listener.

To gain patients' co-operation in their assessment of the patients' state, nurses need to be aware of these thoughts, which may be present in patients' minds, and to respond in the appropriate way.

## The nurse's manner of approach

A research study (Ashworth, 1980, p. 17) refers to the positive effect on human interaction of physical proximity, eye contact, a friendly tone of voice and conversation about personal topics. The nurse establishing contact with the dying patient can make use of these findings as follows:

(1) By sitting close to the patient, by the bed or chair where it is easy to talk face to face. A smile and friendly greeting should be immediate.
(2) By attention to the tone of voice and articulation. The patient may not be able to hear well whether through age or weakness, so that a clear, measured mode of speech helps. Courtesy, shown by addressing the patient by his or her correct title, and warmth of tone, imply concern and interest.
(3) Touch is a powerful source of social bonding, and the nurse should take the patient's hand in the initial greeting. Where it seems helpful, as with a patient who is obviously distressed and anxious, the nurse should not hesitate to hold the patient's hand gently for a time.

These initial steps to establish contact are very important to the dying patient in showing that care will include the unhurried offering of time by his or her professional carers, especially in being prepared to listen.

## Obtaining information

Having established contact, and expended effort in gaining the patient's confidence, the nurse should have a clear idea of the sort of information he or she needs in order to identify problems and plan the appropriate nursing care. This will be done by asking the patient questions, by observation and examination.

Much has been written in recent years about obtaining a nursing history, and the various ways to do this. Flexibility seems to be the consensus of opinion, and that information by verbal questioning must be obtained gradually over a period of time.

The dying patient may be quite unable to answer any but the minimum of necessary questions, due to weakness, pain, confusion or other distressing symptoms, and the nurse may have to rely on the relatives to supply the necessary information.

One factor that is of particular importance for all those caring for the dying patient is the extent of insight that the patient appears to have into the nature and prognosis of his or her illness. Today, many patients are well informed as to their diagnosis, and will volunteer this information readily. Indeed, the patient in the terminal stage of congestive heart failure or chronic bronchitis is only too well aware of years of ill health and many forms of treatment. Patients with a malignant disease are also not unlikely to refer to a growth or tumour, or actually to use the word cancer to describe their conditions. Assessing whether patients understand that they are dying is often difficult and needs time for relationships to be established between patients and carers. On the other hand, some patients will make their thoughts clear at the outset, in direct statements about their approaching demise, or in a firm optimism about an eventual cure. This information should be recorded in the nursing history sheet whether it has been obtained by the nurse or another colleague, so that all the caring team are aware of the extent of the patient's insight into his or her condition.

The nurse will need to find out a number of practical details in order to provide the maximum comfort for the patient. These will include sleeping habits, special likes or dislikes in food and drink, recreational interests and any prosthesis worn, such as hearing aid, dentures or spectacles. In enquiring about the patient's religious beliefs, it should be ascertained if he or she has any special wishes in this respect. Worries may be expressed regarding finance or family welfare, and these should be noted for the attention of the social worker, after assuring the patient that help will be forthcoming.

The help of an interpreter may be needed if the patient does not have a good command of English; otherwise increased anxiety will be an additional burden for the patient, and difficult for the nurse.

## Observation of the patient

The nurse can learn much by observing the patient during the initial contact, as the following examples will demonstrate:

(1) *Facial expression* This may reflect pain, anxiety, apathy, hostility, depression, one of which will give a clue to underlying problems both physical and psychological. On the other hand, the patient may appear serene and smiling. People may mask their feelings so that superficial observation of the face does not reveal the true state of affairs. It is thus helpful to try to see patients 'off guard' before or after actually meeting them face to face.

(2) *Position in bed/chair* Many dying patients prefer to be out of bed for part of the day and even walking about until weakness overwhelms the power of mobility. Posture can again reveal emotional problems such as depression or anxiety, and certainly pain. The patient may

be sitting or lying in an unnatural position with contorted limbs. If walking about, the degree of agility can be noted, and the presence of a limp. The depressed patient may be hunched up, with bent head, or hidden under the bed-clothes. Anxiety or confusion is often accompanied by restlessness and twisting of the hands.

(3) *Odour* On approaching the patient, the nurse may be aware of an odour that gives a clue to a particular problem even before close proximity. The smell of faeces or urine alerts one to a situation of incontinence or a badly controlled stoma. The patient may not actually be vomiting at the time, but contamination of personal clothing by vomit on a previous occasion may not have been dealt with adequately and leaves a typical lingering odour. The presence of a fungating wound is not uncommon, especially in advanced breast cancer, and will certainly have an unpleasant odour that may be apparent even when the wound is not exposed.

(4) *Sounds* Respiratory symptoms are common in the dying patient so that the nurse may hear the patient coughing, breathing noisily or, if death is near and secretions are filling the trachea that the patient cannot expel, the so-called 'death rattle'. In listening to the patient, the nurse may notice a speech impediment such as slurring, or hoarseness of voice.

(5) *Level of consciousness* When first meeting a dying patient, a wide range of mental states will be observed. Some patients remain alert and conscious right up to the last moments before death occurs. This can be the case in the terminal stage of a chronic illness as well as in sudden and unexpected death.

In a chronic illness, most patients lapse into coma during the last few hours if not earlier. A semi-conscious state is common during the last 48 hours, especially during the terminal stage of a malignant disease. The nurse may realize that the patient is confused to some degree and unable to give reliable information by word of mouth.

## Physical examination of the patient

This should be done gently and unobtrusively, and starts with the first attempt to make the patient comfortable in bed or chair, and later when dealing with skin, toilet and other aspects of physical care.

Specific observations will include:

- colour, texture and integrity of skin and mucous membranes;
- presence of swellings in any part of the body;

- oedema or muscle wasting;
- abnormal position of limbs;
- unusual movements such as shaking or trembling;
- incontinence of urine or faeces; and
- level of consciousness and orientation.

The nurse will, of course, gain further information from the doctor's findings, such as the result of rectal or vaginal examination, abdominal palpation and the quality of cardiac and respiratory functions. The nurse should also be aware of the signs of impending death as his or her first contact with the patient may be at a late stage in the terminal illness (see Chapter 6).

## ASSESSMENT OF THE FAMILY

All those caring for dying patients must consider them within the context of a family unit, however small. When patients appear to have no living family or friends, their professional carers must become their 'family' to some extent.

Details of the initial care of the family when patients are at home are given in Chapter 16. The following guidelines are offered for nurses who are dealing with the family when patients are admitted for residential care. A methodical history should be taken to obtain the fullest information possible, including the family's perception of the patient's problems and the part that they have so far played in looking after him or her. As with patients, nurses should be alert in observing signs of anxiety, fatigue and exhaustion, even actual ill-health in family members. The interview may take place while the doctor is elsewhere assessing the patient. A warm, sympathetic approach on the nurse's part and provision of a cup of tea is a good beginning to forging a relationship. Relatives often express guilt that they have allowed the patient to be removed from home, and positive reassurance that they can continue to help in other ways is important.

After the doctor has seen the patient he or she will talk with the relatives and, together with the nurse, a simple, clear explanation of the patient's condition should be given together with the likely prognosis. The relatives should have the opportunity to ask questions and should be told that they are welcome to visit at any time or to telephone. They should be assured that they may stay the night if they wish. A telephone number where the next-of-kin can be reached should be obtained. Enquiries regarding the religious faith of the patient should be made and any special requests carefully noted. Information about the religious practices and beliefs of the main world religions will be found in Chapters 6 and 13. If the patient has been admitted at an already late stage of dying, the relatives should be informed of the likely changes during the next day or hours and asked if they wish to be present at the time of death. Some relatives do not wish to be at the bedside then, and their wishes must be respected.

This chapter has set out the first stages of the process of nursing dying patients and their families, i.e. assessment. A number of subsequent chapters will deal with establishing nursing goals, giving appropriate care and evaluating its effectiveness. Further chapters have been written by professional colleagues who are experts in other aspects of care, such as medicine and social work. There will be some overlap between all the writers, which will serve to re-inforce important points, and also to reflect the fact that, to be successful, the care of dying patients and their families is a team effort that people share for a common goal, namely, death in peace, comfort and dignity.

## REFERENCES AND FURTHER READING

Ashworth, P. (1980) *Care to Communicate*, Royal College of Nursing, London.
Lamerton, R. (1980) *Care of the Dying*, Pelican, Harmondsworth.
Long, R. (1981) *Systematic Nursing Care*, Faber & Faber, London.

# 4. Nursing Care: Planning, Implementation and Evaluation

As with the use of a nursing history sheet, readers will be used to a variety of different nursing care plans, and treatment and evaluation documents. Terminology varies, and the headings used in this chapter are only one example among many in use. Many aspects of nursing care of a dying patient are also applicable to the seriously ill patient who is likely to recover. It is the *special* needs associated with a number of common problems that will be considered here. Evaluation of care is implicit in the discussion and treatment will often have to be changed hourly rather than daily.

## NAUSEA AND VOMITING

The patient feels ill and weak, often with dizziness, headaches and sweating. Constant retching may become a nightmare and cause tenderness and bruising over the sternum. Vomiting causes mental distress, since the patient feels that it is offensive to others, and diminishes his or her own self-respect and dignity. There are many causes of nausea and vomiting in the dying patient. Among these are intestinal obstruction, hepatic metastases and uraemia, and also severe constipation.

### Aims of care

(1) To help in the control of symptoms by administering any prescribed anti-emetic drugs.

(2) To improve the patient's comfort by hygienic action.
(3) To raise the patient's morale.

Patients may have had these distressing symptoms for some time and need assurance that immediate action will be taken to relieve their misery. Any cause that has been identified and can be removed should be dealt with, for instance, severe constipation. Many of the causes of nausea and vomiting in the dying patient cannot be removed and, therefore, the treatment is symptomatic. Special attention to the mouth after vomiting, e.g. a refreshing mouthwash, is helpful, and changing of any soiled linen at least mitigates an increase in nausea that many patients find worse than actual vomiting. Ideas in helping the patient to take fluid and some nourishment in this situation will be found later in the chapter. Anti-emetic drugs are invariably prescribed and the following are some the nurse is likely to administer. A précis of actions and side-effects is given so that the nurse can help the doctor to assess if the drug is unsuitable or the dosage needs to be adjusted.

## Anti-emetic medications

(1) Anti-histamines:

- cyclizine 50 mg three times a day as tablets or by injection
- promethazine 25 mg three times a day – makes the patient rather drowsy.

(2) Butyrphenones:

- Haloperidol 0.5 mg to 1.5 mg three times a day – available as tablets, capsules or in ampoules for injection. Prolonged use causes extra-pyramidal effects.

(3) Phenothiazines:

- prochloperazine 5 mg to 10 mg four-hourly or three times a day – available as tablets, suspension or in ampoules for injection
- methotrimeprazine 25 mg tablets twice a day

These drugs have sedative and analgesic effects as well as being anti-emetic. Prolonged or large doses of phenothiazines may produce twitching – dyskinesia – that usually ceases on reducing the dose. Dryness of the mouth may also be a problem, but is usually dose-related.

(4) Metoclopramide 5–10 mg three times a day in tablet form. Can also be given as a syrup or by injection. It is also available in sustained-release form as Gastrobid Continus 15 mg twice a day. This drug accelerates gastric peristalsis and augments gastric emptying.
(5) Domperidone 10-mg tablets four-hourly. This drug is a dopamine antagonist and also affects gastric mobility in a similar way to that of metoclopramide.

This is not an exhaustive list and according to the cause of the nausea and vomiting, other drugs may be found to be particularly effective. Sometimes a combination of drugs may be used and administered via a Greaseby syringe driver. Sometimes fear and anxiety could be exacerbating the symptoms, and helping patients to talk about their fears and worries may relieve the situation. Even when the vomiting is controlled the dying patient may worry that the symptoms could return, and needs the assurance that a receptacle and tissues are near at hand – although discreetly out of sight. Anxiolitic drugs may be prescribed such as diazepam 2–5 mg three times a day.

## PROBLEMS WITH THE URINARY TRACT

Problems with the urinary tract can cause great distress to a dying patient, particularly incontinence and urinary infection. Urinary retention and frequency of micturition can both be due to intrapelvic tumours affecting the bladder. The patient may be incontinent because of drugs (e.g. diuretics), infection, neurological problems, urinary fistula and anxiety.

### Aims of care

(1) To preserve the patient's independence in using the lavatory or commode for as long as possible.
(2) To pay particular attention to hygiene of the genital area.
(3) To ensure that the patient drinks sufficient fluids for as long as he or she is able to do so.
(4) To be prepared to catheterize a patient as a last resort in order to maintain comfort.
(5) To administer any drugs prescribed by the doctor to alleviate symptoms.

For all patients in their terminal illness it is most important that the nurse does everything possible to maintain continence. Assisting patients to the lavatory or ensuring that a commode is within easy reach are important factors. Seat heights can be adjusted, or rails fixed beside the commode or in the toilet can help to maintain a degree of independence until the end. When bedpans and urinals are necessary these should be readily available and as comfortable as possible for the patient. Sometimes catheterization appears to be the best option, but many patients and spouses find a catheter an unacceptable mechanical device. When given the choice, some patients would opt for a catheter and it should not be withheld because of difficulties of infection experienced by long-term use. Alternatively, a uridom may be used for a man although they do sometimes cause soreness and are difficult to keep in position. Sometimes women will find the St Peter's boat or Subaseal urinal helpful.

When catheterization is chosen, an indwelling catheter should be inserted with 5–30 ml of water in the balloon. The cheap latex type of catheter may be used, although the more expensive silastic catheter is preferable being long lasting and not irritating to the mucous membrane. There is the advantage that the patient may only have to be subjected to one or two catheterizations throughout his or her last illness with the latter type of catheter. There is usually no problem with drainage even when the patient's fluid intake is below average. Bladder washouts are not often required but may be helpful should there be problems with drainage.

Care should also be given to the choice of drainage bag. Small, discreet leg bags are preferred by some with or without a drainage bag at night. Others will use the larger drainage bag but have it covered by clothing. Plastic 'driblet' bags are available and suitable for some men as an alternative to catheterization or other appliances. Both men and women patients can make use of Kanga pants and pads and these are available for all National Health Service patients. The Maxi-plus pants and pads (supplied by Molnlyck) are particularly comfortable and effective. The physiotherapist may be asked to help some patients by teaching them how to carry out pelvic floor exercises to improve control over micturition.

## Urinary infections

These occur frequently in dying patients and the nurse may be the first to observe the onset, remembering that the signs and symptoms may appear unrelated to the urinary tract, for instance rigor, headache. An appropriate antibiotic is usually prescribed to relieve the painful and distressing symptoms often accompanying a urinary infection. If painful urethral spasm is present this may be relieved by one of the following drugs: flavoxate, 200 mg three times a day; or phenazopyridine, 200 mg three times a day.

## Retention of urine

Retention of urine in the dying patient may be due to a number of causes, in particular infiltration of the urinary tract by malignant tumours or impacted faeces due to unrelieved constipation. It is usually necessary to pass a catheter, but in the case of severe constipation, relief of this may solve the problem without resort to catheterization.

# BOWEL PROBLEMS

## Constipation

Again, this symptom is very common in the terminal stage of most illnesses. The patient or relatives may mention the difficulty to the nurse, and rectal examination by the doctor may reveal a state of impacted faeces leading to a distressing and undignified situation for the patient.

Causes of constipation in the dying patient are the inevitable result of weakness and inactivity, diminished intake of food and fluid, and side-effects of drugs, especially opiates. A spurious diarrhoea sometimes accompanies severe constipation, and resolves when the hard faeces are removed. There may be a mechanical bowel obstruction caused, for example, by a malignant growth.

## Aims of care

(1) To deal with the present condition by clearing the rectum and lower bowel.
(2) To take appropriate measures to prevent recurrence of constipation, which can include regular administration of aperients and rectal suppositories or enemas.

(3) To show understanding of the embarrassment and distress the patient may feel, and afford privacy and ready availability of help with commode, bedpan or assistance to the lavatory as appropriate.
(4) To attend to necessary hygiene.

The main aim of the nurse should be to prevent constipation in the dying patient as far as possible. One of the following regimes will be found helpful: Senokot Syrup 20 ml or Milk of Magnesia 10 ml at night; or Milpar 15 ml or Lactulose (Duphalac) 15 ml once, twice or thrice daily; or Normax 1–3 capsules daily.

In treatment of severe constipation a combined treatment of glycerin suppositories, bisacodyl (Dulcolax) suppositories and Microlax enema can give a good result with minimum discomfort to the patient and a saving on nursing time. An olive-oil enema will be necessary where faeces are very hard; this should be retained for two hours if possible then followed by a phosphate enema. Sometimes a manual removal of faeces is the only possible course and a local anaesthetic lubricant such as lignocaine (Xylocaine) gel should be used to minimize discomfort. It may be necessary for the doctor to administer intravenous diazepam (Valium) to relax the anal sphincter before the procedure can be carried out without causing severe pain to the patient.

## Diarrhoea

Unless there is some specific pathological reason, true faecal incontinence is uncommon in the dying patient until the last hours, except where diarrhoea is present and the patient is unable to control this because of his or her weak state.

Causes of diarrhoea may include the following: certain drugs such as some antibiotics; radiotherapy; pancreatic tumours; tumours of the large intestine; bowel infection; and anxiety and nervous tension.

## Aims of care

(1) To give appropriate treatment that will control the diarrhoea.
(2) To carry out the necessary hygienic measures.
(3) To preserve the patient's dignity.

Caring for a weak and ill patient suffering from diarrhoea requires sensitive and skilful nursing. Should the cause of the diarrhoea be due to constipation, the necessary suppositories, enemas or bowel washouts should be promptly given. Drugs prescribed by the doctor may include codeine phosphate 15 mg three times a day or diphenoxylate hydrochloride 2.5 mg and atropine sulphate 0.025 mg; these drugs have an opiate-like action and are usually effective. It is important to ensure that the patient discontinues this treatment as soon as the diarrhoea eases, so that subsequent constipation is avoided. Loperamide hydrochloride 2 mg in a dose of two capsules three times daily inhibits peristalsis. Steroid-retention enemas – prednisolone (Predsol or Predenema) – are useful for persistent diarrhoea caused by radiotherapy or tumour infiltration; the pancreatin preparation Pancrex V is valuable as capsules or tablets given with food for steatorrhoea in this case. The use of a deodorant in the room would also be appreciated by the patient and family.

When present, anxiety and frustration should be recognized and careful counselling given by the appropriate person. Sometimes mild tranquillizers may be necessary, as diazepam 2–5 mg three times a day or lorazepam 1 mg twice a day.

While the diarrhoea still persists the nurse should ensure that the patient has easy access to a toilet or commode. Bedpans, if required, should be given promptly and courteously. A barrier cream should be applied to prevent chafing of the skin in the anal region. Where appropriate, a supply of incontinence pants and pads should be given. Disposable sheeting can be used to save the patient the embarrassment of knowing that soiled sheets have to be laundered.

Diarrhoea is less common than constipation in the terminally-ill patient, but is a distressing symptom.

## Stomata

Care of a patient with colostomy or other stoma will depend largely on how long the patient has had it and his or her ability to cope with it (or the ability of a member of the family who has been used to helping in the matter). A patient with a long-established stoma will have become used to a particular type of appliance and his or her own way of dealing with this, and it is best to continue in the same way during the terminal illness. Obviously as the patient becomes weaker he or she may need help from nursing staff or family. Offering assistance as a patient loses control is always a sensitive step. Having a stoma is for many people a private affair and such matters as disposal of equipment may have been dealt with in a secret way, so the nurse needs to consider the patient's sensitivity here. The nurse should consult the patient as to his or her preferences in attending to the hygiene of the stoma. A nurse may have access to a nurse specialist, i.e. a stoma-care nurse, if advice is needed.

Problems of abnormal stool, consistency, soreness of surroundng mucosa and skin or malignant tissue in the actual stoma or surrounding area may be present. The many firms specializing in stoma care equipment are always pleased to help with information about types of equipment.

Sometimes a patient who has had an abdomino-perineal resection of colon will have a troublesome discharge from the rectal stump. The administration of steroid suppositories and insertion of Proctofoam rectally often gives relief.

## PROBLEMS WITH NUTRITION AND FLUID INTAKE

With progressive weakness, patients in advanced terminal illness may become unable to take a normal diet or sufficient fluids. The nurse must recognize that this fact in itself often causes great anxiety to patients and also to their families.

There are several aspects to this problem, which are as follows:

(1) There may be an obstructive lesion in the gastrointestinal tract (or upper respiratory tract) preventing the normal ingestion and passage of food and liquids. In the early stage of the disease, the patient with such a problem may have commenced artificial feeding by nasogastric tube or gastrostomy tube.
(2) Anorexia eventually becomes a problem for all dying patients no matter what the particular disease. There may be some underlying factors contributing to the lack of appetite, for instance, certain types of therapy (e.g. cytotoxic drugs); nausea; constipation; gastro-intestinal lesions; jaundice; uraemia; anxiety or depression; sore, dry or infected mouth; or inappropriate diet offered.

During the last 48 hours of life it is not unusual for the patient to become increasingly unable to take any nourishment by mouth, except sips of fluids, before lapsing into unconsciousness.

## Helping the patient to eat and drink

In everyday life the average person in reasonable health enjoys meals and 'feels better' for them. There are psychological as well as physical reasons for this. Likewise, the patient who is terminally ill benefits from a balanced intake of food and fluids in the form of ordinary meals for as long as possible, even though the helpings of food will usually be small. The reasons for encouraging the patient to eat and drink are as follows:

(1) Taking regular fluids, if necessary as small, frequent drinks, will help to keep the mouth moist and fresh and thus more comfortable. Fungal and other oral infections are common in the dying patient, and some of the drugs in common use cause dryness of the mouth. Together with oral hygiene, frequent drinks will help to lessen the discomfort of these conditions. It will also prevent concentration of urine and lessen the risk of urinary infection.
(2) Eating a certain amount of solid food, containing some roughage, helps to counteract constipation and, again, chewing of this food encourages salivation and a moist mouth. The risk of pressure sores with their attendant pain and discomfort is ever-present in the dying patient. Regular intake of protein helps to prevent this, in whatever food the patient can best assimilate it.
(3) While the patient remains alert, every effort should be made for his or her life to be as normal and as pleasurable as possible. This includes making meal times enjoyable social occasions. The active involvement of the family in providing favourite tit-bits should be encouraged and they will appreciate being invited to help.

## Helping to maintain appetite

The aims of care are as follows:

(1) Involving the patient and relatives in choosing an appropriate diet.
(2) Flexibility of approach with regard to times of meals.
(3) Carrying out any prescribed medical treatment that may improve the patient's appetite, or any nursing measure to alleviate a contributory cause of anorexia.

The first consideration is to control any distressing symptoms that are preventing the patient from wanting to eat or drink. Pain control is important from this point of view and, above all, the relief of nausea and vomiting. Control of all these symptoms has already been discussed in detail. It should be remembered that it sometimes takes a little while for an anti-emetic drug to take effect, and that it may be necessary to try more than one drug for the most effective result, or even give a combination of two drugs. A sore, unpleasant-tasting mouth will also be a deterrent to the desire to eat.

The administration of small doses of steroids, for example, will usually have a stimulating effect on the appetite and the effect is especially appreciated by patients if they have previously experienced a period of anorexia. Once their appetite has returned to some extent, many patients long for a particular dish they enjoyed in the past. One lady suddenly requested and enjoyed on several days in September a consignment of mince-pies because they had always given her pleasure at Christmas!

It should be mentioned that patients who have been taking relatively-large doses of steroid drugs for a specific medical reason can develop an abnormal appetite during their terminal illness with constant craving for food. This can be distressing and embarrassing for the patient and present a dilemma for the doctor.

Small amounts of alcohol are often enjoyed, as an aperitif such as sherry, or taken with a meal, especially if the patient has been used to this in the past.

## Presenting food and drink

Once the patient's appetite has been restored, he or she will often enjoy small helpings of food at normal meal-times to within a day or two of his or her death.

This is more likely to happen if the patient's particular likes and dislikes can be studied, and the food attractively presented. Small details, such as a tray-cloth, can make all the difference. Too strict an adherence to previous diets for medical reasons is out of place at this stage. Care should be taken to avoid nausea. It has been noted that sweet foods are more likely to cause this than savoury ones.

There will be some patients who have special needs for cultural or religious reasons. They will be grateful for any efforts that can be made to find food to their liking. Most patients like small pieces of fresh fruit if prepared in an easy way for them to handle and eat, and this also helps in moistening the mouth. Patients should not be hurried; the weak individual will naturally be slow in eating.

Gradually the dying patient will only tolerate minimal amounts of food, and it will be a challenge to the nurse to give fluids that will both hydrate and nourish the patient as far as is possible. There are a number of well-known high-protein supplements such as Complan or Build-up that can be used. Egg flips can be offered, although not all patients like these. Virtually any drink that the patient will take should be available. The savoury tang of Bovril or Marmite drinks may be enjoyed, although their saltiness may not be acceptable if the patient tends to have a sore mouth or lips. Fizzy drinks are often useful; if too gaseous they can be diluted with water. The older patient may not be so keen on cold drinks, and prefer the well-loved cup of tea.

Helping patients to take their drink will be an important part of nursing care; the dying patient will eventually become too weak to hold the cup or glass him- or herself and thus need the help of the nurse or a member of the family. Drinks should be provided willingly at any time of the day or night at the patient's request, and also given at frequent, regular intervals when the patient is unable to ask for them. Patients suffering from dry mouths because of certain drugs can benefit from having methylcellulose solution with an appropriate flavour added to sip between meals, while they are still able to eat.

While the aim will be to encourage a fluid intake of about 1 litre in 24 hours for as long as possible, the patient will gradually not manage this, and in a slowly-deteriorating terminal illness will eventually only take sips of fluid, and small ice chips, before lapsing into unconsciousness. There may be some fundamental problem at the beginning of the terminal stage of an illness that makes eating and drinking difficult or impossible. The decision as to whether it is ethically right to institute some form of artificial feeding for certain patients is discussed in Chapter 14.

## PROBLEMS INVOLVING THE SKIN AND MUCOUS MEMBRANE

The skin, being such a vital organ, will reflect many aspects of the dying patient's bodily and mental state and may be the cause of discomfort if not actual suffering. In assessing the condition of the skin the nurse may have observed abnormalities of *colour* – of the face and sometimes over the whole body:

- pallor – possibly due to anaemia, or apprehension;
- jaundice – due to disease of the liver or biliary tract;
- cyanosis – due to cardiac or respiratory disease;
- cachexia – the typical greyish facial hue with gaunt cheeks commonly seen in patients with advanced cancer, and accompanying other symptoms; and
- petechiae – scattered bleeding of small blood vessels – abnormalities common in renal failure and blood dyscrasias.

and of *texture*:

- dryness – due to dehydration;
- sweating – may be due to fever and fear;
- shiny, taut skin with underlying swelling – oedema;
- the puffy, moon-face (Cushing's syndrome) may accompany steroid drug therapy;
- pressure sores – these can occur in the terminal stage of any disease and range from small abrasions to deep cavities; and
- widespread scratch marks – the patient's reaction to intense itching that causes much misery. The underlying cause may be obstructive jaundice, or allergic reaction to drug therapy.

## Pressure sores

Any patient in the terminal stage of an illness is at risk with regard to developing pressure sores, irrespective of the particular disease, as the body systems deteriorate, especially the vascular system. With an inefficient blood supply and diminished metabolic activity in the tissues it is not surprising that sores develop easily. There may be other factors contributing to the risk, such as emaciation or the presence of gross sacral and ankle oedema. Increasing weakness means that patients are less able to turn themselves in bed or to shift their position if sitting in a chair. Once the first signs of an incipient pressure sore appear – i.e. an unhealthy redness of the skin – tissue breakdown can proceed at an alarming rate until the distressing situation develops of a large necrotic area that becomes infected and causes sloughing to take place.

## Fungating lesions

These are most common in breast cancer, but may occur in many other sites, such as lymph node metastases in neck or axilla. They may also occur in mucous membranes such as are in the vagina or rectum. Other situations in which fungating lesions may occur are in malignant melanoma and epithelioma of the skin.

## Stomata

The patient may have an artificial opening onto the skin as a direct result of his or her present disease process, particularly in malignant disease, or incidental to this. Colostomy and ileostomy are common; gastrostomy may also be present. These may be well managed, or present problems of inflammation of skin and mucous membrane.

## Aims of care

(1) To give meticulous care to the cleanliness of the skin.
(2) To try to prevent pressure sores by relieving pressure on vulnerable areas, and protecting the skin.
(3) To relieve the pain and discomfort of lesions of the skin and mucous membranes by appropriate topical treatment and administration of other drugs, e.g. by oral route.
(4) If there is a problem of odour, to take steps to minimize this.

## Care of the skin, and general toilet

Washing the patient's skin should be carried out with due regard for personal preferences. Being immersed in a warm bath can be very relaxing and soothing, and even a very ill patient can find this procedure pleasurable. In the bathroom, a soft appliance in the bath will help the thin patient. On the other hand, there should not be a relentless-routine approach either to giving the patient a bath in bed or in the bathroom. Timing is important so that the patient does not feel exhausted. If an overall wash cannot be tolerated at a particular time, washing the face with special care of the eyes, the axillae and groins will meet the need to make the patient feel fresh and comfortable.

Patients should be allowed to do as much for themselves as they wish, the nurse helping with areas of difficulty such as the feet and back, and assisting with manicure of finger and toe-nails. Women patients will appreciate interest in using their favourite brand of talcum powder and perfume. Care of the hair is vital in both sexes for comfort and appearance; this is something a relative who wishes to help can be asked to do if the patient cannot manage. A visit from the hairdresser when appropriate can be a great morale booster. Men should be helped to shave daily for the same reason.

## Prevention of pressure sores

First, the patient should be encouraged to be out of bed for as much of the day as he or she feels able; this activity will, of course, gradually come to an end. Once the patient needs to be in bed all the time, regular turning and attention to all pressure areas must be carried out meticulously, which will include maintaining cleanliness of the skin and using an appropriate barrier cream if considered helpful. As with other patients at special risk of developing pressure sores, a suitable aid should be used, such as sheep skin, ripple mattress or foam mattress. It should be remembered that the patient sitting in a chair needs to have regular change of position and a pressure-relieving aid no less than the patient in bed. The use of an indwelling catheter for the dying patient who is incontinent of urine will prevent maceration of the skin and lessen the risk of pressure sores developing.

## Wounds

Sometimes the dying patient will have a wound varying from a healing post-operative one to a large ulcerated lesion that includes pressure sores. Patients with cancer may have external growths that require attention, the main cause being breast cancer. These will vary from a dry, undressed area to a large, discharging, open wound, ulcerated and with an offensive odour. This will require frequent cleansing, dressing and reassessing. A swab may be requested by the doctor and an appropriate antibiotic may be ordered. Various types of agent are used to clean the wound, such as chlorhexidine (Hibitane 1/1000); hydrogen peroxide; normal saline; savlon. Various types of dressing material can be used, such as the traditional gauze or gamgee, sometimes soaked in the lotion. Newer agents recently available are Foam Elastomer or Varidase.

If the patient is in a hospital or hospice, he or she may ask to be cared for in a side-room off the ward, and this is understandable. Efforts should be made to lessen the isolation by treating patients like any other – sitting close to them, and talking in a normal way with them. If sinuses or fistulae are present, they need to be well cleansed. The lotion of choice may be noxythiolin (Noxyflex), using a syringe or catheter to irrigate. If the drainage is profuse, a colostomy bag may be fitted. This will reduce the frequency of the dressings, prevent soiling of clothes and reduce odour.

Yoghurt is sometimes used as a dressing for a fungating lesion, being soothing and deodorizing in effect. Such a dressing will need to be changed at least once during 24 hours. If the patient is having antibiotics, this may defeat the result of the dressing because the antibiotics may destroy the lactobacillus. Gauze dressings impregnated with soft paraffin ointment (tulle gras) are helpful in preventing sticking of the dressing and therefore in reducing pain in the area.

Wounds that leak may be sealed in cellophane paper or a colostomy bag adapted to fit over the wound. This will also help to control the odour. For this purpose a deodorant such as Nilodor may be applied to the outer dressing, or charcoal pads used. This problem can be distressing to the patient and relatives and it is worth trying to find the most effective measure to diminish the odour. Occasionally patients may benefit from a surgical debridement of the wound, carried out in an operating theatre. Malignant growths that destroy the bony structure of the face present a challenge to the nurse not only in the physical care needed but because of the severe mental distress that the patient will often experience. While dealing with the dressing of the cavity the nurse should be careful to show no sign of repugnance. Irrigation is sometimes used by pouring normal saline through an infusion set and collecting the fluid.

## Intense itching

If severe, this can cause great distress and misery to the dying patient, whose threshold of tolerance is likely to be low. The nurse will be asked to apply an appropriate topical application according to the cause of the irritation. Oral medication may also be prescribed. Fungal infections are common, especially in the inguinal and perianal regions, and pruritus often accompanies jaundice and uraemia.

## Oedema

There may be many causes of generalized oedema in the terminally-ill patient. Localized oedema may result in massive enlargement of a limb, especially of an arm in women patients following radical mastectomy. This will now only be seen in elderly patients as this extensive surgery is rarely performed today. This is most uncomfortable, and the use of a Jobst pump may be effective. This is an inflatable cushion that is applied to the limb, completely surrounding it. The cushion is connected to a small, electrically-driven motor, exerting continuous pressure for about 20 minutes, which disperses the excess fluid back into the circulation. This gives considerable relief although it does not prevent eventual recurrence of the oedema. The same treatment can be used for oedema of the legs. Any other means to make the patient more comfortable, such as the judicious use of cushions or footstools to support limbs, should be tried.

The nurse may be asked to assist the doctor in removing ascitic fluid in a dying patient if this is causing distress because of distension or breathlessness. The patient is catheterized and when the abdomen is tapped the fluid will be allowed to drain away slowly. Injection of Coparvax (*Corynebacterium parvum*: Wellcome) 7 mg ampoule diluted and injected into the peritoneal cavity after draining away the fluid is effective in preventing recurrence in about 60 per cent of cases.

### Tracheostomy

It is not uncommon for the nurse to care for a terminally-ill patient who has a tracheostomy, usually performed for a malignant condition. The actual care of the tracheostomy site will be the same as for other patients, but dying patients will need special understanding regarding their need for communication as they become weaker. If they have been dealing with the tracheostomy themselves they may feel anxious about having to leave this to a nurse whom they do not know when admitted to a hospital, if they are too weak to continue. Having one or two nurses only to deal with this will inspire confidence as they get to know the patients and their needs. There may be a member of the family who has become skilled in the matter and should be consulted about any detail of information that will be helpful; indeed, he or she should be allowed to continue to help with the procedure if desired.

## PROBLEMS ASSOCIATED WITH LOCOMOTION

Many dying patients have few problems of this nature until the last few days of their illness, when increasing weakness overtakes them. Other patients may become virtually immobile for many weeks or months during the terminal stage of their illness. This may be as a direct result of neurological, cardiovascular or muscular disorders or as a signal to certain forms of malignant disease. Some patients may indeed have had years of immobility due to a chronic neurological disease, such as multiple sclerosis, so that the terminal stage is simply a continuation of the problem.

Dangers of immobility are similar at any stage of an illness, notably: pressure sores, pneumonia; muscle wasting; and joint contractures. Apart from these potential dangers, the patient who is unable to move without help will often become physically uncomfortable, and psychologically frustrated.

## Aims of care

(1) To organize a regular programme of changing the patient's position whether in bed or sitting in a chair.
(2) To ensure that all limbs are gently exercised and placed in anatomically correct positions.
(3) To avoid over-tiring the patient in any therapeutic endeavour.
(4) To co-operate with the physiotherapist in his or her efforts for the patient's comfort.

The patient whose terminal illness is advancing rapidly may become frustrated and depressed at increasing weakness; sometimes considerable patience is needed to tolerate anger and irritation from the patient who has always had an independent and strong personality. Placing everything within easy reach when the patient can no longer walk is important, and appropriate physiotherapy will help to diminish the usual risks of immobility such as stiffness of joints and pressure sores.

The patient should be allowed and helped to move about to whatever extent he or she wishes. The use of a walking-stick or frame can prolong mobility and although at first the patient may be reluctant, a wheelchair can enable the patient to enjoy outside scenery again and visit places of enjoyment such as the local pub or park.

A patient with a malignant disease of the bone is liable to sustain one or more pathological fractures. If this occurs in the pre-terminal stage of the disease it is common for a surgical procedure to be carried out, usually some form of intramedullary pin and plating. During the terminal illness, further fractures may occur, presenting problems of immobility and difficulty in moving the patient without causing him or her excruciating pain. Further surgical intervention may be out of the question, and simple methods, such as applying skin traction or supporting the limb in a sling or on pillows, will be used.

In lifting the patient several people should help, and an unhurried gentle approach is essential. Before moving the patient, it is kind to consider whether an analgesic drug should be administered as a boost to the patient's regular pain control regimen. The advice and help of a physiotherapist will be valuable.

## PROBLEMS ASSOCIATED WITH MOUTH CARE

Good mouth care is important in all areas of nursing and in addition there are extra factors that demand close observation and attention when patients are dying. This section briefly discusses two main subject areas:

(1) The reasons why mouth care may be of special importance in terminal illness.
(2) The components of mouth care for such patients.

Mouth deterioration is not inevitable in the dying patient. Perhaps this is the most important reason for giving the correct care, since mouths may then be kept in a good condition. It has been noted that they may be restored even in the face of rapid general deterioration.

### Problems involving the mouth

Poor mouths have bad physical and psychological effects. A dry mouth will often feel unpleasant and result in difficulty with eating. One dying patient with candidiasis described the feeling as 'If I put my tongue in fizzy lemonade it would go zzzzzzzz'. When a patient knows that his or her mouth is not quite right there is fear of halitosis and consequent withdrawal from others. All these situations diminish the quality of life. Terminally-ill patients are often elderly and have denture problems. If there has been loss of weight these do not fit properly and rubbing may produce open sores that may proceed to infection because the wearing of dentures occludes air from oral surfaces. Patients may have been deteriorating over a long period during which weakness has reduced their ability to care for their mouths. In their last days patients may lack full consciousness and the ability to complain of a distressing mouth condition. They may also be unable to experience the sensation that would warn of trouble. Other reasons why mouth care is especially important in dying patients are as follows:

(1) Terminally ill patients have often had inadequate diets for long periods if they have been experiencing nausea and vomiting for some time or have been living alone and unable to make the effort to obtain a balanced diet. Other patients, for instance, those having steroids, tend to assuage their hunger with excessive carbohydrate intake. Unless the debris is removed adequately there can be a very rapid deterioration of the gingiva, increasing greatly the patient's general misery.
(2) Very sick patients are often reluctant to eat and drink. One of the effects is that the salivary glands are then not stimulated to function. This results in poor clearance of the mouth and debris left as a focus of infection.
(3) Candidiasis is associated with various diseases; among these are malignant conditions, especially the leukaemias, infections and diabetes mellitus.
(4) Many drugs affect the mouth including those given previously to many terminally-ill patients. Examples are immunosuppressive agents, corticosteroids and antibiotics, and also anti-depressants.

## Aims of care

(1) To prevent mouth deterioration by regular observation and choice of the most suitable cleansing agents.
(2) To maintain a clean, comfortable mouth with the patient's co-operation.
(3) To report any abnormality immediately so that the appropriate treatment may be instituted without delay.

## Regular observation of the whole mouth

This should be daily for patients whose condition is weak and deteriorating. It is often a practice to observe the tongue alone but candidal infection and other disorders can affect all the oral mucosae. The most natural and least disturbing time for this inspection is when the patient would normally be receiving mouth care and removing dentures. Many patients are so weak or suffer such nausea that it is a real effort for them to take out a denture, particularly if it is a close-fitting one. Any deviation from the normal appearance of the tissues should be promptly reported to medical staff.

## Encouragement towards self-help

Whenever possible, mouth care is best undertaken by the patient, with assistance if necessary to provide help and confidence. The patient alone will know the tender spots and those where pressure would cause retching. Those who have difficulty swallowing or breathing may find mouth care a very frightening procedure. If in an unhurried way they can be gently helped to control the process then confidence will be gained.

## Care tailored to the needs of the individual

This includes both the timing and the process of care. It may be sufficient for ambulant patients with reasonable appetites to clean and refresh their mouths after meals; the unconscious patient, particularly the mouth breather, will require two-hourly attention. This should be given when he or she is lying on his or her side, great care being taken that he or she does not aspirate any fluid. Other patients who have dry mouths and anorexia have been found to benefit from oral care before meals so that salivary glands and appetite are stimulated.

## The agents of care

There are many different traditions of care that have been derived through the experience of years rather than any systematic and scientific investigation. Research findings will be quoted in this section and they indicate a need for further enquiry. Some research suggests that the process rather than the agent of care is the important factor.

## Removing debris

A soft, small toothbrush combined with unwaxed dental floss is found to be most effective for removing debris from all surfaces of the teeth. The electric, rotating type of toothbrush was found excellent in one study, for use by patient or nurse. Access to all areas was made easier. Toothbrush heads were kept in 1 per cent sodium hypochlorite solution. Foam sticks and a swabbed finger have been found to be the next most acceptable tools by nurse and patient, although more effective for removing debris from the soft tissues than from the teeth. Mouthwashes only remove loose debris.

An effervescent action is necessary to remove mucus and crusts and both sodium bicarbonate (one-half teaspoon to 1 pint water) and hydrogen peroxide 3 per cent (diluted 1:4) are used as mouthwashes. It is, however, suggested that these preparations are only used when strictly necessary as both have potential to damage the oral mucosa and sodium bicarbonate has an unpleasant taste. As a more pleasant provider of mechanical action half a vitamin C tablet may be dissolved on the tongue.

One small piece of research indicated that a mixture of mouthwash, ice chips and tap water applied to the tissues might reduce the surface tension and penetrate the mucous barrier, stimulate the blood flow and, through friction, remove the remaining sordes which could then be rinsed out with the mixture.

## Moistening, softening, freshening, stimulating

Mouthwashes moisten and soften the tissues although their refreshing effect is thought to be very transient. Mild commercial mouthwashes may be used or normal saline. Redoxan mouthwashes have been found to be useful when patients have a fear of swallowing other types. Research indicates that chlorhexidine (Corsodyl) has an anti-plaque effect.

Fruit juices play a part in the care of the mouth, where they moisten, refresh and stimulate. Pineapple chunks may be chewed, grapefruit juice may be sipped and lemon juice, often combined with glycerine, applied to tissues. Lemon stimulates the salivary glands but caution has to be taken over the frequency of application otherwise there may be a 'reflex exhaustion' effect. Chewing gum, preferably the non-sugar type, may also help in the stimulation of salivary glands. When the mouth remains very dry there are various forms of artificial saliva that may be sipped or applied to the mouth surfaces, e.g. methylcellulose with water added to reduce the sensation of dryness.

## Caring for the lips

This is an important area, for dryness can soon develop in very painful cracks that provide sites for candidal infection. Lips may be cleansed gently with saline swabs and KY jelly, vaseline or glycerine applied. Care needs to be taken with the latter two as they are thought to be potentially harmful if aspirated.

## Fluid and diet control

There is controversy at present over the relation of general hydration to moisture in the mouth but one researcher concluded that the patient who was reluctant to eat and drink was more at risk of dehydration and poor condition than the patient having tube feeds or intravenous fluids. When there is a mouth problem high-moisture foods should be encouraged as well as the maximum amount of fluids that the patient can drink. Diet control that is consistent with keeping the patient happy can be attempted with the patient who feels constantly hungry. Less-sweet items may be offered between meals or perhaps the eating of sticky items can be timed shortly before mouth care is due.

## Reporting abnormalities

All abnormalities should be reported as soon as possible, for not only does the smallest lesion create disproportionate discomfort but also when the patient is very debilitated it is easy for candidal infections to take a rapid hold. A variety of antifungals may be prescribed using either a local or systemic approach. In the case of local applications it is important that the suspension or contents of a medicated lozenge be allowed to come in contact with all the oral surfaces. This will not be the case if the patient is wearing dentures. The patient should hold the suspension for as long as possible before swallowing, and twice daily when dentures are cleaned, they should be coated with antifungal. It is important to note any directions that relate to the treatment, for example, sodium bicarbonate should not be used when the patient is receiving nystatin (Nystan), which is thereby rendered less effective. Finally, patients should always be encouraged to complete the prescribed course to help prevent recurrence.

# RESPIRATORY PROBLEMS

There are a number of diseases in which symptoms related to the respiratory tract may become very distressing to the patient during the terminal stage of the illness. The commonest symptoms are cough; excessive, sometimes purulent or blood-stained sputum; dyspnoea; haemoptysis; and chest pain.

Causes of dyspnoea in a dying patient may be the result of a chronic condition such as asthma, chronic bronchitis or congestive cardiac failure, or of a malignant tumour infiltrating the lungs and other parts of the respiratory tract.

Pneumonia is common in the terminal stage of many illnesses. Fear or anxiety may produce dyspnoea which itself leads to further tension and thus a vicious circle of cause and effect. Cough is another problem that may be present in association with dyspnoea, and sometimes from the same cause.

## Aims of care

(1) To provide the most comfortable physical position to ease the patient's dyspnoea or cough.
(2) To administer drugs and assist with other forms of treatment prescribed by the doctor.
(3) To co-operate with the physiotherapist if required.
(4) To try to lessen emotional tension that may be aggravating the dyspnoea.

## General principles of care

### Positioning the patient

Most patients with respiratory problems are more comfortable when sitting upright. They will need plenty of pillows, and some form of backrest. Some patients are more at ease sitting in an armchair than in bed, and may insist on doing so for much of the time until they lose consciousness.

### Mouth care

The nurse should remember that respiratory symptoms are often accompanied by a dry and unpleasant-tasting mouth, so mouth care becomes even more important.

### Fear and anxiety

Some respiratory symptoms arouse great fear and anxiety in the patient, which have repercussions on the family. Patients with dyspnoea may feel that they are suffocating and the panic induced will increase the dyspnoea and thus a vicious circle is set up. Haemoptysis is frightening and unpleasant, and the patient may have several episodes and a final catastrophic one occurring at the time of death. The nurse and the doctor together can do much to minimize this distress, by ensuring that the patient is never left alone, and by the use of medication.

## Special measures

### Cough

This may be dry and unproductive, making the patient exhausted. Steam inhalations may be helpful, and the use of a linctus, such as Phlocodine. Sips of hot drinks are soothing.

A productive cough with mucopurulent sputum may be relieved by a broad-spectrum antibiotic given for a few days, such as chloramphenicol 250 mg four times a day. The physiotherapist will be invaluable in helping with postural drainage and gentle chest percussion.

### Dyspnoea

This symptom often frightens the patient, and the relatives too, and, as pointed out, becomes worse with fear and anxiety. The nurse should make sure that the patient is not left alone, and that a subdued light is by the bed at night.

When patients feel particularly distressed, having them facing an open window and feeling the air on their faces can be comforting. In some cases, administration of oxygen for short periods may be tried although the benefit is likely to be psychological rather than physical; sitting with patients and listening to their fears should accompany these efforts.

Drugs will be prescribed according to the cause of dyspnoea, for instance, diuretics in the case of pulmonary oedema, and if the patient is already having an opiate drug regularly for pain control this will help to reduce the rate of breathing. A treatment that can be quite effective in some patients is inhaling through a Bird nebulizer. The addition of a mixture of ventolin and sodium chloride may be prescribed. When the emotional overlay is high, dramatic improvement may be obtained by an injection of diazepam.

Rarely, if there is a large pleural effusion, the doctor may decide to carry out a partial aspiration of the fluid but this can be distressing for the patient and the nurse will need to give much support before, during and after the procedure.

### Haemoptysis

Patients may have had several small warning haemorrhages, and if in hospital or hospice, it will be advisable to have them in a single room if a final massive haemoptysis is anticipated. Red towels should be available to protect the bed, the idea being to minimize the distressing effect for the patient. A suction machine should also be at hand. Immediately a massive haemorrhage occurs, the doctor should be summoned and will give the patient an appropriate dose of an opiate drug by injection, taking into account what the patient is already receiving. Further active treatment such as blood transfusion is not now appropriate and the patient will lose consciousness and die peacefully. A member of the family may wish to sit by the bed and hold the patient's hand during this time, but a member of the staff should be present as well.

This is a difficult experience for the nurse and doctor when in other circumstances the instinctive reaction is to take heroic measures, if necessary, to stop the bleeding and restore the patient to health as far as possible. The family, if present, will need particular support and assurance that the patient died without pain and further distress.

## PSYCHOLOGICAL AND SPIRITUAL PROBLEMS

If one seeks a definition for both these areas of human life, it becomes clear that they cannot be separated into neat compartments. The *Concise Oxford Dictionary* (1988) includes certain relevant definitions as follows. Spirit: 'Animating or vital principle of a person or animal. Intelligent or immaterial part of a person. Soul.' Soul: 'Spiritual or immaterial part of man held to survive death, moral, emotional and intellectual part of man. Person.' Psyche: 'Mind, soul, spirit.'

Nurses may find some or all of these statements are in tune with their own philosophical beliefs and are, therefore, a useful framework in considering the needs of the patient and family. People who would describe themselves as humanists may not assent absolutely to belief in the immortality of the spirit. They might deny this unequivocally, or say that it is an open question. Dying patients now facing their own deaths may be consciously working out their beliefs for the first time.

It can at least be agreed that the end of life is a time above all when those caring for the dying patient are doing their best for a unique human *person* – whilst that mysterious, vital principle continues to animate and to hold together body and mind.

## Psychological needs of the dying patient

The work of Elizabeth Kubler-Ross in enhancing awareness and understanding of patients' responses to their dying process has been mentioned in other chapters of this book. The role of the nurse in helping and supporting the patient in the light of this research and of others will now be considered. As long as consciousness remains, powerful emotions will affect the patient's attitude and the degree of suffering or discomfort that he or she experiences. In their observation and assessment of this emotional state, nurses play a vital role in relieving the effect of painful emotions and involving the family and other colleagues in these efforts.

The first priority is for nurses to establish a relationship of trust with the patient. This will not develop if they give an impression of wanting to hurry away on every occasion, and avoiding any real contact. By getting to know the patient they will have an awareness of the patient's emotional state, which, of course, can change from day to day. Personality, family attitudes, and the patient's physical condition are among the factors that will influence emotions, and vice versa. The main emotional problems for which the patient needs help will now be discussed in outline, and developed in subsequent chapters.

### Fear

A fear of how the final phase of dying will occur is common and may be linked with anticipation of certain intolerable physical events such as choking to death. If patients can voice their fears to doctors and nurses, so that assurance can be given that these are unfounded, much relief will be given. Fear of the mystery of death and uncertainty as to an after-life may be helped by offering the services of a minister of religion, and this is discussed later.

### Loneliness

This is sometimes linked with fear if patients feel there is no one to whom they can turn to share the burden by listening to their problems.

Nurses should be aware that patients can still feel lonely in a ward full of other patients. Even if nurses are busy, a smile and pause to enquire if the patient needs anything reinforces a sense of personal care. Providing companionship and suitable diversionary activity helps to dispel loneliness.

**Anxiety**

The patient may tend to be already of an anxious disposition and the facts of dying can produce many particular anxieties such as worries about finance and family well-being, and uncertainty about the prognosis of the illness. The nurse can play an important role in enlisting the help of other colleagues such as the social worker. To help the patient who becomes excessively anxious and agitated, drugs may be prescribed such as diazepam 2–5 mg twice or three times a day, or lorazepam 1 mg twice a day.

If dying patients are receiving care in an institution, they may express a great longing to see their homes again, and become restless and anxious. Even if the patients are weak, it may be justifiable to meet this request and arrange for them to be taken home for a short visit. It is found that patients are often remarkably peaceful once they have achieved what they probably know is a last farewell to their homes.

**Sadness**

It is understandable that dying patients who have insight into their condition experience sadness at the impending loss of their lives and all that they value, including those they love. There is no easy remedy to prescribe for this natural reaction, but if the care given by all the caring team is of a high quality, patients will at least be relieved of distressing symptoms that interfere with progress towards acceptance of their coming death. Where there are close family relationships, and both patient and family have reached acceptance together, the remaining span of life can take on a new and precious quality.

**Depression**

It is not always easy to distinguish sadness from depression, but it is important to treat the latter before it becomes severe and very distressing. The observations of the nurse will be vital, as the patient may assume a mask when the doctor visits, and the true state of affairs can be missed at first. A psychiatrist or clinical psychologist may be asked to see the patient, and antidepressant drugs will be prescribed. The timing is important, as these drugs do not usually have any significant effect until the patient has been taking them for about a week; this is a long time in terms of many terminal illnesses. An example of a useful antidepressant drug with fewer side-effects than some is mianserin 20–30 mg taken at night.

Depression may be one cause of insomnia, although, of course, there are many others. The nurse will often be involved in trying to help a patient to sleep, first by investigating the possible causes. There can be a number of physical causes, or simple environmental problems such as noise or over-heating of the ward or room. Specific remedies should be tried first, including sitting with the patient and quietly discussing a possible solution with him or her. Eventually, some patients will need sedation, such as dichloralphenazone 650 mg or chlorpromazine 25–50 mg.

### Weakness and tiredness

One of the symptoms that will often result in the patient who also feels anxious or depressed is the lethargy and weakness associated with the gradual deterioration of the bodily systems. This is particularly noted in the state known as cachexia, which is present in advanced cancer. The administration of corticosteroids – prednisolone (enteric-coated) 10 mg twice a day – is often useful in producing a subjective improvement in a feeling of well-being. If anaemia is the cause of the weakness, it may be appropriate to give a patient a blood transfusion. This symptom can be a trying one for the patient, but if all other symptoms are well controlled it may not worry the patient unduly if the process is a gradual one.

## Cognitive function

Some dying patients appear to retain all their intellectual powers to the end. In others, they begin to fail, the extent varying with the individual. The patient is less able to concentrate and cannot cope with activities such as reading or writing. Decision-making becomes difficult and conversation limited to monosyllables. Some of these problems may be due directly to increasing physical weakness or the effects of drugs. Memory may be retained up to the end, even though the patient may not be able to demonstrate this verbally. The nurse may observe that the patient is restless and anxious about some unfinished business that he or she desires to complete before it is too late. For the patient's peace of mind and for the future well-being of his or her family it is important that the patient has put his or her financial affairs in order and has made a will. The nurse may be asked by the patient or family to help in this matter (see further details in Chapter 6). The tenacity to live to fulfil important events may be extraordinarily strong even in extreme weakness. Such examples as experiencing the happiness of seeing the first grandchild, or the special wedding-anniversary of the patient and spouse – literally hanging on to life by a thread to achieve the highlight of happiness – are common experiences.

### Confusion

The nurse may often have to care for a dying patient who is confused. This can occur from a number of causes: toxic – for instance, pneumonia; cerebral – especially tumours or metastases; and biochemical – for instance, uraemia.

If the patient is elderly, admission to an institution from home may precipitate a mild senile dementia. The patient should be handled gently and calmly, and there should be no attempt to argue if the patient appears to be hallucinated. Sometimes a respiratory or urinary infection can cause confusion, and unless the patient is thought to be near death, treatment with appropriate antibiotics may produce a dramatic improvement. It is not unknown for a dying patient to become confused due to alcohol withdrawal, and this will need skilled handling.

It is usually necessary to resort to medication if the patient is anxious as well as confused. Useful drugs are diazepam 5–10 ml or capsules 1–2. This drug is especially useful for patients experiencing alcohol withdrawal.

## The role of religion

Religion has provided a visible framework of support and guidance to human beings in their endeavour to lead a good life and prepare for a life after death, from the beginning of recorded history and beyond. This rests on a belief in the immortality of the human spirit and the existence of a higher power, namely the deity, or sometimes more than one deity.

Death is seen as a gateway to an eternal life of perfect happiness. These spiritual beliefs, presented here in a simplistic way, have been of great solace to many dying people, although it is said that in Western society their numbers are declining. In Chapter 13 some details are given regarding the role of ministers of various religions in the spiritual care of patients and their families, and how the nurse can assist in bringing this service to his or her patients.

Many people will say that they believe in God and some kind of an after-life, without belonging to a particular religious faith. Others say that they believe that death is the end of the human person. Whatever their own attitudes, nurses should ask such patients if there is anything that they would find helpful if they do not wish to have religious facilities. They may like to read, or have read to them, words from the world's great philosophers or religious leaders, including the Psalms or words from the Christian gospels, or books of other world religions. In some hospices, short prayers are said in the wards at the beginning and end of each day. Comments are often made by patients that they have found this custom a comfort to them. However, it would be intrusive to subject a patient to formal religious services in ward or chapel unless he or she wished to be present.

It should be remembered that in many religions certain physical actions and material objects used as symbols are very important to the believer, and should be respected. Some examples nurses may meet are described in Chapter 13.

## The reality of suffering

'Pain' is sometimes used synonymously with 'suffering', but perhaps the latter word is more vivid in summarizing the total condition of the dying patient that the nurse with other carers is seeking to mitigate. It encompasses all the distressing symptoms of mind and body described in this book, and the close interaction between physical and psychological factors.

Suffering is a reality of life and always has been. It denotes something more than minor discomforts and, indeed, may be so devastating as to be described as intense, agonizing or intolerable. Through modern mass-media, people are daily exposed to suffering on a global scale, some of it man-made but some also natural disasters. It provokes such questions as 'why does this happen to innocent people?' 'If there is a God, why does he allow this?' Suffering through illness and dying also begs these questions, and the additional one, 'Why me?' Many philosophers and theologians have attempted to find answers to these and similar questions, and the wisest will say that there are no complete answers.

Some people profess that there is no meaning at all and would agree with Ernest Hemingway that 'life is just a dirty trick, from nothingness to nothingness'. Others search for meaning and find this gradually through a life-time of experience. Viktar Frankl (1963, p. 63) wrote, after searing experiences in a concentration camp, 'If there is a meaning in life at all, then there must be a meaning in suffering. Suffering is an ineradicable part of life, even as fate and death. Without suffering and human death, life cannot be complete'. Those who have witnessed beauty, love and heroism, demonstrated in suffering human individuals, would agree with him. Those with a strong religious faith will find support to bear suffering in themselves and others, particularly so if they believe in a loving God, and an after-life free from suffering. This does not exclude at times of crisis moments of doubt and anger with God and one's fellow-humans.

## The nurse and suffering

Nurses will feel more confident and comfortable in responding to questions from dying patients in bewilderment, anguish and anger at their suffering if they have thought through their own beliefs and have some knowledge of the patient's religious faith if he or she professes one (see Chapters 13 and 14).

To be present and listening in sympathetic silence, or the quiet answer 'I think I would be feeling angry, too, in your position' is more valuable than attempting any theological or philosophical answer – even if one felt adequate to do so. There are now ample means to reduce physical pain in the dying patient so that this may become virtually non-existent and in turn will leave the patient less fearful and anxious.

However, the sufferings of the family may be at a far greater level than the patient's, both in their anticipatory grieving and subsequent bereavement. Colin Murray Parkes (1975) found this to be more common in such instances as the loss of young children, or where the bereaved person has other stresses both in present life and in the past. Again, the nurse in frequent contact with the family can share in carrying the burden of family suffering by empathetic listening as above, and by co-operating with other care-givers who bring special skills to the bereaved individuals or families. These skills are described in a number of other chapters in this book.

Finally, since the nurse is brought into close contact with suffering in the realm of dying and bereaved people, it is not surprising that there is a considerable element of stress in these care-giving situations and that the nurse him- or herself needs support (see Chapter 12).

# REFERENCES

Ainsworth-Smith, I. and Speck, P. (1982) *Letting Go – Caring for the Dying and Bereaved*, SPCK, London.
Cockburn, M. (1980) 'The dying patient and his family', in E. Pearce (ed.) *A General Textbook of Nursing*, Faber & Faber, London.
Downie, P. A. (1978) *Cancer Rehabilitation – An Introduction for Physiotherapists and the Allied Professions*, Faber & Faber, London.
Frankl, V. E. (1963) *Man's Search for Meaning*, Pocket Books, New York.
Hanratty, J. F. (1981) *Control of Distressing Symptoms in the Dying Patient*, St Joseph's Hospice, London.
Hector, W. and Whitfield, S. (1982) *Nursing Care for the Dying Patient and the Family*, Heinemann Medical, London.
Lewis, C. S. (1957) *The Problem of Pain*, Fontana, London.
McGilloway, O. and Myco, F. (eds) (1985) *Nursing and Spiritual Care*, Harper & Row, London.
Parkes, C. Murray (1975) *Bereavement – Studies of Grief in Adult Life*, Pelican, Harmondsworth.
Twycross, G. (1984) *A Time to Die*, CMF Publications, London.

## Mouth care

Daeffer, A. (1981) Oral hygiene measures for patients with cancer, *Cancer Nursing*, Vol. 4, No. 1, February, pp. 29–35.
Harris, M. D. (1980) Tools for mouth care, *Nursing Times*, 21 February, pp. 340–2.
Hilton, D. (1980) Oral hygiene and infection, *Nursing Times*, 17 July pp. 1270–80.
McCord, F. (1988) Brushing up on oral care, *Nursing Times*, 30 March, pp. 40–1.

## Disfigurement

Collyer, H. (1984) *Facial Disfigurement – Successful Rehabilitation*, Macmillan, London.

## Nutrition

Goddison, S. (1987) Assessment of nutritional states, *The Professional Nurse*, August, pp. 48–50.

# 5. Management of Pain

## WHAT IS PAIN?

Pain is a protective mechanism for the body; it occurs whenever tissues are damaged and it causes the sufferer to react to remove the painful stimulus. It is, then, a dual sensation: one part is perception the other is reaction. In fact, this is an over-simplification of an extremely complex phenomenon and it is the purpose of this introduction to explain some of the basic principles upon which our understanding of pain is based.

### Acute and chronic pain

It is important to distinguish between acute or (transient) and chronic (persistent) pain. They are perceived differently and give rise to different effects requiring distinct forms of treatment. The former is of secondary importance in, for instance, patients with advanced cancer. It is the latter, chronic pain, that most often affects such people. Usually, acute pain is obviously useful, in a protective sense. It is often sharp or pricking in character and may result in rapid physical reaction – as, for example, when the skin is cut with a knife. Frequently, the cause is immediately apparent, relief is seen to be near at hand and the pain holds little threat to well-being. Awareness of this in itself aids relief. In contrast, chronic pain is a threatening experience rather than a passing event. This sort of pain is usually much less localized – burning, throbbing or aching in character – and since no physical reaction is effective in removing the painful stimulus, the pain tends to get worse rather than better. This causes marked emotional reaction in the sufferer, to whom it represents a great threat to well-being. Indeed, such pain may become a patient's sole pre-occupation, impossible for him or her to ignore and pervading every minute of every day. When this point is reached, life seems no longer bearable and some patients will request euthanasia as the only perceived form of relief.

Fortunately, as knowledge and expertise improve and disseminate, largely from the hospice movement worldwide, this situation is becoming less common. Sadly, though, even today such patients are found and vigilance is required on the part of all those caring for the terminally ill in developing skills in the control of pain and in communicating their skills to other workers, to prevent the development of such catastrophic suffering. The use of 'when required' prescriptions for these patients should be particularly condemned, since this always results in long periods of unrelieved agony and decreased pain threshold.

Some of the differences between acute and chronic pain can be explained on the basis of known physiological mechanisms; others are probably psychological. Clearly both types of pain can coexist in one individual and this must not be forgotten. Not all pains in a patient with, for example, advanced cancer are necessarily due to the cancer itself, and not all the pains caused by cancer will necessarily be identical. These are important points to remember when assessing an individual patient's pain or pains because diagnosis of the cause of the pain is always necessary before appropriate treatment can be planned. For example, decubitus and peptic ulcers, and constipation, are all potentially painful conditions from which the dying patient may suffer, and all need to be treated specifically rather than with increased prescriptions of strong analgesics.

## The pain receptors

The pain receptors in the skin and other tissues are all free nerve-endings. They are widespread in the surface layers of the skin and in certain internal tissues such as periosteum, parietal peritoneum and pleura, arterial walls and joint surfaces. Most of the remaining tissues and organs deep within the body are supplied with lesser concentrations of pain nerve-endings. Nevertheless, any widespread tissue damage can stimulate large numbers of receptors and cause severe pain from these areas.

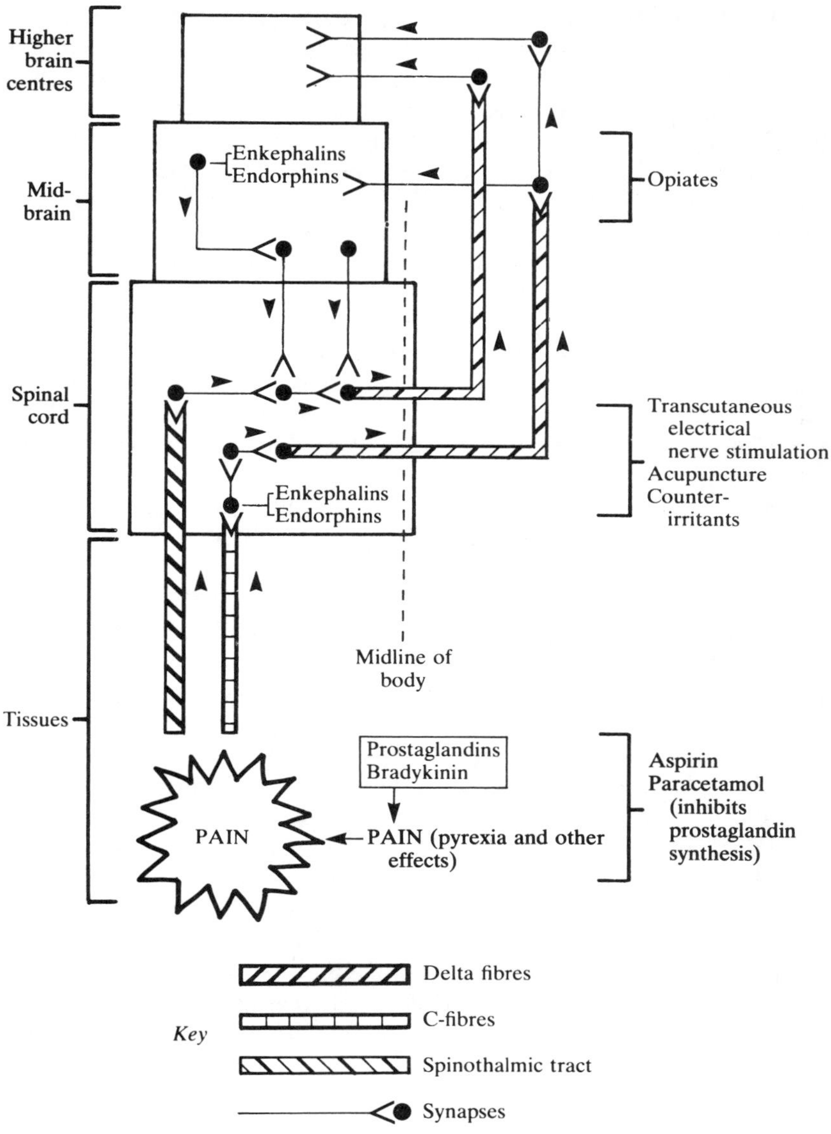


**Figure 5.1** Pain pathways showing where naturally occurring analgesics affect pain transmission, and where drugs and physical methods affect pain transmission.

The exact mechanism by which these free nerve-endings in the tissues are stimulated by 'damage' to the tissue is not known. Research has shown that chemical extracts from damaged tissues can cause pain when introduced into 'normal' tissues and it is almost certain that some chemical substances (which may be bradykinin, a small protein molecule, prostacyclin or some prostaglandins) released from damaged tissues stimulate the free nerve-endings. This goes some way towards explaining the action of some non-opiate analgesics. Aspirin, for instance, is known to inhibit prostaglandin synthesis and some of the effects of bradykinin (see Figure 5.1).

In contrast to most other forms of sensory receptors, pain receptors 'adapt' very little, or not at all, to stimulation. That is, the threshold for excitation of the receptor does not increase with exposure to the stimulus but remains constant, and the pain remains unabated until the stimulus is removed. This contrasts with the adaptation made by the ears to loud sound or the eyes to bright light.

Under certain conditions, continued painful stimulus progressively lowers the threshold of excitation, and these receptors become progressively more active with time, i.e. the pain worsens. This 'negative adaptation' of receptors gives rise to increased sensitivity seen clinically as hyperalgesia or over-sensitivity of an area (usually of skin) wherein pain is elicited by only light touch or presssure.

Pain signals are transmitted from the nerve ending in the tissues to the brain (via the spinal cord) by two different types of nerve fibre. The first and smaller of the two, the delta fibres, conduct impulses very rapidly (3–20 m/s). The second type, C-fibres, are more sluggish (0.5–2 m/s). Therefore, a sudden onset of painful stimulus gives a double-pain sensation, and a fast, sharp or pricking pain is followed a second or so later by a slow, burning or aching sensation. The delta fibres quickly apprise the individual of the presence of a damaging stimulus and play an important role in acute pain in initiating immediate reaction to prevent further damage. On the other hand, the slow, burning sensation delivered by the C-fibres tends to become increasingly painful with time. It is this sensation that gives rise to the intolerable suffering of chronic pain.

## Spinal cord

Pain fibres of both sorts enter the spinal cord and are there connected via one or two short neurones to long fibres that immediately cross to the opposite side and pass upward to the brain. The intensity of pain signals can be modified as they pass through the interconnections in the spinal cord by simultaneous signals transmitted to the cord from non-pain receptors elsewhere in the body, or by signals reaching the spinal cord from the brain. The process is called 'gate control' (a theory proposed by Melzack and Wall in 1965) and is the probable explanation for the common experience that the pain threshold can be raised or lowered by other stimuli either physical or psychological. It may also, at least partially, explain the mode of action of 'physical analgesics' such as applied heat, acupuncture and transcutaneous electrical nerve stimulation. The theory is that these stimuli activate non-pain fibres that are present at interconnections in the spinal cord and block the transmission of signals from pain fibres.

## The brain and perception of pain

(See Figure 5.1.) Once received by the brain, pain signals from delta and C-type fibres are handled differently. Most of the delta input travels via the thalamus to the cerebral cortex and thus potentially reaches consciousness very quickly. The C-fibre input, on the other hand, apparently terminates in the thalamus and parts of the brain that together make up what is called the reticular activating system. This system, which is well endowed with opiate receptors, transmits activating signals into all parts of the brain including the hypothalamus, an area known to secrete beta-endorphin – a natural opiate – in response to painful stimuli. Thus, the C-fibres, because they excite the reticular activating system, have a very potent effect on the entire nervous system; their sustained activity creates a state of insomnia, anxiety, apprehension and urgency.

Many of the actions of opiate analgesics are attributable to binding of the drugs at specific receptors in the reticular activating systems and other parts of the nervous system. This binding then results in modification of both the sensation and the patient's reaction to it, generating the overall analgesic effect. The delta fibres might be expected to avoid these modifications since they have few connections in the reticular activating system. This may explain why opiates give relatively poor relief in certain sorts of pain, for example, bone pain and skin trauma where, presumably, delta fibre stimulation predominates.

Recently, naturally occurring compounds called collectively the enkephalins and endorphins have been discovered. These are produced in the body from various sites in nervous tissue and presumably act as natural analgesics. Acupuncture and transcutaneous electrical nerve stimulation, mentioned earlier in relation to 'gate control', may also act in this way, causing increased secretion of endogenous opiates and therefore analgesia. It has been known for some time that some forms of acupuncture analgesic can be reversed by naloxone (Narcan), a specific opiate antagonist, and therefore by inference acupuncture would seem to be at least partly dependent upon endogenous opiate activity for its effect.

## Referred pain

Often pain is felt in a part of the body remote from the site of the tissue damage causing it. This is called 'referred pain' and arises because the internal organs themselves cannot be localized. Usually the term represents pain arising from an internal organ and being 'felt' as affecting an area of body surface – sciatica, i.e. pain in the leg due to pressure on the nerve roots, as they enter the spinal canal, from a bulging intervertebral disc is a good example of this. Sometimes pain can be referred to another area deep within the body.

A knowledge of the phenomenon of referred pain is useful in establishing the cause that can often be inferred from an analysis of the distribution of the pain.

## Reaction to pain

Even though the threshold for recognition of pain (by receptors) remains roughly constant from person to person, the degree to which each individual reacts to pain varies considerably both between individuals and within one individual in different circumstances. Conditioning, personality and 'gate control' probably all have parts to play in this variability, but more important are factors that can be influenced by those caring for the patient in pain.

*Factors that raise the pain threshold*:

- reassurance and a supportive environment
- sleep
- rest
- distraction

- analgesics – particularly opiate drugs
- anxiolytic drugs

*Factors that reduce the pain threshold:*

- fear/isolation
- anxiety/depression
- anger
- insomnia/fatigue

It follows that there is much to be done for those in pain besides prescribing and administering analgesics.

## CONTROL OF PAIN IN TERMINAL CANCER

In caring for dying patients where pain is a prominent symptom, the majority will be in the terminal stage of cancer. To achieve successful pain relief, health-care workers in this field must have a special understanding of pain and its effects on the sufferer. This section will therefore concentrate specifically on the management of pain due to malignant disease, but much will be applicable to patients dying from other causes and who are also in pain.

The pain of advanced cancer has no protective or useful purpose. It is not like the acute ephemeral pain such as occurs, for example, if a finger is trapped. It is all embracing, unremitting and destructive. It clouds the mind and prevents mental concentration and it interferes with social interests and activities. There is also a spiritual component that may prompt such questions as 'Why me?' and 'What have I done to deserve this?'

The patient's pain threshold may be raised by sympathy, understanding, rest, diversion and a pleasing environment, but most patients will require some analgesic therapy.

*Mild pain* only needs mild analgesics:

- Aspirin is a safe and effective minor analgesic for most patients and it is included in the formulation of a large number of analgesic preparations – mostly in combination with paracetamol and/or codeine. The main disadvantage of aspirin is its tendency to cause gastric irritations in some patients. To overcome this, many formulations have been devised, e.g. enteric coated, delayed release or combinations with antacids.

- Paracetamol does not have the disadvantage of gastric irritation but may cause constipation.
- Codeine is a centrally acting narcotic with approximately one-tenth the analgesic potency of morphine to which it is metabolized in the body.
- Dextropropoxyphene is a weak synthetic narcotic similar to methadone.

*Some suitable mild analgesics:*

- Soluble aspirin 300 mg – 2 four-hourly
- Co-Codamol – 2 four-hourly
- Co-Proxamol – 2 four-hourly
- Paracetamol 500 mg four-hourly
- Benoral (benorylate) suspension 10 ml twice a day
- Ponstan (mefenamic acid) 250 mg – 2 three times a day (may cause diarrhoea)
- DF 118 (dihydrocodeine) 30 mg – 2 three times a day (may cause constipation)

*Severe pain*: as soon as it is apparent that these or similar drugs are ineffective there should be no hesitation in using the stronger opiates. The use of opiate drugs is as follows:

(1) Give them earlier rather than later in the illness.
(2) Give them in sufficient strength.
(3) Give them regularly every four hours, day and night, i.e. not waiting for the pain to recur before giving the next dose.
(4) Side-effects, e.g. nausea and constipation, should be anticipated.
(5) Administer the opiate in a form to ensure absorption.
(6) Monitor the dose frequently.

Opiates are frequently withheld for fear of addiction, drowsiness or respiratory depression. Addiction is an irrelevance in terminal illness. Drowsiness, if it does occur, soon wears off. Respiratory depression is rarely any problem and is insignificant in comparison with the overriding benefit the patient obtains from having effective pain control.

The traditional Brompton Cocktail is not a suitable medium for administering opiates as there are so many variants of its formulation, e.g. morphine, diamorphine, cocaine, various phenothiazines and alcoholic flavourings. There is no flexibility in its use, and should an increase in the dose of opiate be needed there is the consequent increase in all the other ingredients with the risk of undesirable side-effects. Cocaine is no longer used as it has no significant beneficial effect.

There is not much to choose between morphine and diamorphine (heroin) for oral medication so long as it is remembered that they are not equipotent. Diamorphine is a 'pro-drug' as, *in vivo*, it is rapidly deacetylated to morphine, and it is as morphine that it exerts its analgesic effect. Being ten times more soluble than morphine it is absorbed more rapidly and more completely but its analgesic effect is rather shorter. At St Joseph's Hospice morphine is used for oral medication. The approximate oral equivalence of the two drugs is: diamorphine 1.5 times more potent than morphine, e.g. 5 mg diamorphine = 7.5 mg morphine.

Morphine sulphate given orally in an appropriate dose (depending on what medication the patient has been having previously) is the most effective introduction of an opiate. A customary start for a patient previously inadequately-relieved by non-narcotic drugs would be 5 mg or 10 mg every four hours: morphine sulphate 5 mg (five), syrup or appropriate flavourings as required; chloroform water to 10 ml (ten), dose – 10 ml every four hours.

To determine the correct dose, the morphine is titrated against the patient's pain by increasing the four-hourly dose by 5 mg each day. Once the dose reaches 20 mg the daily increments may be 10 mg, and over 100 mg they may be 20 mg. When 24-hour pain relief has been achieved, that is the dose required for that patient at that time.

It is essential to ensure that the patient takes the medication every four hours throughout the 24 hours, although a larger dose at bedtime or the addition of a slow-release morphine tablet (e.g. MST Continus) at 10 p.m. sometimes obviates the administration of a dose during the night.

Should the patient be unable to take oral medication (e.g. vomiting or dysphagia or weakness) the opiate may then be administered *per rectum* in the form of morphine suppositories. These are available in strengths of 15 mg, 30 mg and 60 mg, and provided there is no rectal or bowel pathology preventing administration are almost as effective as by mouth. As with oral medication, the drug must be given every four hours. Prolodone (oxycodone) suppositories are also available in a strength of 30 mg equivalent to 15 mg morphine and are inserted three times a day.

If oral and rectal administration are impossible the opiate will have to be given by injection. Diamorphine is clearly the drug of choice for injections as its greater solubility enable larger doses to be given in a smaller volume of fluid, e.g. 1 G morphine needs 20 ml of water for solution; 1 G diamorphine needs 2 ml of water for solution. By injection, diamorphine is twice as potent as morphine, e.g. 5 mg diamorphine = 10 mg morphine. The potency by *injection* of both morphine and diamorphine is twice as much as when given *orally*. Accordingly, when transferring from oral to injection therapy, the dose should be halved. Injections are given intramuscularly or subcutaneously. The intravenous route is never used.

Patients unsuitable for treatment by oral or rectal medication usually require four-hourly injections that may be unsettling or even distressing. The need for regular injections is now obviated by the use of the Greaseby syringe driver (MS16). A 24-hour dose of the medication (usually diamorphine and an anti-emetic) is drawn into a 10-ml syringe to which a cannula with a butterfly needle is attached. The syringe is fitted into the driver, which is set to compress the syringe plunger at a steady rate and empty the syringe in 24 hours. The butterfly needle is inserted subcutaneously in the suprascapular region or appropriate site and the driver fits snugly into a sling under the arm.

Excellent and continuous pain-control is achieved with this method – often with a smaller total dose of medication. The syringe is re-charged each day and the needle site is altered after 48 hours as localized indurations may develop if the needle is left continuously in one place. Indurations may also be caused occasionally by phenothiazines that have been included as anti-emetics.

Patients at St Joseph's Hospice suffering from severe pain uncontrollable by oral or rectal medication have been given effective relief with this method of administering opiates. The 24-hour dose has varied from 30 mg to 600–3,000 mg of diamorphine and various anti-emetics have been used with it, e.g. Stemetil, Maxolon, cyclizine, Largactil and Motilium although these are often unnecessary. Some patients have had continuous medication with this method for over six months. Others were so effectively controlled that oral medication could be resumed.

Other opiate drugs with morphine equivalence are as follows:

- Diconal (dipipanone HCl) 20 mg (given with cyclizine 30 mg) = 5 mg morphine
- Omnopon (papaveretum) 10 mg = 5 mg morphine
- Narphen (phenazocine) 5 mg = 15 mg morphine
- Dromoran (levorphanol) 1.5 mg = 8 mg morphine
- Palfium (dextromoramide) 5 mg = 15 mg morphine
- Physeptone (methadone) 5 mg = 7.5 mg morphine
- Pethidine (meperidine) 100 mg = 10 mg morphine
- Dilaudid (hydromorphine) 1 mg = 6 mg morphine

MST Continus – slow-release morphine 10 mg, 30 mg, 60 mg and 100 mg given twice a day. Temgesic sublingual (buprenorphine HCl) 0.2 mg is a partial antagonist and should not be used in conjunction with other opiates. Palfium is too short acting (1–2 hours) for routine use, but it may be used as a supplement, e.g. before some potentially painful procedure. Physeptone has a long half-life and a tendency to cumulation – it is not advisable for regular continuous use, but may be helpful as a nocturnal supplement. Pethidine (meperidine) and Fortral (pentazocine) are not suitable drugs for the severe pain of terminal cancer as their action is too short-lasting and they have a tendency to cause confusional side-effects.

The side-effects of opiate drugs are as follows:

(1) Nausea and vomiting are controlled by administering:

- Stemetil (prochlorperazine) 5 mg three times a day;
- Serenace (haloperidol) 0.5 mg twice a day;
- Motilium (domperidone) 10 mg three times a day; or
- Maxolon (metoclopramide) 10 mg three times a day.

The nausea and vomiting are often initiation reactions and wear off after a few days enabling the anti-emetics to be reduced or even withdrawn (*see under* 'Nausea and vomiting' for other anti-emetic medication).

(2) Constipation needs to be anticipated (for more details *see under* 'Constipation').

(3) Other side-effects such as sweating, dizziness, confusion, are not common and usually subside after a few days.

(4) Narcan (naloxone) 0.4 mg by intravenous injection is the appropriate antidote for opiate overdose.

Opiates are the most useful drugs for combating pain but other therapies may be indicated to control special types of pain. There may also be different types of pain due to a variety of causes acting at the same time. It is helpful, therefore, to analyse the pain.

## Pain analysis

- Location
- Severity
- Onset

- Course
- Character

In relation to:

- Movement
- Meals
- Bowels
- Urinary tract
- Emotion

**Visceral pain**
Colic, for example, may respond to:

- Buscopan (hyoscine butylbromide) 10 mg tablets – dose 20 mg four times a day. Also available as injection, 20 mg.
- Merbentyl (dicyclomine) tablets 10 mg or 20 mg three times a day.
- Probanthine (propantheline) 15 mg three times a day.

Continued use of these drugs may lead to troublesome side-effects such as dry mouth and urinary retention.

**Bone Pain**
This usually arises from bony metastases arising particularly from primary cancer of lung, breast or prostate – although other tumours may also metastasize in bone.

- Non-steroid anti-inflammatory drugs act as anti-prostaglandins within the bone and are often very effective in reducing bone pain.
- Froben (flurbiprofen) 50–100 mg three times a day and as 100 mg suppositories.
- Benoral (benorylate) 10 ml twice a day.
- Indocid (indomethacin) 25 mg or 50 mg three times a day, also as sustained-release tablet Indocid R. 75 mg at night, and as suppositories 100 mg twice a day.

All of these may occasionally cause gastric irritation.

- Steroids in the form of enteric coated Prednisolone 10 mg twice a day are also very useful for bone pain.
- Dexamethasone 4 mg twice a day is even better but if this is used, Ranitidine 300 mg at night should be given as well.
- Palliative radiotherapy should be considered if the patient has not already received the maximum dose.

- Immobilization is occasionally helpful, although patients do not usually welcome a plaster or splints.

**Muscle spasm**
This may respond to:

- Dantrium (dantrolene) 25 mg three times a day increasing to 100 mg three times a day.
- Valium (diazepam) 5 mg twice a day.
- Rivotril (clonazepam) 0.5 mg increasing to 2 mg twice a day.
- Nocturnal cramps are occasionally helped by quinine sulphate 300 mg at night or Carisoprodol 350 mg.
- Physiotherapy is often soothing.

**Nerve compression**

- The severe neuritic pains from nerve compression can only be effectively relieved by reducing the compression or ablating the nerve. Sometimes significant relief is obtained by using diuretics and steroids to reduce tissue fluid and inflammation.
- Transcutaneous nerve stimulation using a portable high-frequency, low voltage stimulator, e.g. 'Pulsar' or 'Medaid', is sometimes dramatically effective – especially for brachial plexus lesions. The optimum siting of the electrodes and adjustment of the stimulator may not be obtained at once and there is scope for trial, with the help of the patient, to obtain the best result.
- Nerve blocks – peripheral, sympathetic, epidural, coeliac/ or intrathecal – may be needed occasionally, and the help of an expert, usually an anaesthetist, may be required. If a trial injection with a local anaesthetic is effective this can be followed by a neurolytic injection of diluted phenol or alcohol, which will give permanent relief and permit gradual reduction and even complete withdrawal of analgesic medication. Some blocks may result in permanent, partial or even complete paresis of a limb, or sometimes urinary or bowel incontinence. Patients must be warned beforehand if these side effects are possible in case they consider that the chance of permanent loss of mobility or control is too high a price to pay for complete pain relief. If a tender 'trigger point' can be identified, much ease can be given by infiltrating it with a mixture of Depo-Medrone (methylprednisolone acetate) 1 ml and 2 per cent Xylocaine 2 ml.
- Acupuncture has a place in the control of nerve pain but should only be used by someone trained in its technique.

- Intractable pain may need neurosurgery, e.g. cordotomy or thalamotomy; pituitary ablation may also be considered. These extreme therapies are rarely necessary and no patient at St Joseph's Hospice has as yet required them.

**Neuralgia**

Neuralgia, particularly in the head and neck, often responds to:

- Tegretol (carbamazepine) 200 mg twice a day rising gradually to 400 mg four times a day; or
- Amitriptyline 25 mg to 100 mg at night;
- Epilim (sodium valproate) 200 mg twice a day increasing to 400 mg three times a day.

**Raised intracranial pressure**

Raised intracranial pressure causing severe headaches or neck rigidity can often be relieved by Dexamethasone 4 mg four times a day. After several weeks the dose is reduced gradually otherwise Cushingoid features will develop. The intracranial pressure will eventually rise again as the tumour grows worse but the few weeks or months of relief are well worth achieving. Dexamethasone 4 mg four times a day may be used as a therapeutic trial. If there is an inadequate response within six days it can be stopped at once. If it is used longer than this, withdrawal must be gradual.

Diuretics are not usually of any benefit for raised intracranial pressure.

**Lymphoedema**

The pain of distension and the weight of a massively-swollen limb can often be diminished by intermittent compression using a Jobst pressurized sleeve.

Steroids are occasionally effective in treating lymphoedema, e.g. Dexamethasone 4 mg twice a day.

**Infection and ulceration**

Pain from these causes should be treated by using appropriate antibiotics and drainage of any abscess that has formed. Betadine preparations are useful for sores, ulcers and fungating lesions. (For more details, *see under* 'Pressure sores' and 'Fungating lesions'.)

**Other causes of pain**

A dying patient may suffer great distress from conditions quite unrelated to the terminal disease. Toothache, musculo-skeletal conditions, thrombo-phlebitis, constipation, haemorrhoids and various infections are just some of the potentially painful conditions that may occur. They should respond to specific treatment and such treatment should not be withheld just because the patient is dying.

## NURSING MANAGEMENT OF THE PATIENT WITH PAIN

The nurse has a powerful and responsible position with regard to pain. He or she is often the key person to resolve whether the patient's pain gets better or worse, since nurses provide a continuous service to patients and are thus in a position to convey an accurate picture to the doctor of the pattern of the pain. This entails developing skills of observation in which all aspects of the symptoms are perceived and understood.

### Attitudes and communications

If nurses are to help patients they must accept that pain is a subjective experience. Any sense by patients that the reality and degree of their pain is doubted will have a detrimental effect. Depression will occur, if not already present, and this is likely to intensify the pain, since tension and depression are interrelated. A guiding principle should be '*Pain is whatever the experiencing person says it is*' (McCaffery, 1983). This is fundamental to nursing the patient effectively and is linked with the conviction that pain is affected by the emotions that may be experienced by the dying patient, notably fear. Indeed, fear of pain that will become increasingly intolerable is not uncommonly the most prominent feature in many people's expectation of dying. When the dying patient is actually suffering from unrelieved and severe pain, this becomes a vicious circle with fear exacerbating the pain.

In assessing the needs of a dying patient, the ability to recognize cues regarding pain experience is crucial. There must be time to listen to the patient's description of his or her pain, to watch for non-verbal signs, for example, facial expression, posture and sounds such as moaning, rapid breathing or sighing.

Sometimes the nurse will experience inward distress at witnessing pain not yet adequately relieved in a dying person. In such a difficult situation where, despite efforts by the caring team, the problem is not yet resolved, there may even be a temptation for the carer to avoid the patient because of these painful emotions.

Nurses also have their own individual personalities, and bring to their work learnt attitudes to pain and illness behaviour (Latham, 1987). It is important to recognize this, and the trained nurse could, with benefit, discuss the matter with the student nurse when there is a problem.

The nurse needs to develop a positive attitude towards the availability of resources to control pain. These include not only the use of drugs and various therapies the doctor will initiate and the nurse will be responsible for maintaining, but also a number of other means of relieving pain the nurse can operate alone.

It has been mentioned that individuals all have their own pain thresholds, so that one person will not be able to tolerate easily a level of pain or discomfort that another will find hardly worth mentioning. This difference is influenced by the patient's unique personal history, including cultural factors (Sofaer, 1984). Where it is proving difficult to assess pain in a dying patient, it may be useful for the nurse to use a pain chart such as those developed by J. A. Raiman (1982).

## Some methods of pain relief

It must be accepted that the nature of pain, its causes and relief are not fully understood; therefore it is necessary to work *with* the patient to alleviate his or her pain. New information is constantly unfolding in this field and can enhance understanding of how to manage individual pain control. For instance, it is now recognized that the use of placebos will relieve actual physical pain, and that this does not mean that the patient is a malingerer.

### Being with the patient

Simply staying with patients can contribute to pain relief. This is because anxiety and other distressing emotions may be lessened because of a feeling of confidence in the patients that they are not left alone, especially with anticipatory fears that the pain will return.

It also gives patients the opportunity to gain relief from some of the mental pain that may be afflicting them, and they may choose to unburden themselves to the nurse who is giving his or her company. Thoughts of impending loss of everything that life holds for them, terror at the idea of death coming in a violent manner, or a sense of frustration at what seems in retrospect a life containing little tangible achievement call for compassionate and unhurried listening. 'Physical and mental suffering are closely interwoven and a division into bodily and mental pain is an artificial one' (Lamerton, 1980).

**Achieving comfort of position**

The patient may find it difficult to achieve a comfortable position in bed or chair, due to emaciation and thus pressure on bony prominences. Or oedema may be present, causing painful tension of swollen limbs or abdomen. The presence of pressure sores will add to the problem. In patients with cancer, the presence of bony secondary deposits calls for very careful handling by the nurse both to avoid causing pain and also because of the risk of pathological fractures.

Patients themselves and the relatives may have found the best way of sitting or lying to avoid pain, and the most comfortable arrangement of pillows, and the nurse should accept their advice. A variety of positions may be adopted, and plenty of pillows should be available; the large triangular pillow is often valued. Patients with neck lesions need special attention; sometimes a cervical collar is helpful, or small neck pillows. Other aids to comfort in bed, or sitting in a chair, that are commonly used in nursing for many types of patient can all be of value to the dying patient in helping to relieve pain.

The patient with spinal metastases or spinal cord lesion will need particular attention. A firm-based bed is essential, as is careful positioning of limbs to prevent contractures. Some form of paralysis may be present and therefore, all these points regarding position are of great importance. If the paralysis is of recent occurrence the patient will probably be anxious and frustrated by loss of function, and need a sympathetic and positive approach from his or her carers. The help of a physiotherapist will be an asset to advise on suitable exercises and aids to support of the paralysed limb. These include ripple beds, sheepskins to sit on or place under heels, and footstools.

**Dealing with painful skin and mucous membranes**

Since all systems of the body are linked together, the dying patient will have a number of physical discomforts to contend with, some of which may cause severe pain, and not be directly caused by the main disease. The skin is a potent guide to the state of an individual's health, and inevitably is at risk in the deteriorating dying body. Pressure sores may arise, despite care, or gravitational ulcers in the patient with cardiovascular disease. Preventive measures having failed, nursing care must be planned to minimize the pain and further breakdown of the skin and underlying tissue. This will require judicious topical medication, and relief of pressure on the area.

A painful mouth is very common, and should always be anticipated in the dying patient by frequent topical care, using any special medication prescribed by the doctor. Severe ulceration with haemorrhage may occur, particularly in patients with leukaemia or end-stage renal failure, and is very painful. Dryness of the mouth adds to the discomfort, and the nurse should use all measures to relieve this, realizing that the patient may not be able to draw attention to the problem (see Chapter 4).

The presence of haemorrhoids is another condition that can cause much pain and misery to the dying patient, exacerbated if the patient tries to pass hard stools. Here, prevention of constipation is a serious responsibility on the nurse's part, to avoid this largely unnecessary pain. If haemorrhoids, or anal fissure, are present, local application of suitable ointment or analgesic rectal suppositories should be used.

In women, the vulva may be a site for tenderness and pain if, for instance, a malignant lesion is present. Or a rectovaginal fistula will also result in an inflamed mucosa and be very painful because of the excretions passing over it. The pain is further compounded in the conscious patient by embarrassment and anxiety because of the site involved, and the unpleasant smell that is often present. Here, the tact and gentleness of the nurse is all-important. Local treatment to soothe the inflammation and to maintain hygiene is required, and care that the level of analgesic drugs that the patient is receiving is at an appropriate level to aim at controlling the pain.

The bladder mucosa may become inflamed; cystitis is quite a common and very painful condition. Antibiotic therapy is usually prescribed unless the patient is near death, and the nurse should also take the usual steps of seeing that the patient is taking as much fluid as possible, and handle an indwelling catheter with scrupulous care to avoid further infection.

The patient may have an open wound that is extensive and painful. Malignant skin lesions, such as fungating carcinoma of breast, are unpleasant both for the patient and the nurse. Secondary infection is likely, and offensive odour. This is another example of pain with both a physical and mental component, needing analgesic drugs to control it, plus local dressings and some means of suppressing the odour such as an aerosol spray used in the room.

## Headache

A dying patient may suffer from an occasional headache like anyone else, which clears up quickly following administration of a mild analgesic such as aspirin.

Headaches may, however, have a grave cause such as a brain tumour, or occur in end-stage renal failure. Here the headaches will be intense, prolonged and occur at frequent intervals. The pressure building up within the skull is due to excess cerebrospinal fluid and, in the case of a tumour, actual increase in size of the space-occupying lesion.

Temporary relief can often be obtained by giving large doses of steroid drugs which will reduce oedema in and around the tumour, and thus the intracranial pressure. Unfortunately, a decision eventually has to be made as to how long this palliative treatment should continue.

Whether the headache is from a benign or malignant cause, the nurse can help to relieve the pain by using such time-honoured simple remedies as cold compresses to the forehead, shading the patient's eyes from bright lights and providing a quiet atmosphere.

## Use of relaxation and distraction techniques

Relaxation can be defined as a state of freedom from both anxiety and skeletal muscle tension. Dying patients with pain are likely to be anxious and tense, which lowers their pain threshold. Simple techniques, such as getting patients into as comfortable a position as possible and instructing them to close their eyes and breathe rhythmically and deeply, can be used by the nurse. Sometimes soft, slow music may help, and act as a distraction from the pain.

Distraction as a non-invasive pain-relief method is a kind of sensory shielding, a protecting of oneself from the pain sensation by focusing on and increasing the clarity of sensations unrelated to pain (McCaffery, 1983). Nurses who wish to try this method need to know their patients well enough to judge what distraction would be most likely to help. For instance, if a patient is very keen on sporting events, the topic could be introduced and discussed for a brief period. Music has already been mentioned, and the use of visual images such as showing patients a series of pictures likely to interest them is another example.

This whole field of non-invasive pain-relief methods is a complex one, and is arousing a good deal of interest for patients with chronic pain, including those in a terminal stage of illness. Cutaneous stimulation is another method that includes some ancient techniques, such as use of heat and cold applications to the body, massage and counter-irritants, and transcutaneous electric nerve stimulation. A further step, where the skin is actually penetrated, is acupuncture.

Some of these ideas may be used with benefit to the dying patient by the nurse and doctor working together or singly according to the degree of sophistication favoured. Special training is needed before using certain relaxation and distraction techniques, and details of these are beyond the scope of this book.

### Administration of drugs for control of pain

Since this is the main way of controlling physical pain, it is considered fitting to end this section of this chapter by emphasizing again the crucial role of the nurse in the matter. The basic principles of safe administration of drugs are, of course, as important here as in any situation, especially as most of the drugs used will be opiates, i.e. controlled drugs.

There are other aspects that need special mention:

(1) Oral medication is used as much as possible, and the dying patient often needs help with this towards the end, when weakness is increasing and muscle co-ordination is difficult. An unhurried approach is essential.

(2) Close monitoring of the effects of the drug will mainly fall on the nurse. If the pain is unrelieved or has re-appeared before the next dose is due, this must be reported as soon as possible to the doctor so that action can be taken to improve control of the pain. It is important that the nurse checks the effect of the drug about half an hour after it has been administered, and then at least half an hour before the next dose is due.

(3) When death is near, it should be remembered that if opiates have been given regularly to control pain, they must continue to be given even if the patient becomes semicomatose. If this principle is not followed and an opiate is suddenly discontinued, there may be withdrawal reactions, and the patient may experience pain even though unable to communicate verbally. Drugs that hitherto have been taken orally will now have to be administered by suppositories or injection. The dose of the drug will continue to need careful assessment by the nurse and the doctor. Sometimes the amount may be reduced but occasionally there may be evidence of increasing pain requiring larger doses of opiates.

Patients and their relatives need to be assured that putting up with the pain is contrary to the goal being aimed for, and that there is no question of the patient being considered cowardly or ungrateful if he or she gives an accurate picture of inadequate relief. The qualified nurse also has a responsibility to educate his or her junior colleagues, e.g. student nurses, in the proper approach to pain control. Paying lip-service to the principles is insufficient; attitudes are more often 'caught, not taught'.

Nurses who act compassionately and intelligently with their medical colleagues in striving to reach the ideal situation of complete pain control render a considerable service to their dying patients.

## REFERENCES AND FURTHER READING

Hayward, J. (1981) *Information – A Prescription against Pain*, The Royal College of Nursing, London, research project.

Hockey, L. (1981) *Recent Advances in Nursing I: Current Issues in Nursing*, Churchill Livingstone, Edinburgh.

Lamerton, R. (1980) *Care of the Dying*, Pelican, Harmondsworth.

Latham, J. (1987) *Pain Control*, Lisa Sainsbury Foundation series, Austen Cornish, London.

McCaffery, M. (1983) *Nursing the Patient in Pain*, Harper & Row, London.

Raiman, J. (1982) 'Responding to pain', *Nursing*, November, p. 1, 362.

Sofaer, B. (1984) *Pain: A Handbook for Nurses*, Harper & Row, London.

# 6. Caring During the Last Hours of Life

## SIGNS OF APPROACHING DEATH

It is important to remember that, as always, patients during their last hours are individuals and each one will react in his or her own way; trying to assess what are in fact the last hours may not be easy, even for experienced nurses. There are many occasions when the nurse concerned is convinced that the patient will die before morning but, to the nurse's amazement, the patient survives for several more days.

Some terminally ill patients die suddenly from severe haemorrhage, a pulmonary embolus or coronary thrombosis, but the great majority gradually weaken as their vital functions become less able to cope, and they then pass gently into unconsciousness and finally into respiratory or cardiac failure.

### Changes nurses may observe in terminally ill patients

Nurses who are attending the patient throughout the 24 hours are often the first to observe changes that indicate impending death. These may be summarized as follows:

(1) There may be a gradual loss of interest in what is happening around them – social disengagement – but this is not universal, and many patients retain their interest in life to the very end.

(2) Patients whose symptoms have so far been well controlled may become restless, agitated and obviously uncomfortable. They may start plucking at the bedclothes and a slight frown or tautness of the facial muscles may indicate the presence of underlying pain or discomfort. General weakness or drowsiness may prevent the patient from describing his or her problem. As actual pain may be present, even if the patient is in a coma, analgesics should not be withdrawn, but they may sometimes be reduced.

(3) Mentally, patients may remain very alert until remarkably near the end, and they may voice the knowledge of their impending death with incredible certainty. This may take the inexperienced nurse aback, but it is important that he or she stays with the patient and allows the patient to talk it through, as frequently there is an accompanying fear of how death may finally come and what lies beyond.

(4) Conversely, some patients pass through altered states of confusion, often due to biochemical changes or toxic effects of infection. However, anxiety and fear can play their part too, and a calming, reassuring close relative is often the best able to assist the patient.

(5) Patients become increasingly unwilling or unable to take food or fluids. The mouth is usually very dry, as at this stage patients frequently breathe through the mouth.

(6) Changes in colour may occur, such as extreme pallor, cyanosis or jaundice. In these days, living in a multi-racial society, it is essential to learn to observe the differences in colour that take place in those with 'non-white' skins.

(7) Changes in pulse rate and rhythm are important observations. The pulse may become weak, thready, rapid and irregular – it may no longer be felt at the wrist, but have to be taken at the carotid artery in the neck, or it may be necessary to feel for the heartbeat. With the hand held over the apex of the heart one can actually feel the heartbeat stop completely – quite a dramatic moment.

(8) Changes in breathing are often a sign of impending death and can take various forms. Stridulous or noisy breathing, sometimes called the 'death-rattle', is due to the accumulation of secretions in the larynx and trachea, which the patient is too weak to cough up. Air hunger – gasping for air – may be associated with internal haemorrhage and is also a very distressing sign. Cheyne-Stokes respirations involve periods of apnoea, followed by increasingly rapid respirations that reach a peak and then gradually become quieter until apnoea occurs again. This cycle is often repeated until breathing

ceases for good. The jaw may droop or be tightly clenched. Uraemia may cause foetor and/or hiccoughs.

(9) The eyes may be staring, squinting or have a rather glazed look, and in wasting diseases, where the fatty pads lining the eyeballs have dissolved, there is a hollow-eyed appearance, which is very characteristic. Sometimes the eyes are closed, or they may remain open even when the patient is unconscious – a somewhat eerie effect. Occasionally the eyes may be positively fixed on some object apparently visible to the patient but not seen by others.

(10) Due to relaxation of the sphincter muscles, incontinence of urine and/or faeces may occur, although at times retention and faecal impaction are present and give rise to restlessness.

(11) Increasing coldness of the body can be observed, especially obvious in the limbs, and cold sweat often appears on the face and hands.

(12) Altered states of consciousness are common; the patient may fail to respond to stimuli, then appear to regain some degree of response – twitchings may occur. Then eventually there is a lapse into the coma preceding death. There is often a noticeable change in expression: after an almost agonized look, the calm, peace and serenity of death may be very striking. The patient may also appear younger than in life as after a while lines disappear from the face and a youthful smoothness is seen.

## NURSING CARE OF THE PATIENT

This care will make all the difference to the comfort of the dying patient and must be carried out with great gentleness and understanding. Maintaining an atmosphere that is both peaceful and calm will be very beneficial to both the patient and his or her relatives.

### Pain

As the patient's general condition becomes steadily weaker, the drugs given to control pain continue to be given, as ordered by the doctor. Sometimes the dose is reduced, particularly if renal failure is apparent, and the drugs are best given as suppositories (unless there is rectal pathology preventing administration or pelvic pathology preventing absorption) or by injection. The use of a Graseby syringe driver has done much for the comfort of the terminally ill patient while reducing the necessity of regular injections (see Chapter 5).

## Respiratory problems

Sometimes a patient who is almost comatose may develop a distressing symptom often known as 'death-rattle'. This is due to excess secretions in the trachea, which the patient is too weak to cough up. In the majority of cases this does not trouble the patient but the noise causes distress to the relatives and other patients in the ward. Changing the patient's position, for example from one side to another, may alleviate the problem. If not, drugs will be prescribed such as hyoscine or atropine. It is important to remember the side-effects of these drugs and, therefore, not to give them before the terminal phase. However, at the same time they need then to be given sooner rather than later, as they will be ineffective once the lungs are congested with fluid or the patient is in heart failure. If hyoscine is given for more than 24 hours, tolerance to it may develop rapidly and therefore the dose will almost certainly need to be increased. If there is some pulmonary oedema a diuretic such as frusemide will be given by injection. In extreme cases suction can be used, but this may cause distress to the patient and it must be done with extreme gentleness and skill.

## Hygiene and measures to aid comfort

All the usual nursing care is given to ensure that the patient is kept clean, dry and as comfortable as possible. It is important to change the patients' positions regularly, especially if they appear to be lying awkwardly, and every effort must be made to place them where they are able to breathe most easily and are not putting pressure on any sore they may have. Skilful arrangement of pillows and support for the feet may make all the difference to their comfort and this may need to be repeated at frequent intervals if they are inclined to be restless. A bed cradle may help to relieve pressure from bed-clothes. Gowns that are loose and open easily for treatment to be carried out are convenient and cause less disturbance to the patients although individuality should be maintained as far as possible. A light shawl or bedjacket to protect the shoulders is useful especially if the patient is in a propped-up position. During the last hours care should be taken not to exhaust the patient with over-zealous washing – face, hands and genital areas should be gently washed as appropriate; actual sores or wounds will be dressed as necessary. A compress wrung out of cool water or eau-de-cologne and placed on the forehead often relieves headache and may be found soothing and refreshing. If there is an unpleasant odour, dressings may need to be changed more frequently and charcoal dressings and deodorants such as 'Nilodor' may be useful. For those with anaerobic infections metronidazole is often prescribed orally but when the patient is no longer able to swallow, it can be given by suppository or topically into the wound. The importance of keeping bed-linen clean and fresh and of making sure the patient is comfortably warm, but not overheated, cannot be stressed too strongly. A bed is the patient's last home, so to speak, and must be made in such a way as to provide the maximum rest and comfort for the occupant. Sometimes the patient will prefer to rest in an arm-chair and may die peacefully in this position.

## Mouth care

As many patients at this stage breathe through the mouth and are often reluctant to drink, the care of the mouth is of utmost importance. A dry mouth adds greatly to the patient's discomfort, so frequent attention to the mouth is necessary: glycerine of thymol may be used on foam stick applicators and a soothing cream applied to the lips, especially if they are beginning to crack. This treatment must be carried out with great care as patients frequently resist it and may clench their teeth. Dentures must be removed if the patient is semiconscious. If there are no sores or cracks in the mouth or lips, a small piece of lemon can be given to the patient to suck and is both cleansing and refreshing.

Other methods include giving patients chopped ice, flavoured to their taste, ice-lollies or sweets to suck, or pineapple to chew, or a moisturizing drink (artificial saliva may be used consisting of methylcellulose with a flavouring of orange or lemon – make 1 g up to 100 ml with water and give small sips frequently).

## Eyes, ears and nose

Keeping the nasal passages clear by cleaning with cotton-wool buds may help to alleviate the dry mouth and aid easy respiration. It is also important for the relatives and the dignity of the patient to have such details attended to as the ears, with nails clean and, for men, to ensure that they are clean shaven.

Care of the eyes is also essential, especially if they remain open: bathing with normal saline lotion or hypromellose (artificial tears), instilling soothing eye-drops and occasionally placing soft eye-pads over the lids in the case of unconscious patients whose eyes remain open. This may upset the patient's relatives if they are visiting and a full explanation of why this treatment is being carried out should be given to them.

## Restlessness

It is quite common for patients during the last hours of life, to become increasingly restless and every effort should be made to try and discover the cause. It could be due to withdrawal reaction of the patient's medication when an opiate drug has been suddenly discontinued. This should not happen; if the patient cannot take the medication orally it should be given by injection although a slightly-reduced dose may suffice.

Faecal impaction, urinary retention or incontinence may be the cause of discomfort and restlessness. Measures may be taken to relieve the faecal impaction, or it may be considered best not to disturb the patient at this stage but to give an appropriate sedative drug such as diazepam or chlorpromazine. If the patient has a distended bladder or is incontinent of urine it is kind to insert a self-retaining catheter to drain into a bag.

The 'restless-legs syndrome' in uraemia is thought to be due to disturbed function of brain-stem reticular formation. It does not respond to any drug except Rivotril (clonazepam) given in an appropriate dose prescribed by the doctor. Generalized twitching is also due to uraemia and once again will be relieved by administration of clonazepam. Even if the patient is not thought to be in actual pain, dealing with any problem that may be causing restlessness will not only maintain the patient's comfort, but also ease the anxiety of relatives at the bedside.

Some patients may become restless for no apparent physical reason. They are often those who have expressed some fear of death or a denial of their impending state, although others may not have done. The presence of a relative or nurse may do much to calm the patient but sometimes measures need to be taken to relax or sedate the patient with drugs, e.g. diazepam, veractil, chlorpromazine, promazine or lorazepam. These drugs may also be useful for the patient whose fear of respiratory difficulties leads to extreme panic and dyspnoea. At the same time these patients should never be left alone, neither should they be 'crowded' as they often feel they are being engulfed or trapped.

## Sudden death

There are a small minority who may die suddenly from a severe bleed such as haemoptysis, haematemesis or bleeding from an ulcerated/fungating wound. This is obviously extremely frightening for the patients and therefore they should never be left alone. This crisis is also discussed in Chapter 4.

## Spiritual care

Throughout these last hours, the nurse's approach to the dying person must be one of care, support and sympathetic understanding, all shown as a respect of the individual human being, making every effort to maintain his or her dignity. As has been said, some patients are in great fear and dread of death and have not come to terms with their illness. They should never be left alone when their condition has deteriorated and death is expected soon. A relative, friend or nurse should be at the bedside and available to comfort and support the patient. One cannot stress too strongly the value of touch, which keeps dying individuals in contact with those around them: holding their hands, gently caressing their back and talking to them quietly all may help them in their last moments. One must always remember that hearing is the last sense lost and often patients can hear someone speaking even if they are apparently in a coma. The nurse should never say anything in the presence of the seemingly-unconscious patient that would not be said to his or her face.

## Religious and cultural aspects of care

In continuing to care for the dying patient as a unique person the nurse should recognize the particular importance for the patient and family of religious and cultural aspects during the last hours and at the moment of death. For the family, great importance may also be attached to ritual surrounding the funeral and throughout the period of mourning. It is considered that some measure of ritual helps the bereaved to come to terms gradually with the loss of their relative and a turning-point in their own lives. Whether acknowledged or not, many rituals at this time have a religious element.

There is also the question of giving spiritual support to the large number of individuals in the UK who profess no particular faith, although it may have been assumed that they are nominal Christians. All these matters are considered in other chapters (Chapters 4 and 13) in relation to dying patients and their families, before the patient is actually near to death. The following section concentrates on care during the late stage of dying, and immediately after death, with regard to some of the major world faiths.

## The Christian faith

Practising Christians of all denominations will welcome the ministrations of a priest or minister when they are dying, and the nurse should facilitate this, meeting any requests of the patient. There may be a situation where the relatives are not of the same denomination and tact is essential to avoid any conflict between their views and the clearly-expressed wishes of the patient. When this seems likely, a team approach is advisable rather than the nurse trying to resolve the matter alone. If the particular church has a sacramental system, the patient is likely to have received the sacraments before death is imminent.

If the patient is dying at home, and has one or more relatives, they will be the link between the patient and his or her religious minister and the nurse will simply ensure that there are no difficulties, for example, of communications, with the minister requested. Even so, the nurse might be present at the death, and invited to share with the family in customary prayers at the bedside to console the dying person in his or her last moments (who may still be able to hear). The prayers may be led by the priest or minister, or by a member of the family or the nurse might be requested to read them.

In hospital or other institutions the nurse should ascertain whether the chaplain wishes to be called at the time of death. The chaplain's decision will depend on circumstances such as the closeness of the last visit and the wishes of the family. As at home, it is customary to recite short commendatory prayers for the consolation of the patient and family, if they are present.

## Non-Christian faiths

### Judaism

The saving of life because the body is considered 'the vessel of divine creation' is of the utmost importance to the Jew and this can, therefore, produce some conflict as the patient approaches death. However, with gentle skill and tact and the introduction of a rabbi, much can be done to help patients accept their situation and turn their eyes to the after-life that their faith incorporates. Judaism does not define the form of this after-life except for a belief in reward and punishment. The person near to death, therefore, is encouraged to recite the 'confession on the death-bed', and the words in the monotheistic declaration in the last verse of the Book of Deuteronomy – 'Hear O Israel, the Lord our God is one God' – should be the last words of the dying person, said for them if they are unable. The relatives or friends may wish to read scriptures or lamentations just after death and a single room may make this easier.

### Islam

Muslims are urged to seek forgiveness and mercy from God and to affirm the unity of God before death, but they do not need any 'minister' to help in this matter. However, they will usually want the family or members of the local mosque to recite the holy book, the Koran, with them while they are dying. Allowing patients to face Mecca as they are dying is important to them. This means placing them on their right side with their face towards Mecca, or on their back with their feet in the direction of Mecca and their head slightly raised so that they face it. 'There is no God but God and Muhammad is the Prophet of God' will be their last words or whispered into their ear by a member of the family. Sweet-smelling substances may be placed by the patients but any means of diversion such as music should be kept away from them. It is perhaps important for the nurse to realize that menstruating women and women during the forty-day period after childbirth are considered ritually impure and may, therefore, be kept away from the dying patient.

### Hinduism

Hindus believe in reincarnation. A Hindu prepares for death by leading a calm life, by rejoicing in the things of the spirit and by being detached from all sensual pleasures. As Hindus are dying, money and clothes may be brought to them to touch before they are distributed to the poor. Some relatives or a priest will usually sit with them and read from a holy book, the *Bhagavadgita*. Sometimes the patient may wish to lie on the ground to be close to Mother Earth at the time of death, to have an oil-lamp lit and incense burned. The eldest son will be expected to lead the family at this time and even if he is a small child he will be expected to be present before, during and after the death of his father. The families may often grieve aloud at the time of death, regarding this as a help and in no way unsuitable.

**Sikhism**

As the Sikh is dying, relatives and friends will read from the Sikh holy book, *Guru Granth Sahab*. Sikhs believe in reincarnation and this may make their actual death easier. The Sikhs do not permit loud lamentations at the time of death but are likely to exclaim '*Wahiguru, Wahiguru*' ('Wonderful Lord').

**Buddhism**

Buddhists also believe in reincarnation. Sickness and death are very much accepted as part and parcel of life. Death should be a calm affair and therefore those present may use a text that will induce 'equanimity and fortitude'. A Buddhist monk should be informed as soon after death as possible so that he may perform the necessary prayers that may take about an hour. However, these prayers do not need to be said over the body, they may be said in a temple at some distance away.

Nurses should take the trouble to inform themselves regarding the religious and cultural background of each individual patient and family, so as to be able to give the maximum help and support at this critical time.

## CARE OF THE FAMILY

Although the nurse will take a close interest in the welfare of the relatives of the dying patient from the beginning of their relationship, this reaches its climax during the last hours of a patient's life. The circumstances will be variable. For instance, the dying process may have been a comparatively long one, so the family may have become very tired under the strain either of caring for the patient at home, or making frequent journeys to hospital or hospice. If the terminal illness has advanced rapidly, the patient may be admitted for residential care, literally within the last hours of life.

'Family' may consist of a large number of people of different degrees of kinship, all anxious to do the right thing for a loved member. At the other end of the scale, there may be only one close relative or just a close friend. It is appropriate to remember here the special and sometimes difficult situation for the partner of a dying person in a homosexual relationship who wishes to keep vigil at the bedside during the last hours. Those gathered at the beside may not always be a united, loving family – either among themselves or in their relationship with the dying patient. Because of the variability of the situation, the nurse may be supporting the family in a peaceful atmosphere, or one charged with emotional tension. Nurses need to have a calm, sensitive approach themselves, realizing that conflicting feelings may sometimes cause relatives to act in a way that seems unreasonable and difficult to help.

Cultural background also plays a part. It has been noted that those holding a non-Christian religious faith (predominantly from the Asian continent) may be uninhibited in outward manifestation of grief. The Latin races also have a tendency to this characteristic, as also do Jewish people. In contrast, the British traditional reserve, especially in men, may result in silent, tearless grief, none the less agonizing for that.

## Practical help for the family

Caring for the relatives when the patient dies at home is dealt with in Chapter 16. Consideration will be given here to the situation when the patient has been admitted to an institution, and is in the last hours of life.

(1) It is the right of the close-family members to come and go as they please, whether it is day or night-time. If there are several relatives, they may wish to provide a continuous rota so that the patient is never left alone. If this is not possible a nurse should sit with the patient at the intervening times. In any case, the nurse should come frequently to observe the patient and do anything that is required for his or her comfort, involving a relative if they wish in such actions as moistening the patient's lips. To leave the relatives alone for too long adds to their anxiety and possible fear of the impending death.

(2) Any information that the relatives request should be readily given by the nurse and the doctor. It should be made clear that the patient is expected to die within the next few hours, but that no one can

predict the exact time. If the relatives decide to leave the bedside it should be established whether they wish to be present when the patient dies, and how they can be quickly contacted.

(3) Some provision should be made for a relative to rest at intervals – a comfortable arm-chair next to the bed or a couch of some kind, and facilities in a room near to the patient. Relatives need some light nourishment; even if not hungry, cups of tea or coffee are welcome. Those who are smokers should be able to indulge at this time, without disapproval, away from the patient's bedside.

(4) Whatever is wished by the family (and presumed to be the wish of the patient) regarding religious ministrations should be carried out, as described earlier in this chapter.

(5) Relatives will appreciate the reassurance that the patient is being kept free from pain and to witness concern for his or her comfort. The patient may remain conscious almost to the end, although the majority lapse into coma at some point during the last hours. It is helpful to explain that even an apparently unconscious patient may still be able to hear, and to be strengthened in spirit by the holding of his or her hand, and a reassuring squeeze, showing that he or she is not alone.

Younger colleagues, student nurses or nursing auxiliaries need the support of the trained nurse if they have never witnessed the last hours of a dying patient, and the death itself. They need to participate in the care of both the patient and the family both for their own development and to learn how to give these last services.

## THE MOMENT OF DEATH

Where there has been a gradual progression towards death, there will be progressive dysfunction of one or more of the major systems of the body. Death will be recognized by the cessation of respiration and of the heartbeat (which may sometimes be present even after no pulse can be found at the wrist). The pupils of the eyes will be fixed and dilated, and the skin of the face and extremities feels very cold to the touch.

The time of death should be noted and the doctor who has been treating the patient informed, as he or she must subsequently certify the death. Although the doctor must have seen the patient prior to death, there is no legal requirement that he or she must view the body after death.

In the case of sudden and unexpected death, e.g. due to head injury or cerebral anoxia from cardiac arrest, a doctor must be sent for immediately who will wish to satisfy him- or herself that as well as the classic signs of cessation of respiration and heartbeat, there is also total and irreversible loss of brain-stem function. If not, such a patient may still be alive and able to be resuscitated. Likewise, a patient attached to a ventilator still has his or her respiration maintained but is clinically dead.

## Immediate needs

As soon as the patient has died, the relatives should be allowed to remain with the deceased for a short while in privacy. A nurse should then gently escort them to a room away from the bedside, whilst two other nurses straighten the limbs of the dead body, ensuring the eyes are closed and leaving the bed and surroundings clean and tidy, remembering that some relatives may want to return for a final farewell.

In the meantime, the relatives should be given the opportunity to be alone together for a time, the nurse returning with a tray of tea and his or her sympathetic presence. It is essential to explain to the bereaved that it is perfectly natural in such circumstances to cry and be upset: it is part of the pattern of bereavement and is to be expected. Some relatives may experience feelings of guilt or relief from strain, and may act in totally unpredictable ways that may be somewhat disturbing. The nurse should not appear to be upset by this, but allow the individuals to get rid of their tensions in any way they like, and just to be there to offer help.

Sometimes the nurse him- or herself may be particularly moved by the patient's death, and share in the grief of the relatives in a spontaneous expression of emotion such as putting his or her arms around a relative and shedding a few tears. This demonstration of closeness is often very comforting to the family, but naturally this must be combined with the nurse continuing in his or her role of supporter in a calm and capable manner. There may also be less-experienced young colleagues who need his or her example and help in coping with their own emotions whilst caring for the family. Before leaving, the relatives should have been given clear information regarding the collection of the death certificate the next day, and the personal belongings of the deceased. If any social problems are likely to occur as a result of the death, the relatives will have been referred to the social worker, who will be able to give help and advice. If additional support is necessary, as in the case of a father left with young children or an elderly person left without relatives or those for whom the death has presented complicated psychological problems, a bereavement team is valuable, offering regular visits and the use of their skills to assist in every way possible.

### Sudden and unexpected death

The family of a person who dies quite unexpectedly, having been last seen apparently fit and well, are likely to pass through a series of severe reactions. At first there will be bewilderment and failure to comprehend what has happened, followed by a state of shock. The deceased person may have been found dead at home, or brought to a hospital already dead.

The relatives will need treating with gentleness and compassion, and should not be left alone. A friend or less-involved member of the family who can give warm but calm support will be a great asset to the nurse in his or her efforts to support the relatives at this initial stage. There may be uncontrollable crying, or a feeling of numbness and unreality. Later the relatives will want to talk about the situation with the doctor and nurse, and ask questions about the circumstances of the death. They are likely to ask to see the body, and should be prepared for any possibly distressing features.

One of the most tragic situations is if the deceased person has committed suicide, without any apparent intimation of this. Inevitably the family will question whether they are to blame and could have done anything to avert the tragedy. They will need to talk about their feelings, and their deceased relative, and may need long-term professional support during the process of mourning. In all these distressing situations, careful explanations must be given in simple terms and in an unhurried way.

## LAST OFFICES

In judging when to commence Last Offices, it should be remembered that rigor mortis (contraction of muscles) generally appears 2–4 hours after death, attaining its full intensity within 48 hours and disappearing within another 48 hours.

Last Offices have always been recognized as the final service offered as a mark of respect to the dead person before burial or cremation. Again, it is important to be sensitive to the beliefs of the family as to how Last Offices are carried out. In some instances, the nurse will play no part as the family will do all that they wish. In the case of Christians or those of no particular religious faith, two nurses should carry out the following actions, unless the undertaker is to do all or most of these:

(1) The body is washed and placed in a shroud, unless the relatives have asked for some of the patient's own clothes to be used.
(2) Any catheters or other appliances are removed and any sores or wounds covered with a simple dressing. No safety pins should be used.
(3) The bodily orifices may be packed.
(4) The lower jaw is supported with a bandage if necessary to keep the mouth closed. Dentures, if worn, are usually kept in, but it is best to obtain the consent of the relatives regarding this, and also regarding any rings or other jewellery worn by the patient. In most cases for financial or sentimental reasons the family will wish to keep the jewellery but sometimes it is surprising to note that they even wish to keep the false teeth.

Some families may wish to have a favourite object left with the body although this is often discussed later with the undertaker rather than at this stage. For some, a religious memento is important and for some Roman Catholic families a crucifix or rosary may be placed in the hands of the dead person. The body may be taken to a chapel of rest where the relatives can see it before the undertakers remove it. The body will usually remain at the undertakers until the funeral takes place; sometimes in the Roman Catholic Church the body will lie in the church the night preceding the funeral. This also occurs in the Eastern Orthodox Churches, the only difference being that here the body may be in an open coffin. Burial or cremation is acceptable to all.

## Judaism

'Progressive' or 'Liberal' Jews may permit the body to be laid out in the normal way by the nurses. However, many will join their Orthodox brothers in requiring a strict ritual. The nurse must discover beforehand what will be required. For the Orthodox Jew, the nurse may straighten the body, close the eyes, place the arms straight down the side of the body, and bandage the jaw. Any intravenous infusion or drainage tubes are removed, and the body is then wrapped in a plain-white sheet before being taken from the ward. Some may require that the nurse wears disposable gloves to carry out the above.

A 'watcher' may be designated from the family or local synagogue to remain with the body until burial, although this is often waived aside in large hospitals as they feel there is always someone in attendance. However, if this is the case, facilities should be made available, and the use of a viewing room may be helpful. The body is washed by members of an appointed burial society; men wash men, and women wash women. There are usually three present and prayers are said at the same time. This may take place in the hospital mortuary. There is no embalming, preservatives or cosmetics are not used, and the body is placed in a plain-white shroud in a plain coffin. The burial usually takes place within 24 hours of death after a short half-hour burial service. The family follow this by a strict seven days of mourning and prayers. Reform Jews may occasionally desire cremation.

The body is regarded by Jews as God's gift, and therefore do not accept post-mortems unless legally required. They will donate organs but only on complete death, and not 'clinical death', and only on the grounds that they preserve life when the operation is reasonably established to offer a good progress to the recipient, i.e. it is well beyond the experimental stage.

## Islam

Muslims also have strict washing rituals and these are usually performed by a member of the family designated by the deceased, or if not, the closest relative. Disposable gloves must be used by the nurse who is permitted to straighten the body, bandage the jaw and remove drainage tubes, etc. After the washing, Muslim men are wrapped in three cloths and women in five cloths, and once completed, burial is urged without delay. Cremation is strictly forbidden and if at all possible burial should take place within a Muslim burial ground. In the country of origin, no coffins are permitted, but must be used in Britain. The body is laid on its right side so that it faces Mecca.

Post-mortems are forbidden unless legally required and then careful explanation will be needed. Organ donation is also strictly forbidden.

## Hinduism

Some Hindu families will not follow any specific Last Offices, and the nurses can proceed as usual. However, for others, the relatives will perform the duties led by the eldest son. The body is dressed in new clothes before it leaves the hospital. A Hindu woman wears a marriage cord around her neck and this must only be cut after her death and only by her husband. It is perhaps a sensitive gesture for the nurse to ask for this to be done before a post-mortem, should one take place. Again, Hindus will only accept post-mortems if they are legally required, and even then great sensitivity must be shown and many feel it is repugnant, showing no respect for the dead. All organs must be replaced afterwards to enable the dead person to gain peace in the next life.

Cremation is preferred by Hindus and traditionally the eldest son lights the funeral pyre. However, this is forbidden in Britain, so Hindus here have developed symbolic gestures to fulfil this duty. Children under five, however, are buried.

## Sikhism

Last Offices are usually performed by the family but they must ask if they wish to do so in this country. The nurse may close the eyes, straighten the limbs and wrap the body in a sheet. If the nurse has been allowed to perform the Last Offices it must be remembered that the Sikh is cremated wearing the five 'K' symbols (see Chapter 13).

## Buddhism

There are no specific Last Offices for Buddhists, therefore the nurse can proceed as usual. Helping others is central to their philosophy so there will be no objection to organ transplants. In some countries cremation is the accepted practice, but the Buddhist family may be more flexible in Britain. Committal depends on the lunar calendar and may be within 3–7 days. A Buddhist monk will usually be called for the funeral, and it tends to be a solemn affair reflecting the sadness of the human loss.

## Removal of the body

If the patient dies in an institution, the body will need to be removed from the ward or room after Last Offices have been performed. The nurse has a responsibility to ensure that this is done in a dignified way, not least for the sake of other patients who may be aware of what is happening.

Sometimes relatives may arrive later and wish to pay their last respects. It is helpful if a room is available adjoining the mortuary for this purpose unless the relatives can say farewell in the ward before the body is removed. They will need the same support and sympathetic handling as for relatives present at the time of death.

## STAFF SUPPORT

Nurses who have not been present at a death before may feel rather nervous and anxious at such a time, not knowing what to expect or what to do, and a senior nurse should do all that is possible to guide them practically, to help them understand their feelings, to realize that death comes to us all – that it is a fact we must learn to live with. It should be stressed that by acting in a positive manner with the dying patient, and by using their nursing skills, they enable the patient to die comfortably. Appreciating the place of prayer at the time of death will enable them to see beyond the event. Helping them to see the needs of the family for comfort and support at this time will aid nurses in overcoming any anxiety. Taking the new nurse outside and explaining 'Last Offices' to him or her and taking him or her through it practically, showing respect for the body in gentle and sensitive handling, may all make it into a positive experience, again enabling the nurse to come to terms with death.

The senior nurse should also be aware that many young nurses suffer delayed reactions. They may become quiet, or become emotional over something quite unrelated. Others may not show anything, but it is important that all are given the chance to talk when they need a listening ear. A general atmosphere of caring for each other does much to enable more junior staff to voice their problems over particular deaths.

In hospice wards, a number of deaths in a short space of time can become difficult for all members of staff, and then it can be helpful for both senior and junior nurses to sit down together and talk over a cup of tea. Regular interdisciplinary staff-meetings can also be helpful as a means of supporting one another. For any nurse working full time in the field of terminal care, an active social-life should be encouraged.

## LEGAL ASPECTS

Nurses need to know the principles of the legal aspects involved just before and after the death of a patient. They may be asked questions by the relatives and should be able to answer them.

## Next-of-kin

It is very important to establish who is next-of-kin, and where he or she may be contacted. One would think this was an easy task, but it is not always so, as one discovers through bitter experience. For example, two ladies may claim to be the wife of the patient, or a hitherto unknown relative may turn up and insist that he or she is next-of-kin. Much tact is needed to deal with such situations.

## Time of death

The exact time of death should be noted, and the doctor, if not present, should be informed who was present at the time of death. The names of those present are recorded, both relatives and staff.

## Last Offices

As already mentioned above, the relatives' wishes must be ascertained to avoid possible future litigation as well as natural distress. If there is any question of criminal proceedings there should be minimal interference with the body.

## Property of the deceased patient

Any valuables or large sums of money should already have been deposited for safe keeping with the hospital administrator, and the nearest relative can collect them when convenient. Other belongings normally kept in the bedside locker should be listed by two nurses who then sign the list as a correct record. The property is packed into a parcel or box and may be given to the relatives at a suitable moment, usually when they come for the death certificate.

## Existence of a valid will

Nurses may be questioned regarding the advisability of making a will and should encourage all patients who are terminally ill to do so, as this prevents much friction and even family feuds after the death. If, however, they are asked to act as witnesses to a patient's will, they are well advised not to do so, but to suggest that a solicitor should see the patient and find witnesses. At the same time as this is drawn up, the doctor has to write a statement in the case-notes about the patient's mental state in case the will is later contested. As a valuable document, the will can then be deposited for safe keeping with the hospital administrator, if this is what the patient desires.

## Identification of the dead person in hospital

It is very important to avoid mistakes and the body should preferably be clearly labelled, for instance, by leaving the identity bracelet in place. It is insufficient to mark only the outside of the shroud.

## Death certificate

If the cause of death is clear and there are no suspicious circumstances, the doctor caring for the patient will sign the death certificate, and arrangements can be made for the relatives to collect this and take it to the registrar as soon as possible. If cremation is to take place, the law requires a further certificate signed by two doctors.

## Donation of organs for transplant or research

The nearest relative must act quickly if this was the wish of the deceased person; kidneys must be removed within half an hour of death, eyes within six hours. The nurse's involvement in this matter will consist in making sure that the relatives are in touch with the doctor concerned, and in being aware that, as with a request for a post-mortem examination or a coroner's inquest, this can add to distress and increase the need for support at this time.

For further details of medico-legal matters, see Chapter 7.

# FURTHER READING

Baqui, M. A., Joseph, the late Rabbi B. and Levenstein, Rabbi M. (1983) *Jewish and Muslim Teaching Concerning Death*, St Joseph's Hospice, London, and

*Our Ministry and Other Faiths – A Booklet for Hospital Chaplains*, CIO Publishing, London.

Hanratty, J. (1983) *Care of the Dying – Philosophy of the Care of the Terminally Ill*, St Joseph's Hospice, London.

Hanratty, J. (1985) *The Physiology of Dying*, St Joseph's Hospice, London, occasional paper.

Hanratty, J. (1987) *Control of Distressing Symptoms in the Dying Patient*, St Joseph's Hospice, London.

Henley, A. (1979) *Asian Patients in Hospital and at Home*, King Edward Hospital Fund for London.

Lothian Community Relations Council (1984) *Religious Cultures*, Edinburgh.

McGilloway, O. and Myco, F. (eds) (1985) *Nursing and Spiritual Care*, Harper & Row, London.

Prickett, J. (1980) *Death*, Butterworth Educational, Living Faiths series, Cambridge.

Sampson, C. (1982) *The Neglected Ethic – Religious and Cultural Factors in the Care of Patients*, McGraw-Hill, Maidenhead.

Young, A. P. (1989) *Legal Problems in Nursing Practice* 2nd edn, Harper & Row, London.

## ACKNOWLEDGEMENTS

We acknowledge the help of the Islamic Foundation in Leicester and the Buddhist Society in London.

# 7. The Role of the Doctor

The purpose of this chapter is to outline some of the special facets of the doctor's role in caring for dying patients. The doctor's viewpoint and approach to diagnosis and prognosis in terminal care are discussed. The assessment of the needs of the dying patient and his or her family, as death approaches, are considered, including some practical aspects of medical care at the time of death and of relatives thereafter. It is not the intention to discuss here the treatment of specific symptoms or problems – more details of the management of these will be found in other chapters.

## THE DOCTOR'S VIEWPOINT

The dying patient represents a peculiar problem for modern doctors, whatever their speciality. Doctors today have a long, scientifically based general and professional education culminating in a degree of technical expertise hitherto unknown. This knowledge well befits them for solving the clinical problems of modern medical management of acutely ill patients.

Sadly, though, in all this development something of the human face of medicine has been accidentally left by the wayside. Doctors so trained may have a tendency to see their patients in terms of disease processes with known precipitants and consequences rather than as people with difficulties, often multiple, caused by or causing ill health. The former approach is particularly unsuitable for some groups of patients, and must be seen to be so. It will not have escaped the notice of any health-care worker today that technological medicine does not hold the whole answer for problems of, for instance, the pregnant mother, the unborn child, the handicapped child, the chronically sick, the mentally ill and the elderly.

The dying are one such group, and a very large one, including some 130,000 people dying each year in the UK from cancer.

It is the very unsuitability of modern medicine's management of this group's particular problems that has been the main stimulus to the development of alternative approaches to care for these patients. The hospice movement has fostered this alternative approach, studying and learning from dying patients in a scientific manner and applying the skills of doctors, nurses, social workers, physiotherapists and others to the 'total' care of dying patients. In so doing a wealth of knowledge has accumulated in all areas of terminal care. It is now never true that 'nothing can be done' for a dying patient and such a phrase should be struck from the parlance of health-care workers in this regard. Really it is only another way of saying 'This patient cannot be cured, I can do nothing'. A better approach is 'What can I do?'

Doctors, working with the dying patient, must first reorientate themselves. Cure can no longer be held as their only measure of success. Automatic 'patterns' of behaviour in dealing with patients cease to be appropriate. They must develop alternative techniques.

Investigations will need to be limited, and certain treatments may need to be stopped because they are no longer controlling the disease and are therefore inappropriate. This will necessitate lengthy explanations to patient and family if they are to be at ease with these changes in management; time must be set aside for giving such explanations and for answering the patient's questions, and those of the family. All too often curative treatment is stopped without explanation; the patient may be well aware of the prognostic significance of this and his or her dejection is compounded by the thought 'The doctors have given up on me'.

Even worse, treatment may be continued late into a patient's illness, long after it is appropriate, because those caring for the patient cannot themselves face the difficulty of a direct explanation to him or her as to why it is no longer useful. It is easier just to carry on regardless whilst the patient's deteriorating health is denied by all. Time and flexibility are the keys to managing such patients well. Doctors must learn to be flexible in telling patients and families what *they* wish to know rather than what doctors feel they should be told.

Even if patients appear to have little to say today, time must be spent in allowing them to make this clear. Above all, patients must feel free to talk openly and patients will only feel this freedom if the doctor is attentive, concerned and unhurried in his or her manner (however much else there is to do!).

Doctors must be prepared to befriend their patients, to allow them to voice their fears, discuss their anxieties, and spend much time explaining illness and treatment. It may be that the doctor will be humbled more than once by facing the tragedy of his or her patient's circumstances, or moved to tears of sadness or joy by the patient's comments; such is life, such companionship is itself caring, and will be immediately seen as such by the patient. This relationship between the doctor and dying patient has been compared to that between mother and child, in that, if the doctor openly offers time, concern and explanations, the patient feels a sense of security, protection and trust, which are primordial needs for all of us. The fulfilling of these needs for the patient at the time of death can markedly reduce the pain and suffering of dying. It is the recognition of such needs felt by patients and manifest in many forms, symptoms and problems that is the goal in the hospice approach to the dying person.

## DIAGNOSIS

In Britain today malignant disease is the second commonest cause of death in adults, the commonest being cardiovascular disease. In practical terms the dying are those suffering from an inexorably progressive incurable illness, which is ultimately fatal. Cardiovascular illnesses, even in the elderly, are not inexorably progressive and it would be wrong for them to be viewed as such today. Similarly, multiple-sclerosis sufferers and other handicapped patients should not be seen as 'the dying' or written off. Many such handicaps are compatible with a normal life-span, and rehabilitative care throughout is what is needed for such patients, not 'symptom control'. Thus the commonest diagnosis amongst dying patients will be some form of cancer and amongst these the solid tumours of adult life predominate: these are cancers of bronchus, breast (in women), stomach, colon, pancreas and kidney. Modern treatment can modify the symptomatic course of such diseases considerably, but improves the prognosis little if at all.

The ultimate outcome is virtually uniformly premature death, and a stage is reached in the natural history of all these diseases past which attempts at cure are not only unproductive, but diminish the quality of life remaining for the patient. Some other conditions may also give rise to this sort of picture though they are all uncommon, people dying from motor neurone disease – sometimes just extreme frailty and old age – and those in the terminal phases of illnesses like fibrosing alveolitis. Chronic renal or respiratory failure and, more recently, acquired immune deficiency syndrome (AIDS) are all groups with which the doctor should be prepared to consider openly the symptom-control approach.

Those with AIDS or its complications give rise to special practical difficulties for health-care staff. They also have enhanced needs because of youth, the 'stigma' of diagnosis and the – sometimes bizarre – social consequences of this illness. The means of providing sensitive terminal care for these patients are only now beginning to be developed in the UK with patients themselves, their relatives and carers often providing the motive force.

## Malignant disease

Lymphomas, leukaemias and reticuloses – the so-called 'diffuse' or 'blood-borne' tumours – have a much better response to medical treatment than their solid counterparts. Some of these tumours (all rare) are now classed as curable in some patients but dying patients with these diseases are encountered and they may sometimes be very young children.

Doctors caring for the dying patient must have a sound knowledge of oncology – that is, the study of malignant disease – and understand the natural history of all these illnesses. They need not have specialist expertise in the specific treatment of the illness causing death but they must know and understand the range of therapeutic techniques available and in what circumstances they might be used so that they can confidently advise patients and relatives and call on other specialist services as needed.

It is impossible to consider in detail here the particular illnesses from which dying patients may suffer but it is worth while to consider further some physical aspects common to such patients.

## Some effects of widespread disease

In most patients a primary tumour will have been identified and treated directly by surgery, radiotherapy, chemotherapy or a combination of these. In many instances, and where the initial treatment has been successful, dying patients show little evidence of the primary disease. The problem has become one of disseminated disease and, in fact, some patients already have metastases at the time of diagnosis.

Metastatic or recurrent disease may be 'local' – near the primary site – or more often distant and spread via lymphatics to lymph nodes and via blood to lungs, liver, bones and brain. Multiple metastases are a common finding and sometimes, if the primary tumour cannot be easily diagnosed, it is undesirable to subject the patient to complex and uncomfortable investigations when the prognosis is clear – the diagnosis is then carcinomatosis from an unknown primary site. The most common primary sites for these minute tumours are bronchus, breast, testis, ovary, thyroid and kidney.

## Hypercalcaemia

A raised level of serum calcium is a common complication of widespread malignant disease. Sometimes the levels are so high as to induce vomiting and other symptoms, and in this case the symptoms are generally relieved by treatment to reduce the serum-calcium level. This treatment may involve steroid drugs, intravenous fluids and phosphates and a cytotoxic antibiotic, mithramycin.

The cause of the hypercalcaemia is not known. Often it is associated with bone metastases, but many patients with such metastases do not have raised calcium levels. The underlying cause appears to be abnormal endocrine effects of the tumour and its products.

## Cachexia

There is frequently progressive weakness and weight loss in malignant disease. The results in wasting and other biochemical abnormalities are together termed 'cachexia'. This situation is caused by many factors and bears some relation to the weight of tumour present in the body. The tumour itself consumes vital nutrients and also produces waste products that interfere with normal metabolism. The presence of anorexia, vomiting, ascites, fistula, haemorrhage, infection or ulceration often adds insult to injury and there is increased metabolic rate with protein and calorie malnutrition leading to wasting. Such patients are weak, tire easily and are often depressed; even if food intake is adequate, weight gain is unlikely.

## Anaemia

Progressive anaemia is a common finding – malnutrition, recurrent blood loss, altered iron metabolism and infection may all be contributory factors. Progressive marrow infiltration may result in leucoerythroblastic anaemia, and in patients with carcinoma of the stomach vitamin $B_{12}$ deficiency may also occur. A mixed picture is usual. Blood transfusions are sometimes used to relieve (temporarily) the anaemia of malignancy; good results can sometimes be achieved but each patient must be assessed individually. It may be inappropriate to offer transfusion as temporary respite for no useful purpose (as judged, preferably, by the patient) since the treatment once offered has marked psychological effects on patient and family – usually being seen as life sustaining – and thereafter will be requested again even if no longer of use. Facing the issue of the patient's deteriorating health may be postponed, but it cannot ultimately be avoided; conversely, transfusion may be a valuable adjunct to radiotherapy and surgery in these patients and is widely used as such.

## PROGNOSIS

The prognosis of patients who will benefit from the symptom-control approach to management is variable and can never be assessed very accurately. In general, it can be said to be less than six months. The actual length of estimated life remaining is unimportant. It is necessary for each patient to be assessed individually and the question asked, 'Has the time for terminal care of this patient been reached?'

Doctors need to consider this point carefully as they must introduce the patient to a new symptom-orientated approach. If doctors themselves feel this approach is inappropriate then the patient is unlikely to be put at his or her ease. In trying to judge what is appropriate for an individual patient at a specific stage in his or her illness, doctors must consider several factors:

(1) The patient's symptoms.
(2) Diagnosis and evidence for progressive disease.
(3) Failure of response to curative/conventional treatment.
(4) The psychological state of both patient and family.

Positive findings in all of these areas would indicate that the patient is likely to benefit from the care-orientated symptom-control approach, but the decision to adopt such an approach may often be complicated by the patient's and his or her family's psychological attitude being one of denial. Some patients may have severe symptoms but with little or no evidence of active disease.

These people need some support outside hospital, but it is probably more appropriate that this comes from their general practitioner rather than a 'terminal-care team'. In other instances patients may have evidence of metastatic disease with few or no symptoms, and it may be that such a patient would be confused by apparently (to the patient) unnecessary alterations in his or her care. Some such patients live for many months and it is important for the physician-in-charge to be aware of this; he or she may wish to offer a little advice, but then have no further involvement until a later date when the patient's difficulties increase.

## CARE AS DEATH APPROACHES

As the patient's illness progresses, the doctor must deal with new or changing symptoms or problems as they arise. He or she must also try to pre-empt, where possible, the needs of the patient and family by providing advice and support and frequently re-assessing the situation.

In practice, whatever the primary diagnosis the terminal event for most patients will be bronchopneumonia – infected infiltration of the lungs due to synchronous inactivity, debility and immune failure. This will be preceded by a variable period, perhaps a few weeks, of rapidly-increasing weakness culminating in bedfastness with, after a short time, collapse, coma and then death by cardio-respiratory arrest. (Deaths by acute asphyxia, haemorrhage or other cataclysmic event are all so rare as to be of only anecdotal importance.) This sequence of events implies that as death approaches the patient will need increasing time, help and support from family, friends and carers and, in the last days, will need continuous nursing care.

The doctor supervising care at this time needs to be sensitively aware of the feelings of patient and family in order to allow choice for the patient in electing where to die. For some this event can only occur in hospital and their needs and wishes should be respected. Others will wish to continue at home with family and friends through death, and this will have consequences for the family, the doctor and all involved in care. Relatives, in particular, need much help, reassurance and support in order to continue to care for their loved one, at home, in the last days. Apart from the physical and emotional demands of the task – which can have many positive benefits in bereavement – in some instances, if unsupported, relatives may be left with an enhanced feeling of guilt and despair at 'having failed them at the last'. This can have a profound detrimental effect on the bereaved that can colour the whole of the rest of their lives and, in some instances, pass into the 'family folklore' in a way that damages other family members' capacity for accepting bereavements in their own lives.

## AT TIME OF DEATH

With deaths in hospital, the doctor is unlikely to be present at the moment of death. A member of the hospital nursing, and perhaps pastoral staff, are likely to be present with one or more relatives, at the bedside. The junior hospital doctor will be called to confirm death (often at night). This doctor may not know the patient well, or at all, and quite often it falls to nursing staff to answer the questions of relatives and provide support. When a death occurs at home, the family doctor is likely to be the first person called to the house and may sometimes be present at or shortly before death.

Wherever the death should occur there are certain steps to be taken and the guiding principle for the attendant should be unhurried calm. Time should be given for the relatives to pay their respects in a setting that allows quiet and freedom from disturbance. Relatives should be encouraged to show their feelings without embarassment and offered support and encouragement to allow children (often, unhappily, 'protected' from these events) to experience the family's loss. Due respect should be shown for the religious and cultural beliefs of the patient and bereaved, and facilities provided so that ritual washing, dressing or adornment of the body can be carried out. Some religions, e.g. Judaism, prefer the funeral to follow quickly after death and all administrative procedures should, where possible, be facilitated so that the funeral can take place unhindered.

## MEDICO-LEGAL ASPECTS

In the UK, the death must be certified by a registered medical practitioner who must have seen the patient alive in the two weeks before death. This certificate is free, and must be delivered to the Registrar of Births, Marriages and Deaths, who in turn issues a burial certificate authorizing the undertaker (or anyone) to bury the remains in a public cemetery. If cremation is chosen, the doctor issuing the death certificate and a second, independent, doctor must sign cremation certificates to exclude non-accidental or suspicious deaths – to allow cremation to proceed. These papers are normally handled by the undertaker and both doctors charge the estate a fee.

If the death cannot be certified, because no doctor has seen the patient recently, or there are suspicious circumstances, or the patient has a proscribed disease (usually industrial, e.g. asbestosis, mesothelioma), the coroner's office (or, in Scotland, the Procurator Fiscal) will be involved and a post-mortem may be carried out. In the event of, say, mesothelioma it is wise to be prepared to discuss this with both patient and relatives. (A post-mortem is sometimes also requested for research purposes by a hospital doctor.)

### Disposal of the body in special circumstances

Sometimes the patient may have made a bequest of their body, or parts of it, for medical research or therapeutic purposes. Acts of Parliament have been passed at different times to ensure proper safeguards for such procedures. The most recent is the Anatomy Act 1984 that came into force in 1988 and combines the rules of several other Acts. Donor cards are in common use today and cover the requirements of the Act. Doctors, of course, must be conversant with the medical responsibilities when dealing with such situations. Finally, the organs of patients who have died from malignant disease (other than those with isolated brain tumour) are unsuitable for transplantation. This is not because the disease is 'infectious' – simply that micrometastases could not be excluded. Some bereaved families need assurance on this point.

## CARE OF THE BEREAVED FAMILY

After the death, some immediate problems may arise. Relatives may faint or become agitated and angry; extreme adverse reactions are rare but memorable and careful preparatory care will often ameliorate them. If either occur the doctor should proffer explanation, advice, help and support as indicated in a calm, unhurried and non-judgemental way. Occasional prescriptions of tranquillizers or hypnotics may be requested for relatives. These are very rarely essential but can sometimes be helpful for short periods following bereavement, and advice and practical suggestions are usually more important. Commonly the patient and relatives share the same general practitioner and he or she is in an ideal position to co-ordinate his or her response to their individual needs. Hospital doctors involved in a death should not undertake the treatment of relatives if asked.

It cannot be over-emphasized that thoughtful, sensitive, supportive care for the patient and family in the final days of illness, at the moment of death and the immediate aftermath, is of utmost importance in preventing bereavement difficulties in relatives and children. In turn this may prevent distress in future generations as these people face their own death.

## FURTHER READING

Hinton, J. (1972) *Dying*, Pelican, Harmondsworth.
Lamerton, R. (1980) *Care of the Dying*, Pelican, Harmondsworth.
*The Lancet* (1980) Changing the face of death, editorial, vol. 1, pp. 1,340–1.
Parkes, C. Murray (1978) Home or hospital? Terminal care as seen by surviving spouses, *Journal of the Royal College of General Practitioners*, No. 28, pp. 19–30.
Saunders, C. (ed.) (1984) *The Management of Terminal Disease*, 2nd edn, Edward Arnold, London.

### Medico-legal aspects

DHSS (1988) *What To Do After a Death*, D. 49, Department of Health and Social Security, London.
NCVO (1988) *Citizens Advice Notes System, Stop Press,* Vol. 2, Ref. 15 (34), p.15118 & 8A, The National Council for Voluntary Organizations, London.
SHHD (1988) *What To Do After a Death*, Scottish Home and Health Department, Edinburgh.

# 8. The Role of the Social Worker

'Social work is just common sense, isn't it?' is probably how most people view the role of the social worker, and to some extent this is understandable. In all of the caring professions maturity, experience of life and a pragmatic approach have a great part to play; certainly this is so in social work. In this chapter, however, the role of the social worker will be discussed in some detail, and in particular how he or she operates in a multi-disciplinary team looking after the terminally ill.

Everyone who works in such a team, regardless of their professional background, will know that people who are seriously or terminally ill are not only having to cope with the physical effects of their disease but also with a plethora of other concerns about themselves, their friends and family. Simple matters can become complex issues of great concern about themselves, their friends and family. Discussions have to be faced where there is perhaps just not a viable answer to be found. Such issues need to be shared, listened to, acknowledged as important to the person concerned and unique to their individual life-experience. These concerns can range from anxiety about practical matters such as financial security, to deep-seated emotional and psychological reactions such as fears about mortality and guilt about previous life-experiences.

Social workers view this range of work as pertinent to them. They are able to advise on the spectrum of welfare benefits and in general what is available in terms of legal and social services. Additionally, their knowledge of these areas is placed within the context of a thorough training in counselling, which means they are available to help with the individual's reaction to the various stresses they may be facing. It is in these areas where common sense may not be quite sufficient to support the individual asking for help. Life experience and maturity that leads a 'caring person' to say, for example, 'Oh, yes, I know, I had the same problem with my husband', does not help the terminally ill person with his or her own problems. This is because the corollary of such a remark could be 'Oh, if she coped, I ought to be able to too, so why can't I?' Thus the helping person can actually make the person in trouble feel worse. Guilt and inadequacy can then be added to anxiety.

This chapter is, therefore, addressed to the issue of how social workers can deal with the range of issues that affect the terminally ill person and their family. So first, some of these issues need to be identified.

## TERMINAL ILLNESS AS LOSS

An individual and his or her family coping with terminal illness are facing loss of a dramatic and permanent kind. The ill person is facing loss of function, of finance through loss of employment availability, of independence and of control of him- or herself and those around as he or she faces death. The family are experiencing the same range of loss, augmented by the fear of the future and of survival without the person they love. This can add up to one of the most difficult times with which the family has ever had to deal.

Some families have faced loss and crisis before – perhaps many times. Even if it is the first time a death has occurred, the family may well have had to deal with redundancy, unemployment, ill health, moving, etc. Such families may be able to manage more easily though it will depend on how they have coped with previous loss. If they have come through the crisis, letting themselves feel it, and absorbing it into their understanding, then they will be able to face the current trauma with some strength. If, however, the family have never faced a serious crisis before, or have not really coped with a previous one, then they are likely to be overwhelmed with this one.

Mrs B was 29 when her husband was diagnosed as having terminal cancer. They had four children under the age of 10 and were living away from their country of origin, and so were isolated on the council estate where they were housed. At the time of Mr B's death, Mrs B expressed actively suicidal ideas, neglected the children and in general was quite unable to cope. Over the next year, in interview sessions, she talked about the death of her mother when Mrs B herself was 13; how she had had to take care of her father, until she 'escaped' by marrying Mr B at the age of 17; how they had come to England, where Mrs B then suffered a series of five miscarriages. Now, at 29 years of age, her husband, whom she described as 'the best man in the world – totally devoted to his family', had also died.

In these sessions it was necessary to deal with the many losses in Mrs B's life, starting with the first, before we could look at the death of her husband. We needed to talk of the significance of each loss to Mrs B and how she had reacted, denying the problem because of her other responsibilities; how she was unable to 'carry on' this time; and how this inability to carry on had to happen if the compound grief of many years was to be absorbed. Clearly, the story is a long and complicated one. Mrs B eventually arrived at the stage where she could consider her present position, and look at the possibilities open to her. She could make some sense of her bereavements to the extent that she could recognize how they have helped make her the person she is today.

It would be a mistake to feel that Mrs B's story is unusual. Many people faced with a crisis today shudder, thinking 'here we go again', and try to cope, getting through it, but needing all of their physical and emotional strength to do so. Mrs B just had to let go at the particular time in her life when her husband died. It is the social worker's job to try to assess the needs of the people they meet; what their reaction to loss might be; and how it can be shared and acknowledged.

## The experience of grief

Commonly, families dealing with grief – either at the impending death of a member of the family or at the actual death – will say that they feel ostracized by the community around them. Neighbours, friends, even relatives are embarrassed, awkward, and say to themselves, 'Oh, I expect they want to be alone'. In fact, this is usually the last thing that people, either when anticipating bereavement or when experiencing it, want. They need to talk about their loss, over and over again, because this is one way it becomes a reality. They will be sad, tearful, often withdrawn, but greatly appreciate care extended by anyone coming to share the grief with them.

People usually stay away because they feel that such a weight of sadness must be a 'private thing' and that it is an intrusion to contact the bereaved person. This is a rationalization stimulated by embarrassment and awkwardness. They feel they do not know what to do, so it would be better to do nothing. At all events, keep to a safe distance. Often a neighbour will cook a meal but leave it on the doorstep. Contact must be avoided. They mistakenly feel that grief is a private thing that cannot be understood. However, loss is something everyone has experienced, no matter how slight. The component parts are the same.

## Stages of reaction to loss

Dr Elizabeth Kubler-Ross (1970) has suggested that these component parts are denial, anger, depression, bargaining and acceptance. Such a list is not exhaustive; neither is loss experienced in such a tidy, catalogued way. However, when one is attempting to meet with someone who is grieving, it is useful to keep such a list in mind to use as an indicator of what stage the person may have reached in the process.

So let us test the theory with an example of loss that most of us have experienced – having a tooth extracted! First, there is the niggling pain of toothache, which persists as we deny its existence. We say, 'I must have eaten something particularly sweet' or 'I shouldn't eat ice cream after drinking tea' – anything to deny we have a bad tooth. Second comes the irritation, the anger: 'What a time for this to happen, I can't possibly fit in a trip to the dentist, they charge the earth', etc. Probably we'll be irritable with those around us, they wonder at our tetchiness and so stay away from us. Next comes depression: 'But I don't like going to the dentist, it hurts, my face will be swollen, I don't want to go, I just want to hide and go to bed with a hot-water bottle!' Then the bargaining: 'Well, if I go to the dentist, I could just look in that dress-shop next door, and perhaps buy that skirt I liked' or 'I deserve a treat if I go, that video centre is just along the road . . .'. Finally acceptance: the dental appointment is made, it wasn't so bad as it had been feared and the possibility of a future after the extraction can be considered. What was an overwhelming experience, dictating one's behaviour for a few days, has become an absorbed experience that can be accounted for.

I apologize for labouring this point but it is so important to understand. The process of loss that an individual experiences following the death of someone they loved is the same process as coming to terms with the loss of that tooth, only the depth of reaction and length of time it takes will be different.

Many other commentators on this subject have also identified a series of reactions, and probably the most well known of these commentaries is the work of Colin Murray Parkes (1986). He describes four stages. The first one is of shock and numbness where the individual is quite unable to absorb the reality of their situation and is worried by the fact that they feel immune to anything that is happening around them. Often they will say 'it's as though there is a glass wall between me and the rest of the world. I can see and hear everything that's happening but it doesn't impinge on me at all'. Second, a stage of acute grief, crying and pining and feeling prey to overwhelming surges of emotion, often rages and feelings of great anger. Third, a time of apathy and aimlessness where it seems that the whole of life and living is useless and has no point at all. Too much has been lost that cannot be recovered and the future doesn't exist. Fourth, the final stage, where the individual begins to feel that it is possible to recoup something from the experience they have gone through and that a future can once more be considered and life can assume some sort of pattern again.

These reactions are the same for the patient and the relatives. Contemplation of one's own loss of life or of the death of someone close has the same effect. Having looked at what these reactions might be, the next step is to decide what help can be offered.

## PRACTICAL ISSUES

First, there is much in the way of help that can be offered. For the ill person and his or her family, probably one of the biggest problems is one of reduced finances. It is the social worker's job to advise on the benefits available to terminally ill people, especially when they are being cared for at home. Most of the benefits are handled by the Department of Health and Social Security (DHSS), and particular ones I have found to be most applicable are as follows.

### Attendance allowance

This can be paid at the 12-hourly or 24-hourly rate to the ill person who must have been in need of attention for all personal needs for six months or more. It is non-taxable and does not count in assessment for things like Housing Benefit or Supplementary Pension. This allowance stops if the patient is in hospital or residential care for longer than four weeks.

## Mobility allowance

This is paid to people under retirement age who go out but cannot use public transport. This allowance is again non-taxable and does not count when being assessed for other benefits. It should also carry on for a 'period of time' if the patient is hospitalized or in residential care.

## Invalid care allowance

This allowance is paid to a carer if the person they care for is in receipt of Attendance Allowance and if the carer is not working more than 12 hours a week. This allowance *is* taxable and it *does* count against other benefits of the carer or other members of the household.

There are other allowances such as the 'Constant Attendance Allowance' payable where the disability is assessed at 100 per cent or the 'Exceptionally Severe Disability Allowance' where the disability is assessed as total and permanent, but these are less frequently used. Most pensions, such as Retirement Pension, are payable in full for the first eight weeks of a patient's admission to hospital and from that time they are reduced. It is thus always helpful to inform the relevant DHSS office when someone in receipt of benefits is admitted. A person in receipt of Supplementary Benefit is entitled to have visiting fares paid when they attend the hospital either as a patient or to visit a relative.

Any individual circumstances should always be discussed with the DHSS. However, because there are many variations and the benefit system is constantly being reviewed, the social worker should also be able to advise and suggest which benefits it would be appropriate to apply for. Additionally, it is often possible to contact national charities on the family's behalf. Amongst these, the National Society for Cancer Relief is very generous and helpful. It helps in two ways: first, with a special grant for a particular need, such as an outstanding heating bill or travelling fares for treatment, a holiday, etc.; and second, with a regular weekly grant to help towards the increased cost of caring for a seriously ill person – again, especially at home. Another charity to contact is the Malcolm Sargent Cancer Fund for Children, which helps with the financial needs of families where there is an ill child.

The alleviation of the financial stress that can be obtained from these sources should not be under-estimated. If the patient is in hospital or other institution the ward staff may notice that the family is not visiting regularly. It is useful to consider that this might be because the cost of travelling is proving prohibitive.

As a family realizes that one of its members has a limited time left, there often emerges a particular aspiration, a goal that needs to be met. It can be useful for the social worker to discuss whatever these issues are, and facilitate a positive outcome where possible. Practical problems are important and once dealt with can allow more time for the patient and relatives to talk over more difficult matters. Arranging for a telephone to be installed as an emergency in a patient's home, so that the family can keep in touch and summon help easily, can do just as much to relieve tension in a family as many hours of intensive counselling!

There are an increasing number of patients referred with prescribed industrial disease, for example, mesothelioma caused by asbestos exposure. To claim Industrial Disease Benefit or compensation, the industrial link must be proved and this is a complicated and protracted business. The Society for the Prevention of Asbestosis and Industrial Disease (SPAID) is a national self-help organization established to put such people in touch with each other and is helpful in negotiating this process.

After the patient has died the practical involvement continues. Quite often families will need help with arranging the funeral. Paying for it can often be a real problem, and families may need advice about 'public funerals' and the resources of the DHSS. Since April 1987 the £30 death grant has been abolished and families in reduced circumstances, but not necessarily receiving Supplementary Benefit, can apply to the Social Fund, administered by the local DHSS office, if they do not have sufficient funds. Help may also be needed dealing with probate, widow's allowances and pensions, building societies for rearranging mortgages, etc. Widows often need help with the disposal of a car, finding the gas and electricity meters, even how to get onto a bus, which hitherto had never been done alone. Widowers ask for help with simple cooking recipes, the mysteries of the launderette and the supermarket.

## Social and emotional help

Social workers can give considerable emotional support to patients and their families. They are often the only non-medical member of the terminal-care team, and thus have a unique contribution to make. It is by no means the social worker alone who can help by listening to the patient and his or her family: the whole team is involved in this, but the social worker will often be seen by the family as the one who deals with doubts and worries, precisely because of this obvious non-medical role. However caring and considerate the medical members of the team, families are often embarrassed to ask what they imagine to be stupid questions. It is easier to ask someone they understand to be a lay person like themselves.

Mrs C looked at the social worker in a puzzled way, and asked how she was supposed to administer suppositories to herself in what was clearly an anatomically impossible position. Once she had the explanation, the cause of Mrs C's continuing and puzzling constipation became clear! She felt she could not ask for further instructions when she had first been prescribed the medication and so had tried to administer them as she had understood from the directions. Unfortunately, her understanding did not extend to the relevant orifice!

The same sort of approach is needed for discussions on diagnosis and prognosis, etc. Individuals and families often feel that their questions must sound stupid. All members of the multi-disciplinary terminal-care team can forget that although they are dealing daily with issues of life and death, and recognize many anxious questions from patients as commonplace, to the individuals involved they are trying to face what can be a shattering event in their family's life. Relatives do not always have the relevant vocabulary, may not know how to phrase the questions they need to ask, and may feel the team is too busy and should not be expected to deal with such worries. Thus it may be that the social worker, who is not involved in the clinical work-management of the patient on the ward or at home, may be able to make him- or herself available to patients and families as they come to terms with the bad news they have received.

As previously discussed, the social worker can often be a great deal of help and support to a patient who has been overwhelmed by their impending loss of life. Referring back to the stages of loss, some patients will deny their illness to a disabling degree, so that no honest communication can be carried out by the family at all. Others will become embittered, asking 'Why me?' and remain there, instead of moving along the spectrum to a 'Well, I don't like it but I know it's going to happen and I can't stop it' approach. In actuality it seems more likely to be the family that is denying rather then the patient.

Miss D, a patient living with an elderly mother, resolutely refused to agree that anything was worrying her at all. She would soon recover from this 'virus' and then continue to look after her mother. She became very angry and distressed as efforts were made to discuss with her the fact that her level of obvious anxiety must be connected to concern for herself: 'No, it's not, it's you that upset me', she would say, and then would plaintively add, 'You must be able to do something to make me better'.

The most usual situation is that the family needs to be reassured that nothing catastrophic will happen if they discuss diagnosis with the patient. Often he or she has already conveyed to the team that 'they know' but are afraid to talk it over with the family, who they feel 'won't be able to take it'. On the other hand, the family have conveyed exactly the same thing! What a tragedy that miscommunication should enter a family's history at this stage, especially if there has always been open discussion before. The job is to explain to both sides that the other is waiting to talk things over, and that no one is going to collapse if the shared worries are talked about. What a difference open communications can make, and in bereavement follow-up work the family will particularly remember that conversation. A sizeable proportion of patients, however, are alone in the world, and as such need the team to become their 'family'.

## FOLLOW-UP CARE

Bereavement follow-up is a team task, not just the social worker's. It is essential that the team is concerned for the whole family, not just the patient. However, it is often the social worker who has had most contact with the family, by nature of the tasks that have been covered.

When making a home visit, the social worker is often whisked into the kitchen straight away, without catching sight of the patient, to discuss the family's worries – their fears of not coping, their anxieties about how death will come, how they will manage when it does. The worries can seem endless. It is often only after these feelings have been talked through that the family will ask 'Oh, did you want to see my husband/wife/mother?' with the implied notion that they are not expecting it as they have assumed the visit to be for them. The relationship established at this time can carry through to much of the bereavement follow-up work.

The emotional vulnerability of grieving people is well documented. The surviving relatives, especially if old, young, isolated or weighed down by other worries, are likely to become ill, have an accident or a breakdown. For a few, suicide is a real risk, the survivor feeling that life is totally meaningless and just cannot be tolerated.

Immediately following the death of the patient there is a great deal of activity. There is much to arrange, with callers and relatives arriving for the funeral. Often the survivor is advised to take a holiday, or invited to stay with relatives. Sometimes they return to work straight away – anything to be absorbed in activity of some sort or another. This may be necessary but usually it has the effect of extending the first stage of grief, i.e. denial. After things quieten down, the survivor may find him- or herself sitting alone in the home that had been shared, and becomes aware of a desolation and a loneliness that can be quite overwhelming. Some respond by feeling they must move, change jobs, 'do something', but they seldom find it helps. There are no short cuts through grief. Sharing it with a trusted friend can be so healing. In my experience it takes about 18 months to come to terms with the loss they have experienced and this, of course, does not mean that it has been forgotten. It is useful to have come to know the family before the death of the patient because it makes it easier for the person undertaking bereavement follow-up to become that 'friend' for a period of time: to talk through, as many times as it takes, what has happened. The qualities of the deceased person are pondered upon and, especially important, what part the surviving relative played in the final illness. It greatly helps in the grieving process if the relative is able to say realistically 'I did everything I could to look after him'.

Many relatives who have had their relative die in hospital will feel guilty that they did not look after them at home, however inappropriate it would have been for them to do so.

A timely word of caution is appropriate here. Many relationships are not totally loving. (Such a statement will not surprise the reader, I am sure.) Some families take care of a sick relative for many motives other than selfless loving, and it is no part of the social worker's job to judge what those motives might be. It is, however, important to understand and to listen to what they are, because they can affect crucially the grieving process. For some survivors, the overwhelming feeling is of relief.

Mrs T had been a 'battered wife' for eight years, and although her husband was very considerably weakened by his terminal illness, she was still in great fear of him. Mrs T nursed her husband motivated by this fear, not by care, and she unhappily confessed she was praying for a release from this torment by her husband's death. The complex emotions that follow on a bereavement of this kind need careful handling. It is an old adage 'don't speak ill of the dead', and when an individual such as Mrs T feels she has somehow willed the death to happen, the future life that she thought would be a releasing one quickly turns to a guilt-ridden one.

Gradually, the year of bereavement continues. The first Christmas, birthday, wedding anniversary, and eventually the anniversary of the death, are important milestones – generally very sad ones. Hospices usually send a card on the anniversary of the patient's death, saying simply that the staff are thinking of the family on a difficult day. If it is known that the surviving relative is going to be alone on that day, personal contact is attempted.

After this crucial first anniversary when the bereaved person can begin to realize it is no longer 'this time last year' but 'this time the year before', the raw grief gives way to an absorbed sadness that, of course, still hurts, but it is more likely to be seen as part of life's dealings; and it is at this time that the social-work task may be completed. There may still be the need for follow-up support that may well be provided by an organization such as Cruse, a national organization for widows and parents that have had a child die. Unfortunately, such groups are in short supply, especially in inner-city areas. Bereavement counselling services are beginning to grow, and referral to them may be entirely appropriate. Friendships are made, grieving people realize they are not alone in feeling as they do, and that is an important step along the bereavement process.

## THE SOCIAL WORKER AS A TEAM MEMBER

The particular kind of social work I have tried to describe – in a terminal-care team – is a demanding one. Of course, at times the team members find their individual roles stressful in various ways. As the social worker one is often called upon to listen to other members of the team, and to share the concerns that such a job can produce. This seems to me an entirely valid social-work activity. We are perhaps uniquely qualified amongst the health-care team to understand something of the way pressures can distress and overwhelm a colleague, however experienced he or she may be. As has been suggested, often the social worker may not be so actively involved in the preliminary symptom-control function of the team. What they are available for is to talk with the team members who are thus involved, recognizing the need for such work to be constantly reviewed and assessed.

# REFERENCES

Kubler-Ross, E. (1970) *On Death and Dying*, Tavistock, London.

Parkes, C. M. (1986) *Bereavement: Studies of Grief in Adult Life*, Revised edn, Penguin, Harmondsworth.

# 9. Physiotherapy and the Dying Patient

'If by treating the patient with simple therapeutic measures he is helped to be more comfortable, then proceed' Patricia Downie (1983). The role of the physiotherapist in the care of the dying is a relatively new one. It is only in the last ten years that the place of the physiotherapist in the multi-disciplinary team caring for the dying patient has been established. Pioneering work was done by the British physiotherapist, Patricia Downie, in the 1970s, and it was she who first identified, established and documented the principles of physiotherapy care for the dying in Britain. Currently there are a growing number of physiotherapists working with the dying, and contributions to the literature are growing.

Caring for the dying patient is a team effort. The patient's needs can be complex, and the hospice philosophy of 'living until you die' means a sensitive approach to the changing needs of the patient, as day succeeds day, in order to give him or her the best quality of life possible. The physiotherapist participates in team consultation and decision-making to this end.

## MAINTAINING QUALITY OF LIFE BY PHYSICAL MEANS

The physiotherapist's job is to maintain by physical means the patient's quality of life as far as is possible. This means that not only must he or she help patients to maintain their mobility and independence as far as is practicable, but also he or she will help them with relief of various forms of discomfort caused by their disease process. Physiotherapy treatment starts with careful assessment of the patient and mutually agreed goals are set. Treatment may be geared to improve or maintain function, relieve symptoms or give support. As with other members of the caring team, the physiotherapist will provide a listening ear and a supportive presence during his or her treatment.

## Pain control

With the impressive expertise in the control of severe pain achieved by the hospice movement, there are still lesser areas of pain and discomfort that can be relieved by physiotherapy. Stiffness, aching limbs and tense muscles can be eased with gentle passive and assisted active movements, massage and positioning. Pre-existing conditions presenting alongside malignant disease can be treated using the usual therapeutic modalities. Heat in various forms, ice, ultrasound and gentle exercise may be appropriate. Transcutaneous nerve stimulation (TNS) is useful in relieving nerve-root compression pain, and also post-herpetic neuralgia. Acupuncture, too, can be used by some physiotherapists for pain relief.

## Oedema

A proportion of dying patients suffer with severely oedematous limbs, caused by obstruction of venous or lymphatic drainage due to surgery or tumour. Such limbs are heavy and unsightly. Effective treatment can be given by the physiotherapist using intermittent pressure-pumping apparatus. Gray (1987) describes a regime using a pressure-pump programme in conjunction with elastic-containment garments, thus achieving an excellent result in the majority of cases. The resulting decrease in size and weight, and increase in mobility, help to improve the quality of life for the patient.

## Mobility

Loss of mobility as the result of severe illness is to be expected. If effective pain control is achieved, it may be possible to mobilize a terminally ill patient. The physiotherapist will teach the patient how to transfer from bed to chair, chair to toilet and back, help in regaining walking skills; and he or she will prescribe the appropriate walking aids for the patient. Mobilization of stiff joints and gentle strengthening exercises are given as appropriate. Again, all treatment is undertaken in line with the patient's wishes, in order to enhance the quality of life remaining. The preservation of joint mobility also makes nursing care easier. In cases with hemiparesis or paraplegia, rehabilitation may be initiated if the patient is in a stable condition.

### Splinting

Appropriate splinting can add to a patient's comfort. A collar may be needed to support a painful neck or a splint to support a hand or foot. The physiotherapist can usually supply or make simple splinting. Advice on suitable footwear is also within his or her remit.

### Chest conditions

The dying patient is prone to chest infection. Pneumonia is known as the 'old man's friend', but by treating the patient's chest the physiotherapist's aim is to enhance the patient's comfort without using unnecessarily vigorous techniques. Routine physiotherapy for conditions such as chronic bronchitis, bronchiectasis or asthma can be given as tolerated. Treatment by nebulizer, breathing exercises, gentle vibrations and percussion may all be used as the patient can tolerate it. When no further advantage can be gained from active treatment, assistance in clearing secretions can add to the patient's comfort, particularly to help relieve persistent cough that is exhausting to a weak and ill patient. Steam inhalations may help to loosen sticky secretions; breathing exercises with relaxation help to relieve tension. Physical contact gives comfort even if very little actual treatment is possible.

## TEACHING

The physiotherapist is a resource for other members of the team as well as for the patient and the family. He or she is expert in the use of lifting and handling techniques, and is always ready to show how best to move patients or how to position them for comfort. He or she is concerned about the prevention of back injuries amongst those who are lifting the patient, and can be called upon to lecture and to demonstrate lifting techniques as part of his or her job. Of equal importance is the teaching role with the patient. Most physiotherapy treatments given to a patient involve a teaching element, i.e. transfer techniques, exercises, walking methods, etc. The physiotherapist uses a goal-oriented approach so that following assessment, treatment is aimed towards an agreed goal decided between physiotherapist and patient. Goals will decrease in magnitude as the patient's condition deteriorates. Sensitive discussion between therapist and patient will be needed to help the patient to come to terms with his or her loss of function.

## COMMUNICATION SKILLS

All members of the team caring for the dying patient and family need to develop and use listening, counselling and communication skills to facilitate the helping process. The physiotherapist along with the other members of the team uses these skills when he or she is with the patient. In a time of distress and loss, a skilled listener will try to help patients towards peace of mind, so that their last days with their loved ones can be lived to the full. Referral to the appropriate source of help is important for both patient and family.

The role of the physiotherapist in the care of the dying patient and the family is as a member of a multi-disciplinary team. As such, he or she is concerned not only with assessment and treatment of the patient, but also with holistic care, always aiming towards the optimum quality of life, physical, mental and spiritual, for the patient, and comfort and support for the family.

## REFERENCE AND FURTHER READING

Chatterton, P. (1988) Physiotherapy for the terminally ill, *Physiotherapy*, Vol. 74, No. 1, pp. 42–6.

Davies, B. (1980) Physiotherapy in the care of the dying, *Physiotherapy Canada*, November/December, Vol. 32, No. 6, pp. 337–42.

Doutre, D. Stillwell, D. and Ajemian, J. (1982) Physiotherapy in palliative care, in I. Ajemian and B. Mount (eds) *RVF Manual on Palliative/Hospice Care*, The Ayer Co., Salem, NH.

Downie, P. A. (1983) The place of physiotherapy in hospice care in, C. A. Corr and D. M. Corr (eds) *Hospice Care – Principles and Practice*, Faber & Faber, London.

Doyle, D. (ed.) (1984) *Palliative Care: The Management of Far Advanced Illness*, Croom Helm, Beckenham.

Gray, R. C. (1987) The management of limb oedema in patients with advanced cancer, *Physiotherapy*, Vol. 72, No. 10, pp. 504–6.

Michel, T. H. (1985) *International Perspectives in Physical Therapy 1: Pain*, Churchill Livingstone, Edinburgh.

O'Gorman, B. (1985) *Handling the Handicapped: A Guide to the Movement of Disabled People*, Chartered Society of Physiotherapists, Faulkner Publications, Cambridge.

O'Gorman, B. (1987) Pain: Management and control in physiotherapy, in P. E. Wells, V. Frampton and D. Bowsher, *Management of Cancer Pain in Terminal Care*, Heinemann Medical, London.

Ong, K. (1986) Handling the patient in pain, *Physiotherapy*, Vol. 72, No. 6, pp. 284–8.

Saunders, Dame C. (ed.) (1984) *The Management of Terminal Malignant Disease*, 2nd edn, Edward Arnold, London.

Shanks, R. (1982) Physiotherapy in palliative care, *Physiotherapy*, Vol. 68, No. 12, pp. 405–7.

Speck, P. (1978) *Loss and Grief in Medicine*, Baillière Tindall, London.

Wells, P. E., Frampton, V. and Bowsher, D. (eds) (1987) *Management of Cancer Pain in Terminal Care*, Heinemann Medical, London.

# 10. Caring for the Dying Child and the Family

## THE ROLE OF THE NURSE

It is humbling to be entrusted with the care of a sick child, most especially one who is dying. As nurses, we may become deeply involved with members of the family and may see them at times when their defences are down and they are at their most vulnerable. We may be taken into the confidence of one or more members of the family and allowed an insight into problems and anxieties and patterns of family life that have not previously been shared. We are there not only as professional carers, but also as fellow human beings in whom there must be implicit trust and with whom there need be no pretence.

Whilst the care of the dying child will have special features depending upon the age of the child, for example, in the first two weeks of life, and the nature of the terminal illness, it is hoped that the following principles will be helpful to nurses in their care of the child and the family. The second part of the chapter describes the particular model of care provided at a hospice for children – Helen House – illustrated by several case studies. It is hoped that the reading of the experiences described here will also be helpful for those working in hospitals or caring for dying children at home.

### Basic physical care

Nurses must give meticulous attention to the physical needs of the child. Their standard of care can make all the difference between constant discomfort and nagging reminders of the child's plight and the possibility of freeing the child to focus his or her attention on positive and outgoing thoughts and behaviour.

Care of skin and hair needs to be extended to help the child to feel attractive; well-fitting, pretty or 'fun' clothes, which the child enjoys wearing, are also a boost to morale and these should be chosen or adapted with a view to the ease of dressing or undressing.

Diet needs to be imaginative and varied according to what the child can manage. If only fluids can be tolerated there are many palatable milk-based drinks and fruit juices that are usually pleasing to the taste. With loss of normal physical activity, bowel function is often impaired and if this is ignored it will cause added discomfort and anxiety to the child. Before resorting to large doses of aperients, it is good to try added fibre in the diet, if this is possible.

Hydrotherapy, even just on the apparent level of play, can bring great relief to a child who has muscle contractures, paralysis, or who is emaciated. At its simplest, this can just take the form of the nurse allowing extended play-time in the bath. Indeed, many forms of treatment or routine care can be transformed into fun-times if the nurse is prepared to adopt this approach.

Cleaning the teeth, despite difficulties that may be present, and keeping the mouth clean and comfortable, is all-important.

## The need for mental stimulation

Boredom and feelings of frustration may be over-riding problems for children whose activities seem so limited, and a good nurse will enable them to explore positive avenues of interest that will stretch them, and will not be shocked by displays of anger that may be a direct result of their frustration, but rather will help them to channel their energies. Education and mental stimulation are vital for the child who is capable of benefiting to whatever limited a degree. Continuing relationships with peers can be a lifeline for the dying child, and with a little wise encouragement, the well child will be enthusiastic to include him or her in many ways to the benefit of both.

## Psychological needs of the child

Small children have a natural capacity for being able to live for the present moment, and recognizing this can be used to advantage by those caring for them. If they are free of pain and discomfort and are surrounded by people they love and trust, they are less likely to be fearful for the future. The older child will have taken on more of the fears and complexities of an adult in facing dying and death. It must be categorically stated that there are no hard and fast ways of answering the child's questions or set methods of helping him or her come to terms with the truth. So much depends on our own ability to absorb the impact of the emotional and spiritual implications and to cope with them ourselves. Platitudes and pat answers are less than helpful. At times when there seems to be nothing to say, it is better not to use empty words but rather to try to communicate reassurance through physical presence – just being there through it all. It is often remarked how protective sick children feel towards their parents and to what great lengths they will go to spare them further pain, whereas someone they trust who is less-closely related, but has some authority, may be taken into the child's confidence.

It is vital to listen carefully to what the child is actually saying or asking – adults easily fall into the trap of assuming that he or she is asking a more complex question than he or she really is. A cardinal rule is never to lie to a child. This does not mean to say that the child must be given the whole stark truth in one blow, but one is often able to give truthful reassurance and allay the child's fears about the actual process of dying and death itself always, of course, using terms the child understands, and being careful not to contradict beliefs held by his or her family.

## Symptom control

With great advances in the right use of drugs for symptom control, pain and other distressing symptoms associated with the terminal phase of illness need no longer be a feature. In spite of the development of these skills, it must be admitted that there is still room for research into pain control in paediatrics, for it is an acknowledged fact that the child's absorption of, and response to, drugs is different from that of adults. Optimum use of drugs depends not only on the doctor's skill in prescribing and titrating, but also on the nurse's awareness of his or her responsibility to be acutely observant of symptoms and changes, and to be prompt and accurate in reporting them. It should be remembered that optimum results in the use of drugs in pain control can only be achieved through regular and punctual administration.

The family can be spared some distress by seeing their child relieved of suffering and, even where the child's level of consciousness renders him or her apparently unaware, it is important to continue to minimize symptoms, for example, the use of hyoscine can prevent the 'death-rattle'.

### The need to be observant

There is a danger in caring for the dying child that we may not be sufficiently observant of changing needs, which may come about very gradually. We need to be constantly assessing the child as he or she is, and questioning whether our care remains appropriate. There is scope for imagination and resourcefulness, but always with consideration for the home situation, if this is relevant.

### Staff support

Staff support is extremely important in this emotionally charged work. It cannot be denied that it is draining and there must be a regular opportunity for team members to share some of the joys and sorrows, perplexities and misunderstandings that inevitably occur.

## THE FAMILY'S INVOLVEMENT

The importance of the family's involvement throughout the child's illness cannot be stressed enough, but it is never more important than in the terminal phase. Communication between family and professional carers must be open and honest. The family may well feel particularly inadequate at this time, and will need constant reassurance and encouragement to be involved on every level as far as they are able. Many people are afraid of how death itself will actually occur and relatives should be told as far as possible how the end may come. They may well have fears and fantasies unrelated to reality and if these can be dispelled, some of the anguish may be removed.

There are so many small, unobtrusive ways in which the sensitive nurse can help at this stage. The room can be kept fresh and comfortably tidy, the bed-linen clean yet the atmosphere homely, and the child cherished and tended lovingly.

Change in treatment may sometimes provide the opportunity of helping the parents to accept further deterioration in their child's condition, which they may have not noticed or, indeed, which they may have wanted to ignore or deny. They may not realize that hearing is one of the last faculties to be lost and the child may continue to hear long after he or she has ceased to be able to respond, so they and others should be warned not to say things that may distress the child. To talk to the child, even though there may be no apparent response, to hold the child, or just to hold the child's hand, or stroke the child, is natural and right.

## Prolonged anxiety and grief of the family

However imaginative and understanding we are, we can only begin to be aware of the strain and anguish the family experiences physically and mentally. With an acute illness or accident followed by death, the grieving process and mourning have the potential of being resolved over a period of time, even though it may be a long time. Objectively, at least, others accept this process. With chronic sickness or handicap the grief is terribly prolonged and may often begin from the moment of diagnosis, when it is recognized that there is no known cure and there is not the same possibility of resolving or completing the mourning. Every stage of diminished ability or independence, every loss of function and each new sign of deterioration, is a further cause of mourning to the family and needs the acknowledgement of those around, not least those professionally concerned. This grieving may bring with it the feelings of denial, anger, remorse and guilt, as well as sorrow, common to all bereavement, and the need for the nurse to foster an honest and accepting relationship through all this is crucial.

There will often be times when we have nothing wise to say and when all we can do is stand alongside, not trying to set ourselves up as having the answers. Simply by sharing in the pain we may help to dissipate it a little.

## The place of death

I believe that for most children, home is the right place in which to die, given enough support. However, it must be stressed that for a variety of reasons this is not always the choice of the family, or indeed of the child, and their choice must be respected. Where a child has received care on a number of occasions in a children's hospital or paediatric unit, the parents and child may choose to return in the last days of life because it is a familiar and trusted environment, with the staff and family as 'old friends'. Similarly, a children's hospice may be the right place for the comparatively small number of children whose irreversible life-threatening condition progresses slowly over a period not of days and weeks, but of months and years. The families of such children suffer the strain not only of providing the necessary care for them, but also of cruelly prolonged grief.

### Reflection on the death of a child

The moment at which you are told that your child is going to die is the moment at which your bereavement begins. You are bereaved of the future you have believed was your child's by right, bereaved of the future you had assumed you and your child would share. Hope and optimism die at that instant. Life will never be the same again. There are many families who have little warning of their child's death and indeed for some, death is so sudden that there can be no warning. Perinatal and neonatal death, accident and acute infection claim the highest percentage of young lives in this country. For many children with cancer, including leukaemia, the period between the cessation of aggressive treatment, with the attendant hope of cure or at least of remission, and the death of the child will be brief.

Although families in previous generations faced the same kind of tragedy much more often, the existence of the close-knit extended family and the greater involvement of the local community provided the kind of support that is lacking in our contemporary society. Today's nuclear family, not infrequently a single-parent family, can suffer terrible feelings of loneliness and isolation.

As in many bereavement situations, just when friends are most needed, the family whose child is dying or has just died may find that friends of many years' standing are not around because they feel unable and inadequate to help in such a particularly distressing situation of grief.

## A HOSPICE FOR CHILDREN

Helen House, Oxford (a hospice for children), opened in November 1982 to offer respite care and terminal care on a home-from-home basis to children with life-threatening diseases. It aims to ease the strain for those families who care for their child at home by offering respite care at intervals; by trying to be sensitive in responding to their individual needs and to enable both child and family to achieve the optimum quality of life; and to help the child to live and to die with dignity and then to help the family to live on after the death of their child.

## The building

Helen House is set in three acres of well-established and beautiful gardens. It is a minute's walk from shops and a bus route to the city centre, which is one-and-a-half miles away. The house has accommodation for eight children at any one time and provision is made for parents and siblings to be resident also if they wish. Of the eight individually-designed and furnished children's bedrooms, two pairs of two have intercommunicating double doors, making it possible to have two double rooms in place of four single rooms. Six of the bedrooms have a window-seat that converts into a comfortable divan where a parent may choose to sleep, but most parents prefer the appartment designed for their use upstairs, with its two double bedrooms, sitting room, kitchen and bathroom. The main playroom has glass doors opening out into the garden; a small hobbies room has easy-clean surfaces for messy activities and another playroom is used for reading and listening to tapes or as a dayroom for a child confined to bed. The jacuzzi, a gift from the Royal Air Force, is not only a pleasure to children who are mobile and alert, despite their disease, but is also of tremendous benefit to those suffering varying degrees of paralysis, immobility or emaciation, and often evokes delighted response from children rarely known to respond to any kind of stimulus. The kitchen with dining-area is designed in farmhouse-style and is a natural focal point of the house: children, parents and staff, who eat together, often share in the preparation of meals and the washing of dishes! A room resembling an ordinary bedroom, but with a cooling system, is available for use when a child dies in Helen House and parents and relatives are able to spend time there with their child, often remaining until the funeral.

The staff of Helen House are all non-resident. This is a deliberate policy as it was felt to be important that they live away from what is inevitably emotionally taxing and often draining work. Every possible emphasis has been laid upon making the house resemble home rather than hospital or institution, both in architectural design and in the choice of fabrics and furniture.

## The team

The team caring for the families in Helen House consists of approximately 20 full-time (or equivalent) members of staff. These include registered nurses with specialist paediatric training, teachers, a nursery nurse, social worker, physiotherapist, a chaplain and others, some of whom are parents themselves. There is minimal emphasis on hierarchy although there is a head nurse and deputy head nurse. No one is employed specifically as cook or cleaner – each person shares these activities.

Two doctors in general practice give medical care, each visiting the house regularly once a week, with frequent shorter visits during the week, and otherwise by request. With only a small number of the children suffering from malignant disease and requiring pain relief and symptom control, part-time medical input is sufficient. Members of staff do not wear a uniform and are known by their first names. In selecting the team, it was recognized that it was essential to have people with the right qualifications and experience, but the greatest emphasis was laid upon their personal qualities and on whether they 'spoke the same language'. The final selection relied heavily upon the intuition of the selectors.

## Liaison with other agencies and with families

One member of staff, a trained social worker, is employed to work part time in the house on the ordinary duty rota and part time in the community, visiting children and their families at home or in hospital, and liaising with other agencies involved in caring for the families. Where, for example, a family doctor, home tutor or physiotherapist who cares for the child when he or she is at home is willing to continue to be involved on a practical level during the child's visits to Helen House, they are encouraged to do so, continuity being seen as vitally important for both child and family. However, distance and other practical difficulties often make this impossible.

## Home care

A home-care service has not yet been developed on a formal basis and at present Helen House works in liaison with the existing domicillary paediatric nurses employed by the NHS. Where distance permits, members of the team do give help and support in the child's own home when the need arises, but this is on an informal basis.

It is important that communications between members of the community health team and the hospice team should be good. To encourage overdependence on the hospice team to the exclusion of those professionals offering support in the child's own home can do serious disservice to the family, not only during the child's illness but also after the child has died.

## Staff support

A consultant child psychiatrist acts as a facilitator at a weekly staff-support group, offering an opportunity for open discussion among members of the team about matters of mutual concern.

## The selection of children

Priority is given to children in the final stage of illness. In the West, statistics show that a high percentage of children who die do so in hospital. In cases of acute infection or accident this is clearly the right place, with all the facilities for saving life where this is possible and appropriate. However, in other situations it is very often the wish of the family to have their child die at home and, given the right kind of support, this is both possible and desirable. On the other hand, it is important that we do not generalize when assessing the best course of action for any individual family as each one has different reactions and needs. No family should be coerced into having their child at home to die against their wishes. Sometimes parents feel they could not bear to continue to live in a house where their child has died and would have to move house if the child died at home. Others may have seen other people's children, with the same disease as their child dying by haemorrhage or in convulsion or with pain, and may prefer to be in an environment where they feel totally supported and surrounded by people who will know how to meet all eventualities. Sometimes children themselves will feel more secure in a place where they know there are people who will know what to do in an emergency. We have known each of these situations exist, even when home-care support has been available, and the feelings of child and family must be respected. When a child, who is in the final stage of illness, comes to Helen House, any members of the immediate family are also welcomed and encouraged to stay and to be with their child and to care for him or her as much as they feel willing and able to do.

Babies in the first weeks of life are occasionally referred to us from special-care baby-units of hospitals. If it is recognized that a baby has a condition that is not compatible with life, and curative therapy is either not attempted or is abandoned at any early stage, it is conceivable that an intensive-care unit ceases to be the appropriate environment for the infant and his or her parents. The parents may not feel sufficiently confident to take their baby home and the solution can sometimes be a half-way house such as Helen House is able to provide.

The family can teach us how best to care for their child, especially if he or she is unable to communicate him- or herself, for without doubt, they are the people who know their child best and we have much to learn from them. In getting to know the family we hope to establish a relationship of friendship and trust. Irrespective of race or belief, children who can benefit from this type of hospice care are welcome; the ages range from birth to 18 years, and the catchment area covers the UK.

Children coming for respite care either come at regular intervals (for example, two weeks in every two months or one week in every six weeks), or by arrangement with the family. Some ask only for occasional help in order to cover a holiday or a period of crisis at home. A child would not normally come for more than a month on any one visit unless the circumstances are exceptional, as long-term institutional care is not provided. It is important for children to believe that they belong at home with their families and just come to visit Helen House from time to time, as they might visit friends.

## Referrals

Initial enquiries come from many sources including the family, doctors, nurses, social workers and others in the health team, and sometimes from teachers. All that is required, when it is decided that there is a family to whom help can be offered, is that the parents wish to accept the offer and that the doctor responsible for the child's care is in agreement, and is willing to pass on details of the illness and treatment.

## CARE STUDIES

How the aims and objectives of Helen House work out in practice are best illustrated by care studies of some of the young visitors.

### Michael

Michael was diagnosed at birth as having cystic fibrosis. This was a devastating blow to his parents, both nearly 40 when he was born. They already had six daughters and Michael was their longed-for son. The family was poor, socially deprived and lived in a rough district on the outskirts of a large, sprawling city.

When the family was first referred to Helen House Michael was 12 years old and the disease was far advanced. His mother could see no future for her son, while his father, unable to articulate his feelings, simply could not accept the inevitable outcome. Helen House was so totally different from their own home environment that the parents reacted in a predictable way on their first visit – they surrounded Michael with fierce protectiveness and made his room a safe fortress for themselves. With the agreement of the staff his drugs were kept in his room and administered by his parents, as was his physiotherapy.

It took several stays at Helen House before the family began to relax. Gradually they learned to trust the staff and to allow them more contact with their son. The mother began to talk freely and at length about her feelings, depression, the trials and tribulations of her life, and family. They began to enjoy their visits and were encouraged to go on various trips and excursions, usually organized by the staff. Always, though, their over-riding concern was Michael and their determination to do everything for him themselves was understood and accepted.

More and more they began to lean on the staff for support and comfort in their grief over Michael's deteriorating condition. The father, although by this time more comfortable and relaxed in Helen House, suffered silently from his helplessness to alter the inexorable progress of the disease and found his only relief in constantly entertaining his son, buying him expensive toys and games and bringing him whatever he thought would please him. The mother's grief was more overt, expressing itself in bouts of depression; during one visit she was taken to the local hospital suffering from angina and heart failure, aggravated by gross obesity.

The staff began to recognize their role with this family. Family togetherness was everything to them. Fiercely loyal and bonded together, in spite of the enormous problems of each individual member of the family, they still needed the staff and turned to them constantly for support, strength and friendship. Initially, the mother had vehemently denied that Michael had any conception of the true nature of his illness but, as the months went by, she felt able to accept the truth that Michael was well aware of the implications and she passed over to the staff the task that was too painful for her – that of answering Michael's questions honestly. Finally, she herself was able to tolerate his remarks about death, although she could never actually bring herself to admit the certainty of it to him.

When Michael was in the terminal stages of his illness the parents telephoned in great anguish feeling they could no longer cope despite the excellent support of their social worker and general practitioner. They came to Helen House and Michael, now bed-ridden, always had at least one of them with him. His mother slept in his room, older sisters travelled down frequently to be with him, and his room became their home where they clung together for support. They were now quite comfortable with the staff and reached out to them for warmth and support. Finally the father's reserve broke and he was able to weep.

As the days passed and Michael became weaker, the father became greatly agitated; he had an overwhelming desire to take his son back to where he belonged – home. He felt it was not right to deprive Michael's sisters of these last days, and after initial opposition, the mother came to be in full agreement. Immediately the staff arranged an ambulance and staff escort. The father went on ahead and when the ambulance arrived at home it was moving to see the whole family waiting at the door to receive their brother home. They had prepared his room with tender care and surrounded him with their love. He died ten days later.

With his family the staff's work was not so much with the child (with whom the staff were allowed only minimal contact), but with the parents, enabling them, perhaps, to get through the last painful year of Michael's life, and providing the moral support and friendship that helped them to find the strength and confidence to care for him in their own home at the end.

## Trusting instinct

One beautiful autumn day a 10-month-old baby boy died. The staff knew that he could not live very long but his actual death came on a day when he seemed particularly alert and happy. When he died his mother carried him into the garden, walked and sat with him in her arms for a couple of hours, often with one of the staff beside her, occasionally alone with him. She cried gently and talked to him. She remembered the day that he was born, also a beautiful sunny day; she talked of the joy that he had brought into life and of the pain. Then, in her own time, she carried him back into their room and lay down with him still in her arms and slept for an hour. Then, and only then, was she ready to wash and dress him with very great love and care and without any sense of hurry. She chose the clothes he was to wear and the toys he was to have with him. She had already seen the small room, furnished much like a bedroom but able to be kept very cold, where he was to lie for the next few days. She carried him there.

The little boy's mother and father visited him often in that small room, sometimes brushing his hair or rearranging his toys, sometimes lifting him out of his cot and sitting with him, uncurling his fingers and looking again at his hands, kissing him in the nape of his neck, lost in grief and in the wonder of the miracle that was their son. All they needed was the staff's permission, spoken or unspoken, to do it their way, the way they knew instinctively, and the staff's presence in the background, and the knowledge that the staff felt pain and wonder too and were not afraid to show it.

## Sammy

Sammy was diagnosed at the age of four as having a stage-IV non-Hodgkin's lymphoma involving the ileum, with secondary deposits in the bone marrow. At the time of diagnosis he had a six-weeks' history of intermittent abdominal pain with severe occurrences 10–20 times a day, associated with vomiting 1–5 times a day. He underwent a course of chemotherapy, but in view of the high likelihood of disease relapse on standard chemotherapy, it was felt that the only possibility of long-term survival would be with bone marrow transplantation following total body irradiation. However, it proved impossible to find a perfect match and he therefore underwent an autologous bone-marrow graft.

Initially he did well, apart from two brief episodes of right facial palsy, but one month later he complained of headache, vomiting and lethargy, and lumbar puncture revealed numerous blasts. It was concluded that there had been a focal deposit of lymphomatous cells that resisted radiation treatment and rapidly recurred. Sammy's young parents were fully involved in discussion about his prognosis and future management. His central nervous system relapse during the period of marrow regeneration was only partially controlled with intrathecal chemotherapy and a course of palliative cranial irradiation. Acute-care hospital ceased to be the appropriate environment and it was suggested that the family might like to visit Helen House to see if it was a place they would choose to come to if the situation became unmanageable at home.

Sammy, his parents and three-year-old sister, spent a day at Helen House. Sammy had kept asking if they could have a holiday, but his parents had never been able to afford this. When he saw Helen House for the first time he exclaimed 'It's a real holiday camp! Can we stay here?' and cried miserably when his parents told him they could not stay here this time. His condition deteriorated rapidly over the next few days and the whole family returned to Helen House for the last five days of his life.

Pain control was one of the most urgent problems and this was achieved fairly satisfactorily after a day or two. Sammy improved a little and was able to enjoy playing and being taken out in a pushchair. There were many moments of real pleasure interspersed with the times when he clearly felt very ill indeed. His parents took it in turns to be with him day and night. He developed minor nose bleeds and haematuria and was given platelets to prevent fatal haemorrhage – the form of death witnessed by his parents in another child and which they dreaded more than anything. Sammy died suddenly and peacefully the following morning, having been fully conscious to the end.

His grandparents came the next day to see him for the last time, to be with his grief-stricken parents and little sister, and to see the room and 'holiday camp' that they knew Sammy had loved. At the end of the day they took the little girl home with them and Sammy's parents asked if they could stay during the three days until the funeral. Sometimes alone together and sometimes with the staff, talking of Sammy before he was ill, of his illness, of the future without him, crying with the staff, sharing meals with them, and sitting up with them late into the night, they now talked of those days as a time when the healing began. Two of the staff went with them to their home town on the south coast for Sammy's funeral. The staff knew that returning home was hard for them.

The staff keep in touch with the family with fairly frequent telephone calls, and they, like all the bereaved families, accepted the invitation to visit the staff and to plan to spend part of their summer holiday in Helen House.

## Reality is gentler than fantasy

Children's fantasy and imagination are highly developed. I believe that the reality of seeing a dead brother or sister is easier to cope with and kinder to the child's sensitivities than the ordeal of experience by fantasy. On seeing her dead sister and showing no emotion and making no comment, it was several hours before a six-year-old said, 'I thought when you were dead all your skin peeled off'. And then, still later, 'Where is she? How can she be in heaven when she's still in that little room?' I have found that the analogy of a shell or a chrysalis or a house can be useful. The important part, the living part, has gone and this is all that is left behind. An exceptional eleven-year-old spoke of his body as a reflection. 'It is how you recognize me for who I am. When I die I will leave my reflection behind but the real me won't die; when I die the real me will go to that very special place.' Many children have experienced the death of a pet. 'When my dog died he left his skin behind' was the comment of a seven-year-old. A four-year-old girl was trying to come to terms with the death of her three-year-old cousin. Helping her mother to clear the coal fire at home she said, 'He's gone like the coal. Just the ashes left behind.'

We must guard against using the adjective 'peaceful' indiscriminately when describing death or the face of the child after death. If it is untrue it may distance us from the family who sense that this is one of the games people play. It is true, however, that an hour or two after death relatives will often be comforted by the fact that the dead child does indeed look peaceful and even seems to smile. They may spend time with the child, greatly comforted, despite their grief, with the thought that 'she looks so like herself'. Then almost imperceptibly after two or three days a change comes about and the relatives will remark on how it's 'not him any more', or on how 'he's gone'. Here nature itself takes its share in bringing about acceptance of what has happened and in carrying those who grieve a stage further on.

I hesitate to write about religion as a separate issue. Two things are clear to me. One is that mystery and a sense of awe surround death and whatever lies beyond it. The second is that an effect of love and grief exposed, the soul laid bare, is to bring forth reverence in the beholder. Here we find ourselves beyond the realms of reason crossing all barriers of different faiths. I would say that we share the experience of treading on holy ground. However much they may have ignored any kind of formal religion in the past, I do not think that there are many parents who do not wonder about the existence of a God when their child is dying. I have yet to meet a father or mother who has believed, at the moment of death, that their child ceased to exist. Many parents will want someone to pray with them when their child is dying, or after death. Speaking as a Christian, I know that there are times when I can only say 'I do not know' in response to questions about the meaning of it all. Yet for myself, I hold fast to the conviction that death is a beginning, rather than an end.

## The days following the death

The choice of clothes is intensely personal. For some it will be a traditional white shroud, for others a jogging suit or jeans, for yet others the clothes worn for First Communion or for parties. One little girl wore a ballet dress and new pink ballet shoes; a boy was dressed in his treasured Batman outfit. What matters is that it is right for this particular child and family and it can happen only if we provide an assumed permission to do it their way. I have a haunting memory of the distress a mother experienced when she was taken to see her child after he had died unexpectedly under anaesthetic. He was in a white shroud with his hair neatly brushed forward. She hardly recognized him. She longed for him to be in his jeans and sweatshirt with his hair rumpled back as it had always been. In her grief she was grateful to the person who had taken such care to make him look nice, but he wasn't any longer her son.

Here, I should add that although I write from the context of a children's hospice, many of 'our' children die, quite rightly, in their own homes. Most of what I write is, I believe, equally possible and helpful there. I have been privileged to be with several families when their child died at home and the child has remained in his or her own bedroom until the day of the funeral. Nothing has been hurried, everything has been spontaneous and natural.

Some parents will want to register the death of their child themselves, others will be grateful to be relieved of the responsibility. For many the decision between burial and cremation is a painful one. Either alternative may seem intolerable to contemplate – the gradual decomposition of the body beneath the ground, or the rapid consuming of the body by flames. The thought of the child's hair and face being burnt is especially distressing to many parents. One mother asked to tour the crematorium before deciding. The director of the crematorium could not have been more helpful, showing the visitors behind the scenes and explaining the whole process, answering all questions honestly and straightforwardly. Children who know that they are going to die will often express an opinion. One boy who had a progressively handicapping disease wanted his body cremated because, he said, it hadn't been much use to him in life. Another child wanted to be buried because she knew her parents would want to visit her grave. For some, of course, religion will be the deciding factor.

Parents will often want to choose their child's coffin, and they must not be hurried in their choice or indeed of making any of the arrangements for their child. Toys or special treasures may be put in the coffin, though there will be others who take the view that such things are trivial and inappropriate. Letters or cards written to the child after death and placed in the coffin may be another step towards healing and wholeness for the one who writes. The planning of the funeral service is a personal thing and the parents' need is for someone who will give gentle guidance and perhaps the suggestion of some sort of framework allowing plenty of opportunity for the choice of music and words appropriate to their child. Just as the clothes the child wears are a matter of personal choice, so are the clothes worn by the bereaved at the funeral. We may be horrified at a young couple, whom we know to be very hard up financially, going out to buy new black outfits for their child's funeral. But for them this may be an integral part of their own instinctive ritual of grieving.

Many people say how much they dread the day of the funeral itself. In the event most will say that they found it a much more helpful experience than they had dared to hope. 'Is it awful to say I enjoyed it?' asked one mother, 'I didn't know how many people loved him and cared.' Attendance at the funeral comes to be seen as a tribute. It is also a token of love and support to the parents and the family.

Saying to parents whose child has died, 'You will get over it', is like saying, 'One day it will seem as if he never existed'. Nothing could be more hurtful. They don't want him or her written out of existence. But, given time, given permission to be who they are, given reassurance to behave instinctively, given love and friendship, I believe that they will have the best chance to adjust to what has happened and to grow towards healing and wholeness. Despite society's fear of death and ineptitute in the face of death, I believe that every individual has the potential within to meet death with a severe beauty that in no way denies grief. Being alongside such families you absorb some of their grief. But you also share some of the good things – learning to think of time in terms of depth rather than length; enjoying the swift growth of real friendship; by-passing the usual obstacles of class, creed, colour, age, education; and having 'all one's sensitivities heightened', as one father put it.

In all this it is important to remember that although the families' needs are immeasurably great, families needing hospice care are few. To encourage the proliferation of children's hospices across the country would be unnecessary and wasteful. If there are resources to spare, let us channel them into more support at home for the children and their families, remembering in any case that hospice is not a building but a philosophy of care.

## STILLBIRTH

Stillbirth is defined as a birth after the 28th week of pregnancy in which the baby does not breathe or show any other sign of life after being completely expelled from the mother.

The loss of the baby may be a profound shock and tragedy to the parents, and over the last few years there has been an increasing awareness of the grief reactions involved in this special situation and the importance of allowing space for these reactions to take place. Bourne (1983), in a perceptive article on the psychological impact of stillbirth, states (p. 54) that stillbirth is accompanied by all the ordinary problems of death and mourning but one of the special grieving difficulties the parents of a stillborn baby have is that 'the death of someone known and cherished is painfully real whereas a stillbirth is painfully unreal . . . the baby cannot become known, remembered or forgotten normally'. In one study on mothers' reactions to stillbirth Lovell *et al.* (1986) noted that women said they felt emptiness, disappointment, failure and guilt following such a loss and spoke of their need to grieve without knowing what to mourn for. It is obviously important that parents are helped to mourn their baby fully as it has been shown that relationship difficulties and problems with subsequent children may develop if grief is not acknowledged and expressed. Thus, the profundity of this experience should be recognized by all personnel involved in care and efforts should be made to establish the reality of the event and the baby's existence.

## Supporting the parents immediately following delivery

It is obviously important that the parents have the reasons for the baby's death fully explained to them and be given the chance to express their immediate feelings and to ask any questions they may have. It is now considered valuable to ask parents if they wish to see and hold their baby following delivery and spend time alone with it. If the baby is not physically perfect it is usually possible to wrap it up in an acceptable way so that the parents may see it. If the parents are denied this opportunity it may lead to exaggerated fears that the baby is badly disfigured. If the parents do not wish to see their baby a photograph can be taken and kept in the records, and the parents told of this in case they wish to see it at a later date. The parents may be asked to give consent to a post-mortem examination, and once this is carried out and the report received, it could be used as an opportunity for the doctor to go over the circumstances leading to the loss again, when explaining the result, as the initial explanation may not be fully absorbed. The parents are advised by the hospital staff about the registration of the baby and subsequent funeral arrangements. These arrangements can be undertaken by the hospital but it is thought to be of value to the parents in coming to terms with their loss to arrange this themselves and also to name the baby.

Following delivery, mothers of stillborn babies have spoken of their sense of shame and embarrassment at being in an environment with mothers who have had live babies, and a decision on the most satisfactory environment for a bereaved mother is undoubtedly not easy. It is important that the woman does not feel she should rush home when physically able to if this is not truly what she wants as her family may, in their own grief and anxiety, discourage her from mourning fully, and it also denies her a place as a mother in a situation meant for mothers. Therefore, a suitable placement in hospital should be offered. Hughes (1987), in a review of studies on this subject, noted the diversity of opinion regarding ward placement. It is interesting to note, however, that in Hughes's subsequent study women state that the most upsetting thing about the environment in which they were placed was the inability of people, including midwifery staff, to communicate effectively with them. One criterion when deciding environment should, of course, be that it provides easy access for the mother's partner so that the two may have the opportunity to be together, both day and night if possible.

### Continuing care at home

Obviously the family doctor, community midwife and health visitor should be notified of the situation before the mother goes home and the community midwife will initially visit the parents at home. The parents may well need continued support and this can be provided by professional personnel or a support group such as the Stillbirth and Perinatal Death Association. An ordinary postnatal clinic is not usually an ideal place to carry out the six-weeks' postnatal check and some hospitals arrange for the mother to be seen at a special counselling or gynaecological clinic. Genetic counselling is usually given, if appropriate, together with advice about future pregnancies. Couples are generally advised not to embark immediately on another pregnancy so that time to grieve fully is allowed. As with the loss of any loved one, the parents are unlikely to 'get over' the loss of their baby or forget him or her, but with help may come to terms with their sad loss.

### Reactions of professional carers

There is now a realization that stillbirth is a tragedy to the couple and the families but there is perhaps still a need to recognize that the event may spark off feelings of shock and anger and guilt in the mother's professional attendants. Unless medical and midwifery staff recognize and deal with their own feelings about such losses it may be difficult to help and support the parents fully. Therefore, in an ideal situation, some outlet to enable the professional personnel involved to acknowledge their own feelings should be provided.

## ABORTION

### Spontaneous abortion

Many couples experience grief, pain and disappointment following a spontaneous abortion. This form of bereavement should also be treated with respect and parents given the opportunity to express their hurt.

Advice regarding other pregnancy and genetic counselling may be given but it is important that those involved in the mother's care realize that for the couple concerned, this is perceived as the loss of their baby and that it is not viewed as a gynaecological and obstetric event.

## Termination of pregnancy

Another situation where grief may be very real is following a pregnancy that has been terminated. There is often either no opportunity to express this or the woman will hide it away, feeling that she cannot admit to her sense of loss. There may be guilt feelings immediately after the termination and a form of puerperal depression. Failure to cope with her feelings at this time may cause guilt and grief in a subsequent straightforward pregnancy and, therefore, sensitive support and counselling at this time may be very helpful.

# REFERENCES AND FURTHER READING

Burne, S. R. (1982a) Hospice care for children, *British Medical Journal*, Vol. 284, pp. 1,400.

Burne, S. R. (1982b) Helen House – a hospice for children, *Health Visitor*, Vol. 55, pp. 544–5.

Burne, S. R., Dominica, Mother Frances and Baum, J. D. (1984) Helen House – a hospice for children: an analysis of the first year, *British Medical Journal*, Vol. 289, pp. 1,665–8.

Corr, C. A. and Corr, D. M. (eds) (1985) *Hospice Approaches to Paediatric Care*, Springer, New York.

Hunt, A. M. (1986) Open house, *Nursing Times*, August, pp. 53–7.

McCarthy, G. T. (ed.) (1984) *The Physically Handicapped Child*, Faber & Faber, London.

## Stillbirth and abortion

Bourne, S. (1983) Psychological impact of stillbirth, *The Practitioner*, Vol. 227, pp. 53–60.

HEA (1979) *The Loss of Your Baby*, Health Education Authority, London.

Hughes, P. (1987) The management of bereaved mothers: what is best? *Midwives Chronicle*, August, pp. 226–9.

Lovell, H., *et al.* (1986) Mothers' reactions to a perinatal death, *Nursing Times*, 12 November, pp. 40–2.

# 11. Care of Dying Patients with AIDS (Acquired Immune Deficiency Syndrome)

## WHAT IS AIDS?

Until recently AIDS patients were nursed either at home or in specialized wards and units. All this is gradually changing with the increased incidence of the disease. There will come a time when every nurse will at some time care for a patient with AIDS in a general hospital. It is, therefore, essential that nurses acquire an accurate knowledge of what is now known about the disease, and the skills to care for affected patients.

The terminology is becoming very complicated, and inevitably abbreviations are becoming common practice. A glossary is given to assist in following the thread of the text, and for referring back:

AIDS = Acquired Immune Deficiency Syndrome
HIV = Human immunodeficiency virus
PGL = Persistent generalized lymphadenopathy
ARC = AIDS-related complex
PCP = *Pneumocystis carinii* pneumonia
HSV = Herpes simplex virus
AZT = Azidothymidine

AIDS is caused by a virus called human immunodeficiency virus (HIV), and it infects the lymphocyte cells of the blood that are responsible for the body's immune system of protection against infection. The virus is spread by:

(1) sexual intercourse via contact with infected blood and semen;
(2) from infected blood products via blood transfusion or from using needles and syringes shared with infected drug-users; and
(3) mothers, who are HIV-positive, passing it on to their unborn child during pregnancy.

Many people infected with the virus are healthy but can pass it on – they are referred to as being asymptomatic. Some people have enlarged lymph nodes – persistent generalized lymphadenopathy (PGL).

A type of illness may arise known as AIDS-related complex, which is very debilitating. The patient feels very unwell, there is fever and general malaise and fatigue, and often candidal infection and diarrhoea. Sleeping hours are disrupted by night sweats.

# OPPORTUNISTIC INFECTIONS

It is recognized that someone has developed AIDS and is not simply a carrier of the virus when what is described as 'opportunistic infections' arise. The person may suffer a number of such episodes, and yet live quite a full life and feel healthy in between these bouts of illness. It is estimated that of people infected with HIV, about 25–30 per cent will develop AIDS within five years. Another 10 per cent will have ARC, while the remainder will be asymptomatic or have PGL.

## Opportunistic infections of the lungs

A number of infections and lesions may affect the lungs, e.g. tuberculosis, Kaposi's sarcoma and *Pneumocystis carinii* pneumonia (PCP). The latter condition is developed by 50 per cent of all AIDS patients and is a common cause of death. However, most individuals who are HIV-positive are aware of how that condition presents and the importance of seeking early treatment.

### *Pneumocystis carinii* pneumonia

If this is the first infection, leading to the diagnosis of AIDS, the doctor will discuss openly with the patient the diagnosis, possible prognosis and the treatment involved. The patient may be admitted to hospital or cared for at home. The doctor will commence intravenous antibiotic therapy such as high doses of cotrimoxazole and oxygen therapy.

### The patient's problems

- Shortness of breath
- Rapid respirations
- Dry, unproductive cough
- Mild chest pain
- High temperature with rigors and profuse sweating
- Dry mouth
- Fear and anxiety
- Low blood $O_2$ level leading to confusion and restlessness

### Nursing care

(1) Patients are nursed in a position that they find comfortable and that assists good respiratory function.
(2) Oxygen therapy should be continuous rather than intermittent to maintain a constant arterial pressure of $O_2$ of 60–80 mm.
(3) Having continuous oxygen can cause a very dry mouth, so frequent mouth care is necessary, including prevention of dry and cracked lips, for which Vaseline is useful.
(4) Since high fever is usual, the nurse needs to keep the patient as clean, dry and comfortable as possible. Tepid sponging is performed and frequent changes of bedclothes. Antipyretic drugs such as paracetamol are usually prescribed every four hours.
(5) Plenty of fluids should be encouraged, and iced drinks will be appreciated.
(6) Care must be taken of the intravenous infusion site, and the administration of drugs as prescribed.
(7) The nurse has a most important role in supporting the patient through a time of fear and anxiety, which may include the fear of dying. These emotional problems are likely to exacerbate breathlessness, and the nurse should take time to sit with the patient, ready to listen and to give gentle reassurance. Anxiolitic drugs may be prescribed, such as lorazepam. In severe breathlessness, small doses of diamorphine given via a syringe driver can alleviate the situation.

## Opportunistic infections of the mouth and gastrointestinal tract

Any part of the system from the mouth to the anus may be infected.

### The mouth

Because of immunosuppression, the AIDS patient is prone to a number of lesions and infections.

(1) Kaposi's sarcoma is a tumour of the skin and mucous membranes, and appears as a purple-bluish lesion on the hard or soft palate. It is often symptomless, but secondary infection may cause ulceration and pain.
(2) Oval hairy leukoplakia, which appears as white elevated lesions on the underside of the tongue.
(3) *Candida albicans* – a common fungal infection to which AIDS patients are very prone.

### The patient's problems

- Dry mouth
- Pain
- Bad breath
- May have difficulty in swallowing and eating

### Nursing care

Keep the patient's mouth moist at all times. Encourage the patient to clean the teeth twice a day and also after meals. Pineapple chunks can be chewed, and drinks of Coca-Cola are refreshing; plenty of fluids should in any case be taken. Where fungal infection is present, nystatin suspension will be prescribed and is usually effective. If the infection persists and spreads to the oesophagus, it can cause pain and difficulty in swallowing and eating. The drug Ketaconazole is then prescribed. The patient should be offered a soft diet until the condition improves. Many AIDS patients are prone to infection of the peri-oral area by the *Herpes simplex* virus. It is important to look out for these lesions as they can be treated and kept at bay with an antiviral drug, Acyclovir.

## Gastro-intestinal tract

The main organisms that infect the tract are:

*Candida albicans*
*Cytomegalovirus*
*Salmonella*
*Shigella*
*Cryptosporidium*
*Mycobacterium tuberculosis*

## The patient's problems

- Diarrhoea
- Weight loss
- Colicky abdominal pain
- Electrolyte imbalance
- Nutritional loss

One of the opportunistic infections that can have disastrous consequences is that caused by *Cryptosporidium*, an intestinal protozoan parasite. It may ultimately prove fatal as there is no definitive treatment, so symptom control is of the essence of care. Large amounts of watery diarrhoea may be passed about five times a day.

When this is a terminal illness, the patient may express a desire to die at home, and this is possible if there is a supportive partner or family, and sufficient back-up from all the community services.

## Nursing care

(1) If in hospital, the patient is nursed in a single room for privacy and comfort, especially if diarrhoea is profuse. A commode is kept in the patient's room.

(2) The nurse must always wear an apron and gloves when dealing with body fluids such as stools. The careful and thorough washing of hands should always be performed. While the patient is still able to tolerate a bath, care should be taken to cleanse this thoroughly after use.

(3) The patient will be dehydrated and this will entail administration of fluids intravenously as long as this is appropriate. Fluids by mouth should be encouraged, and also small helpings of food with high-protein supplement, e.g. Complan, Build-up.

(4) Anti-diarrhoea drugs are prescribed and administered, e.g. Imodium (loperamide).

(5) When the patient becomes too weak to get into a bath, a bed-bath is given, and linen changed frequently. Care of pressure areas is very important; skin must be kept clean and dry and a barrier cream used. The patient should be turned every two hours.

(6) For patients who are passing large amounts of watery stools almost continuously, it may be advisable to insert a catheter such as a Foley's catheter into the rectum, using lignocaine gel and connecting it to a urinary drainage bag. This will enable the fluid to drain through the tube and will save the patient from the distressing situation of either continually sitting on a commode or having bed-linen changed.

(7) Morphine slow-release tablets (MST) are usually prescribed for patients when they complain of colicky pain and abdominal discomfort. In patients with malabsorption, diamorphine via syringe driver is commenced.
(8) Because cryptosporidiosis causes some of the most undignified symptoms, patients may suffer psychologically, feeling they have lost all dignity and they can become extremely depressed. In this case, gentle handling and reassurance is most definitely called for, requiring complete sensitivity to the patients' feelings by the nurses.

### Anus–rectum

Many adults (including a large proportion of homosexual men) have been exposed to *Herpes simplex* virus (HSV) and consequently harbour these latent viruses. In AIDS, herpes is frequently re-activated and can cause severe ulcerations, for example, around the perianal area. Ulcerating lesions around the anus may spread into the rectum and can be very painful. The nurse should be alert to observing any lesions round the anus. The antiviral drug Acyclovir is prescribed and saline baths given if the patient is strong enough. If the condition is very painful, lignocaine gel applied around the anus can ease local symptoms.

## The central nervous system

The main types of infection that affect the central nervous system are cryptococcosis and toxoplasmosis.

(1) *Cryptococcus* is a yeast-like organism, and causes meningitis. Patients will complain of headaches, blurred vision and difficulty in balance. They will have a fever and are often confused. The diagnosis of cryptococcal meningitis is confirmed by lumbar puncture.
(2) Toxoplasmosis is a protozoan infection causing a brain abscess, which will be clearly visible on a CT scan. The patient will have similar problems as in the cryptococcal infections, and may also have focal neurological signs, e.g. hemiplegia. If untreated the general condition of the patient can deteriorate rapidly.

Appropriate drug therapy is commenced for both types of infection for a period of four to six weeks. Whilst patients are receiving medication, their level of consciousness should be observed regularly. The nurse needs to assist and to help patients with washing, and helping at meal times when required, and all assistance should be given to patients to prevent them from falling over and being a danger to themselves. If patients respond to treatment, there should be a marked improvement in their general condition, and their neurological symptoms should gradually disappear.

## Eyes

*Cytomegalovirus* (CMV) can affect the eyes, causing CMV retinitis.

### Problems

Blurred and failing vision occurs, and haemorrhages and white areas of retinitis can be seen on the retina. CMV retinitis poses a serious threat of blindness and may be bilateral. The treatment for this condition is a course of an antiviral drug, Ganciclovir, followed by a maintenance dose after the course.

## AIDS encephalopathy

A most distressing condition that occurs in people who are HIV-positive is a condition called AIDS encephalopathy that leads to symptoms very similar to presenile dementia. Patients suffering from this condition in its most severe forms will have difficulty remembering where they are, and they will be unable to concentrate or follow a conversation. This condition is untreatable although AZT (zidovudine) may provide help in some patients.

Any condition or illness where there is neurological disturbance can cause hardship and stress to the partner, family or friends of the patient. These people need much support and guidance, i.e. a voluntary support-group such as 'Buddies' who can visit and stay with the patient allowing the carer to have some free time.

## General points regarding opportunistic infections

The role of the nurse throughout the period of time that the patient is suffering from opportunistic infection is of vital importance, as possibly over a period of months to years the nurse has been looking after the patient from the time they first developed an opportunistic infection or were even first diagnosed as being HIV-positive.

Due to confusing and conflicting reports appearing in the Press – some unnecessarily alarmist and damaging to patients and their families – health-care workers were beginning to believe that the patient suffering from AIDS was highly infectious, which, of course, is most definitely not the case. The nurse caring for the patient must be in possession of all the facts of the virus, how it is contracted and spread in order to nurse the patient in a relaxed atmosphere without feeling socially isolated. The nurse must be aware that because the patients' immune systems are so badly damaged, they are more prone to cross infection if a high standard of nursing is not carried out.

At the moment, the majority of people who are HIV-positive or have full-blown AIDS are homosexual. Again, because of the unwarranted and destructive comments made in some newspapers, they may have been made to feel guilty about their sexuality. It is very important to realize that we as nurses are not dealing with a sexual situation but with a human being dying from a disease; we must show them all the respect and dignity they deserve irrespective of their sex or race.

If the patient is being nursed in a general ward the precautions taken are similar to those for hepatitis B, i.e. the nurse and other staff in close proximity to the patient should wear gloves when handling any body fluids and should observe the hospital policy regarding disposal of such fluids and bed-linen. There is no reason for other patients in the ward to be aware of the patient's diagnosis. Again, the patient's right to confidentiality must be stressed.

## CARE OF THE PATIENT IN THE TERMINAL STAGE

As has been stated, patients suffering from opportunistic infections are acutely ill, so acute medical care is carried out. In these circumstances it is often very difficult to cope with someone who is now in the terminal stages and not responding to intensive medication. It is important for a nurse caring for these patients to have time to talk to other members of the multi-disciplinary team about what they find stressful.

In the final stages of life, there are many duties that must be performed for the patient's peace of mind.

(1) If they have any particular religious beliefs, they may desire or need to see a particular religious leader.

(2) Hopefully prior to this stage, they will have executed their wills, especially bearing in mind the case of a homosexual patient who has lived with a partner for many years, which is not dissimilar to the marital institution. In so many cases where there is no will, the patient's immediate family have intervened and the door has been slammed in the face of the partner.
(3) In the case of the homosexual patient whose family is completely unaware of the patient's life-style, complete confidentiality is called for on the part of the professional staff. At all times, the patient's wishes must be of vital importance. Due to the social stigma attached to AIDS-related disease, some but not all patients request that nurses and doctors should not reveal to relatives the true state of affairs to prevent their families from also suffering from the stigma.

Having dealt with all these social issues, we once again come back to the nursing care of the patient, which really consists of the basic nursing care needed by any dying patient.

The partner and family should be encouraged to participate, i.e. giving sips of water or if the patient is unconscious dipping a foam stick into fluids and applying it to the patient's mouth to prevent the patient getting a dry mouth. If patients are unable to close their eyes, partners can gently swab their eyelids with cotton-wool soaked in normal saline. The partners, families and friends of patients should be encouraged to touch and hold the patient. This time is a very important time for grieving partners and relatives, because after the death of their loved one's, they seem to draw a lot of encouragement from the fact that they played an important part in caring for them in their last hours and indeed their loved ones die knowing that they have been loved and that they are not alone in the face of death. The nurse who has been particularly involved with a patient may wish to attend the funeral service and this should be encouraged.

The following care study has been included to illustrate and, it is hoped, bring together the various principles of care described above.

# CARE STUDY

## Paul – a patient with AIDS

### First stage of the illness

Paul, a 34-year-old school-teacher, attended the sexually transmitted diseases clinic on 8 February 1986 with a purple lesion on his upper arm. A skin biopsy revealed Kaposi's sarcoma; he was very shocked on hearing this news. Despite knowing what the results might be, he could not comprehend that he had an incurable disease that could result in his death. The doctor sensing this decided to arrange for Paul to see him and a health adviser a few days later. Paul attended with Bob, his partner of four years. Paul feared losing his job, thinking he could be infectious to the school children. The doctor had a lengthy discussion with Paul, telling him that the prognosis for Kaposi's sarcoma in AIDS is considerably better than patients with opportunistic infections and that no one can give a definite time for death.

It was explained that having the virus would not cause any risk to the children because the HIV is a particularly vulnerable virus. Its thin, buttery envelope gives it very little protection against the 'outside' world. This means not only that it is easily destroyed when outside the incubating protection of the body, but it is also a very difficult virus to acquire.

Paul's parents had no idea he was gay and, aware of the implications of them knowing his diagnosis, he decided not to tell them. The health adviser discussed with Paul and Bob other matters that were causing them concern:

(1) After discussions, he decided he would be very careful whom he would inform regarding his diagnosis.
(2) Guidelines for safer sex.
(3) Basic hygiene.
(4) Eating a well-balanced diet.
(5) Paul should live life positively and to the full, and that he may go through periods of depression requiring much support.
(6) They were both given phone numbers of helpful support groups, i.e. the Terence Higgins Trust and Frontliners.
(7) A sister from the home-support team introduced herself to them explaining that the support team could care for Paul at home whenever he required help. She would provide a continuity of care between the clinic, ward and Paul's home.

Paul's general practitioner was not very keen to look after him now that he had acquired the virus, so the home-support sister found a sympathetic doctor and Paul registered with him. Over the coming months, Paul continued to work full time. Outwardly things appeared normal, whilst inwardly Paul still had fears about losing his job should his colleagues discover he had the virus. Bob was anxious that he, too, may have the virus, even giving it to Paul in the first place. At their request, it was arranged that he would see a clinical psychologist who would enable them to come to terms with Paul's diagnosis.

In October 1986 he developed diarrhoea, *Cytomegalovirus* (CMV) was diagnosed and a course of an antiviral drug, Ganciclovir, was commenced intravenously followed by a maintenance dose three times a week to prevent CMV from recurring. A port-a-cath device was inserted to enable Paul to administer Ganciclovir himself. He was instructed and observed by the doctor on how to perform the administration of Ganciclovir using aseptic technique, finally feeling confident to perform this task himself. The home-support sister visited Paul at home and found that he was coping adequately. Having the port-a-cath inserted enabled Paul to visit his sister in Australia for Christmas, continuing to administer the Ganciclovir. His sister was aware of Paul's diagnosis and was very supportive. They both discussed their parents and decided to tell them that Paul had leukaemia.

On his return home, Paul received a new drug zidovudine (AZT), which is a synthetic thymidine analogue that inhibits the reverse transcriptase enzyme of human immunodeficiency virus. It was stressed that there might be side-effects with this drug such as anaemia, which would require frequent blood transfusions. There may also be a reduced white-cell count, leading to the drug dosage being reduced.

## Further deterioration

In April 1987, Paul was admitted to hospital complaining of shortness of breath on exertion and fevers. A bronchoscopy was performed, *Pneumocystis carinii* pneumonia (PCP) was diagnosed and treatment was commenced. During his stay in hospital, Paul became very distressed at the thought of dying and received much support from the ward staff and the Anglican minister. Paul also made a will and appointed an executor. He had an uneventful recovery from PCP, going home two weeks after admission. Once at home, Paul felt very weak and lethargic. He decided to resign from his employment and became a private tutor, teaching part time. He found this type of employment less stressful. As a result of the Zidovudine, he required blood transfusions about every six weeks.

On return from holiday in Spain with Bob in November 1987, he complained of blurred vision. *Cytomegalovirus* (CMV) retinitis was diagnosed and a course of Ganciclovir was commenced via a port-a-cath which improved his vision.

## Management of the terminal illness

Having spent Christmas with his parents and the New Year with Bob, Paul started to lose his memory and concentration; he found he was unable to carry on working. A CT scan revealed AIDS encephalopathy. He had also had several bouts of diarrhoea throughout the day that were due to Kaposi's sarcoma in the intestinal tract. Paul did not wish to be admitted to hospital, requesting to be cared for at home, so the home-support sister arranged for the appropriate community services to become involved with Paul's care. A joint visit was arranged with the district nurse to meet and to assess Paul and his needs; although the district nurse was fairly knowledgeable about HIV she still had some doubts about it and required guidance from the home-support sister:

(1) Cuts and abrasions on hands must be covered with waterproof dressing.
(2) When dealing with body fluids, she should wear gloves, thoroughly washing her hands afterwards.
(3) Infected and soiled dressings and waste should be placed in yellow bags and secured. Refuse-disposal services were arranged to collect the yellow bags.

The district nurse visited Paul every other day, supplying Inco-pads, a commode and anything else he required. She also helped Paul with his bath. Paul was still receiving his maintenance dose of Ganciclovir but because he was becoming more vague and forgetful, the home-support sister administered the drug via the port-a-cath. His GP visited frequently and prescribed codeine phosphate for diarrhoea. Paul and Bob possessed a washing-machine/spin-dryer, so any soiled linen was washed in this way. A home-help was arranged. Again the home-support sister discussed with her any fears she may have had about caring for Paul.

(1) No disinfectants are required when cleaning around the flat.
(2) Use disposable cloths, separate cloths for the kitchen and bathroom.
(3) If spillage of body fluids occurs, Paul or the home-help should use household bleach 10 per cent diluted one-part bleach to ten-parts warm water using paper towels, then discarding the towel down the toilet.
(4) It was also stressed how important it was for complete confidentiality so that Paul's illness should not be discussed with anyone.

The home-help visited Paul everyday, and she also did Paul's shopping for him. The occupational therapist visited and arranged for various devices to help Paul around the flat.

### Support for the family and partner

Paul's parents visited frequently. They were asking leading and probing questions about Paul's illness, so Paul decided to tell them the truth. The sudden realization that their son was gay came as a terrible shock to them and not having time to think or accept the situation in hand, they had no other choice but to give Paul the impression that they had accepted Bob for Paul's sake. The home-support sister spent long periods listening to Paul's parents – she also arranged for them to see a clinical psychologist. During this time, Bob required a lot of support and reassurance. He decided to work from home, so that he would be near at hand if Paul needed him.

Over the next couple of weeks, Paul's condition deteriorated quite rapidly, his diarrhoea continued despite all treatment. On 10 March 1988 Paul died peacefully in his sleep with Bob and his parents at his bedside.

### After the death

The GP came and certified Paul's death. He contacted the undertakers and asked them to provide a plastic cadaver bag. The home-support sister was present when Paul died, so she performed the Last Offices wearing a disposable plastic apron and disposable gloves. She washed Paul's body, packing any leaking orifices. She then attached identity bracelets to Paul's ankles and wrists. A label with 'BIO-HAZARD – Danger of infection' tape was also placed around the ankles and wrists. She put a pair of pyjamas on Paul and placed his body in the plastic cadaver bag. A notification-of-death label was attached to the outside of the plastic cadaver bag with BIO-HAZARD tape.

A nurse from the ward, the home-support sister and the district nurse attended Paul's funeral, which was conducted by the Anglican hospital chaplain.

Paul's parents still continued to be in touch with the clinical psychologist. The home-support sister visited them regularly in the home. Bob found much support from his friends, coming to the bereavement-support group at the hospital occasionally.

## FURTHER READING

Green, J. and Miller, D. (1986) *AIDS—Story of a Disease*, Grafton Books, London.

Miller, D., Weber, J. and Green, J. (eds) (1986) *The Management of AIDS Patients*, Macmillan, London.

Miller, D. (1987) *Living with AIDS and HIV*, Macmillan, London.
Pinching, A. and Weber, J. (1986) *Management of AIDS*, Macmillan, London.
Pratt, R. J. (1987) *Strategy for Nursing Care*, Edward Arnold, London.
Weber, J. and Ferriman, A. (1986) *AIDS Concerns You*, Pagoda Books, London.
Woodcock, J. (1987), Drug management of an AIDS patient, *The Pharmaceutical Journal*, 18 July, Vol. 239, No. 6,440, pp. 75–7.

## ACKNOWLEDGEMENTS

I would like to acknowledge the helpful suggestions and support given to me by Doctor Anthony Pinching, Senior Lecturer and Honorary Consultant in Clinical Immunology, St Mary's Hospital, Paddington, and also by Ms Ann Smith, Co-ordinator, Home-Support Team, St Mary's Hospital, Paddington.

# 12. The Needs of Staff

This chapter will consider the needs of staff, particularly nurses (both qualified and in training) when they are caring for dying patients and their families. For these purposes, nursing auxiliaries are included, since they are often involved with the care to a significant degree. Certain aspects will be intensified when such care is the nurse's exclusive function, for example in a hospice, in a continuing-care unit of a hospital or as a Macmillan nurse in the community.

However, it has already been pointed out that there are very few situations where any nurse will not sometimes be providing care during a terminal illness, however brief. It is therefore hoped that senior nurses will find the ensuing discussion helpful in considering responsibilities towards their staff, and that individual nurses will be encouraged to develop their own professional responsibility for themselves and their colleagues.

## EMOTIONAL NEEDS AND SUPPORT

As with many other spheres of work, terminal care carries its own type of emotional stress. The closer the relationship between nurse, patient and family, the greater is the potential strain. This should be borne in mind when allocating student nurses to care for individual patients, during one or more spans of duty. Adequate support and supervision by trained nurses should be readily available at all times, not only because the patient's condition may change quickly and unexpectedly, but also to support the student emotionally.

In hospices, where it is unusual to have student nurses as part of the caring team, nursing auxiliaries often give a considerable amount of the care. They, too, will need careful orientation when newly appointed, continuing supervision and support from the trained nurses, and confidence that their observations and ideas are valued.

## Recognizing stress and strain

Tolerance to stress is an individual matter; some people will exhibit strain as a response to a stressful situation very soon, whereas another person will appear not to be affected. Continuing strain is a sign that the stress being endured is excessive and can be a danger signal that actual illness will occur. Stress is not a disease – protective responses like grief, anger, fear, are needed when there are threats to physical and psychological well-being. It is the prolongation of these responses that is the danger, resulting in intolerable strain. Evison (1986) suggests that it is useful to know of some means of self-help to prevent the build-up of stress. For instance, people need to 'get things off their chest' after an upsetting experience. One should find someone to talk to, but should in turn be willing to listen, otherwise someone else's stress-level may be increased. Natural emotional discharge such as crying, laughing, or 'storming' are means to natural healing processes. If it is inappropriate to allow this release at the time, it could be done later. If feeling tense, actions such as stretching, yawning or loosening the shoulder and neck muscles by gentle movements will aid in relaxation.

The term 'burnout' is a recent one in this country although commonly used in the USA for a number of years. It is described as an extension of stress particularly applicable to members of the caring professions – teaching, health care, social work – when the person experiences a depletion of energy through feeling overwhelmed by other people's problems (Iveson-Iveson 1983). The person becomes increasingly fatigued, hating to go to work, and various physical symptoms may become manifest. A feeling of depression and futility is common; also headaches and sleeplessness. In desperation, even alcohol or drug dependence may start in some cases. In the place of the original high ideals and enthusiasm to serve others, a feeling of apathy and disillusion sets in, and eventually an opting-out, in a psychological if not in a physical sense, from the working group.

This tragic outcome is preventable where colleagues, and particularly those in authority, really care for each other as well as for their clients or patients. Certain personality types are more vulnerable than others, but the main factor lies in good working conditions and ready support for those helping to carry the burdens of others – often quite appalling in terms of human inadequacy and misery.

A change of job is sometimes the answer but, regrettably, talented and sensitive people are sometimes lost for ever from their chosen profession because of insufficient awareness and help from others at a crucial time. Nursing is not exempt from this potential hazard. Those who are exclusively involved with dying and bereaved individuals should be aware of their vulnerability, and that of their colleagues; some of the ideas in this chapter may be helpful as practical measures to counter-balance the particular kind of stress involved.

Where dying people are being cared for under conditions as near as possible approaching the ideal, there is great satisfaction for the staff, compensating for the emotional stress involved. It is when there are constant anxieties and frustrations about inability to provide for a comfortable and peaceful death and continuing care for the family that the burnout syndrome is a distinct risk, especially if other factors are involved such as personal problems or a low threshold-tolerance to stress.

## Staff meetings

When a patient is dying, or has just died, the sharing of relevant information at a reporting session between members of the nursing staff is bound to be emotionally charged to some degree, however matter-of-factly it is conduct. This will depend on the circumstances of the patient's illness, its length, the age of the patient, and how long the individual nurses have known both patient and family. The senior nurse leading the report session should be aware that one or more nurses may be feeling particularly affected because of their closer involvement than other members of the staff.

It is important to make an opportunity for staff to talk over their own feelings, either privately with a sympathetic listener of their choice, or in a group brought together to talk over matters of mutual concern and interest outside the normal report session when time is inevitably limited because of the amount of factual information to be covered. Such a meeting can be appropriate to a general hospital ward, a hospice, a residential home for elderly people, or a home-care team. It can be most valuable in bringing together members of different disciplines, each with their own expertise and problems encountered, and should promote better understanding of individual roles. Those attending should represent all those involved in caring for the dying patient, or patients, for instance all grades of nursing staff, doctors, social workers and paramedical staff. In discussing certain matters, it will be helpful to have the psychiatrist or clinical psychologist present if such a professional worker is regularly involved.

The meeting needs an appropriate leader, who could be a member of any of the disciplines mentioned, but the atmosphere should be as relaxed as possible to encourage participation by anyone who wishes to speak. Like all meetings, if it is to be successful it should begin and end promptly at stated times and should be kept to a reasonable length. The aim of the meeting should be stated – it may be to discuss a particular patient and family because of certain problems that have arisen. Another aim might be to clarify policy on a certain issue, such as the timing of admission of a patient for terminal care. Where a patient has recently died, it may come as a relief to share feelings of doubt and anxiety as to whether the care was as adequate and well managed as possible, and to find reassurance, or at least to admit some sense of failure and learn from it.

Good communications among staff are very important to foster appropriate attitudes. In becoming aware of the different emotional stages through which dying people and their families may pass, it becomes easier to understand that such an emotion as anger may be projected onto an individual member of staff. This may cause a natural reaction of hurt and impatient feelings in the nurse, doctor or social worker. However, in talking over the problem with others, relief is experienced that one need not feel guilty or a failure but can absorb the emotion in the team task of caring and trying to find the best way to help the patient and family. This will forestall the unfortunate sequel of the patient being avoided to some extent by some staff. Because of the variety of pressures at work, it may be difficult to hold such a meeting in a general hospital, although psychiatric hospitals will be accustomed to this means of communication. Informal exchange thus becomes very important at all levels of staff.

## Working conditions

Unless the nurse is working in a hospice or other purpose-built unit, the environmental conditions may be far from ideal for the care of a dying patient. This in itself will be a strain for staff even though the patient and his or her family will feel more than compensated for any inconvenience of surroundings by a high quality of personal care. A major problem may be lack of a room set aside for use when privacy is essential. Doctor and ward sister frequently need to talk with close relatives, or a patient; families want to talk together and relax when spending long periods with a dying relative.

A nurse, too, needs some privacy during or after an emotionally traumatic time. Ingenuity can usually produce a temporary haven, and a short break away from the ward for a cup of coffee will be appreciated and enable the nurse to recover his or her equilibrium before resuming care of the patients.

Nurses caring for patients in their own homes learn to accept that even though the physical environment might be considered less than ideal and comfortable, the psychological advantages for patients who choose to die at home will far outweigh any inconvenience. This will also be the viewpoint of the family where home care is also their wish, as long as they have adequate professional support.

Those nurses who are in continuous or frequent involvement with dying patients should be particularly aware of the need to balance their professional life with family, friends and recreation. Senior nurses will be mindful of the need to see that their staff have reasonable off-duty arrangements, and the occasional long break.

## PROFESSIONAL PREPARATION AND CONTINUING EDUCATION

A nurse who chooses to work in a hospice or Macmillan service needs a thorough period of orientation and teaching in the special aspects of care. Adjustment is required from the different approach in a hospital, away from 'cure', and a trial period of employment – perhaps three months – is a good idea to allow for a mutual decision to be reached between the nurse and his or her employer that he or she is suited to the work. Experienced district nurses joining a Macmillan service team need time to build up relationships with other colleagues in the community, and to learn how their special training and skills will fit into the wider team.

It is usually considered essential for such nurses to undertake a post-basic clinical course, such as the ENB course, No. 930/931,

'Continuing care of the dying patient and the family'. This six-week course is also very useful for nurses who wish to extend their expertise in any field of work that includes care of dying patients. An advanced ENB course No. 285, 'Specialist course in the continuing care of the dying patient and the family' is available for nurses who are to specialize in this work, particularly if they are to hold a position of responsibility such as head of nursing care in a hospice. The nurse should normally hold the Statement of Attendance for course 930/931. Centres offering either of these courses will tailor the course programme to the needs of the individual student. Further developments are taking place with regard to the preparation of Macmillan nurses. In future, all newly appointed nurses will undergo a training course at the Macmillan Education Centre, Dorothy House Hospice, Bath (funded by Cancer Relief).

## Continuing education

Continuing education in one's work is just as essential in terminal care as in other spheres. There is a responsibility for employing authorities to provide reasonable opportunities for their staff to attend appropriate courses whether one day or longer in order that they may be helped to maintain and improve professional knowledge and competence. This is reflected in the UKCC Code of Professional Conduct (1984). The provision of such opportunities will eventually become mandatory as a requirement of the UKCC for eligibility of the nurse to practise. The Code of Practice also charges the individual practitioner to take every opportunity him- or herself to maintain and increase professional competence. Self-directed learning has a place here because nurses cannot attend an unlimited number of courses. It is also useful because of its association with both problem-solving and with the nursing process.

Apart from facilities organized by individual nursing-education departments for staff working in a particular health authority district, many bodies are regularly offering courses and conferences throughout the country. These include Cancer Relief, the Marie Curie Foundation, individual hospices with education departments and others. The Royal College of Nursing Association of Nursing Practice has a forum, 'Symptom control and care of the dying', open to nurses who are involved in such work, to provide support and educational opportunities.

There is, of course, room for multi-disciplinary learning and this already takes place in many ways. A study in Scotland (Doyle, 1982) into the education in terminal care received and perceived to be needed by 343 nurses reported that 87 per cent stated a preference for multi-professional training.

Considerable interest is shown in developing knowledge and understanding of terminal care by nurses working in areas where this is not the main feature but where the right of each individual to a peaceful and comfortable death is recognized. Study days and short conferences are always well attended, and applications to attend the longer course are numerous. This eagerness to learn how to improve patient care should result in student nurses receiving good support and teaching when they are involved in giving terminal care.

## THE NURSE AND OTHER COLLEAGUES

In a multi-professional setting there is always a risk that each group feels it has a monopoly of problems, so that it may not be sufficiently aware of the difficulties of other colleagues, and their needs. Some of the inadequacy of care and mismanagement of terminally ill patients – now recognized and increasingly being improved – can stem partly from a lack of preparation during basic training.

Medical students can still find that low priority is given to the subject during their training. The fact that the medical student first learns the practical aspects of death in the dissecting room can lead to a defensive barrier being erected to enable the student to cope emotionally. This may affect future attitudes to dying patients. The student nurse, in contrast, is exposed at an early stage to physical and emotional contact with such patients and their families, which can help to establish more personal relationships although, of course, this carries its own stress.

Other health-care professional staff such as physiotherapists and occupational therapists, whose work normally has much emphasis on rehabilitation, will also need preparation for seeing the different value of their work in contributing to the comfort of the dying patient. Social workers are better equipped by their training and experience to assist patients and families emotionally, although some feel that they are not so well prepared to deal with bereaved families at home. Theological students sometimes feel that they do not have sufficient training in the practical aspects of death and bereavement for which they will later have to take responsibility – conducting funerals and facing the intense grief of relatives.

One of the nurse's functions is a co-ordinating one in the caring team. Consideration of the above factors should help in understanding and assisting colleagues who are also doing their best to help patients and their families at a critical time.

In hospices, voluntary workers give valuable help to patients and staff in a variety of ways. They, too, need some orientation and training in order to play their part in the service.

## REFERENCES AND FURTHER READING

Doyle, D. (1982) Nursing education in terminal care, *Nursing Education Today*, Vol. 2, No. 4, September, pp. 4–6.

Evison, R. (1986) Self-help in preventing stress buildup, *The Professional Nurse*, Vol. 1, No. 6, pp. 157–9.

Hector, W. and Whitfield, S. (1982) *Nursing Care for the Dying Patient and the Family*, Heinemann Medical, London.

Iveson-Iveson, J. (1983) Banishing the burnout syndrome, *Nursing Mirror*, 4 May, p. 43.

Iwasiw, C. L. (1987) UKCC discussion paper – mandatory periodic refreshment for nurses and health visitors, *Nurse Education Today*, Vol. 7, pp. 222–7.

Parkes, Murray C. (1986) The caregivers' griefs, *Journal of Palliative Care*, Vol. 1, No. 2, pp. 56.

# 13. Religious Beliefs and Practices

## THE SPIRITUAL DIMENSION

Pastoral care is based on the existence of God (whatever be His name) and the spiritual dimension of humanity. It is an anthropological fact that humanity, by its very nature, is prone towards a divinity, towards a God; this can also be seen from basic observation. This tendency can be found in humanity in whatever age and set of circumstances; it is common right across the spectrum of human kind. If this is true and if our total care of the dying patient is to be really 'total', then we must face up to and 'nurse' the spiritual dimension of the patient.

There are particular times in life when these concepts take on a particular urgency – times of joy and sorrow; and times of danger and risk. Among these occasions, periods of sickness, and of course, terminal illness, bring us face to face with destiny, with inevitability, with the unknown. For better or worse the patient grapples with the meaning of humanity, the meaning of life and death and the possibility of a life hereafter; all take on, in a new and very personal way, a significance that is both immediate and relevant. Death as a phenomenon or indeed as a reality for other people, becomes very personal and has to be approached in a very personal way. Death is not just at *a* doorstep, it is at *my* doorstep. Such a realization causes the mind to concentrate. At this stage we are at the heart of the spiritual dimension and the chaplain is part of it. It is for the chaplain (as part of the overall caring team) to stay with the patient, the all-important person whose past is over, whose present is limited in time and whose future is filled with a newness never experienced before. At this stage, thoughts of the past – guilt feelings, regrets, bad self-image – can crowd the mind. Is this a punishment, an abandonment by God? This is the situation into which the chaplain arrives.

Conscious of their own struggles with the mysteries of life and death and with the mystery of God, chaplains are both a symbol of strength and at the same time a witness of finality and helplessness. While it may be true that they have come to grips with their own faith, and with faith answers to the problems of life, they cannot presume faith to guarantee the answers to another's problems. Experience shows that with faith it is indeed possible to face up to death and all its implications, but this may be stated more in hindsight than *a priori* in the case of any individual person. The success over the years in dealing with the challenges of life and of faith can also contribute greatly to a balanced and positive approach to death. But a constructive approach is not confined only to those who have had a successful and balanced life. Chaplains everywhere (and other carers too) continually meet those with a resilience and an inner strength where none would have been anticipated. The spiritual dimension is one area that does not permit generalization.

## THE CHRISTIAN RELIGION

All Christians have a common belief in the meaning of the death and resurrection of Jesus Christ. For the Christian, Jesus came that we may have life and have it to the full (John 10:10). Death contains within itself the moment of resurrection and it was for that rebirth that Christ came on earth. That was the death, leading to the resurrection, that gives meaning to our death and also to our life. 'We believe that having died with Christ we shall return to life with him' (Romans 6:8). This clear and resounding statement is the core of the Christian declaration about death. Well tested over the centuries, it continues to provide solid comfort to the dying. For the Christian, the dead are no longer dead but living in Christ.

The Christian chaplain is there to be available to any who wish to 'talk things over'. When the comment is made that it is good to have someone who is there for that purpose, it is a sign of reassurance and relief that comes not from one who presumes to solve the patient's problems but from the patient him- or herself feeling the support and back-up from another human being who declares gently the normality of human sickness and death. What is beautifully human is already a step into the spiritual. The chaplain's easy pace and presence to the patient can in itself be a witness to a living and caring God. Patients need such an opening and experience shows that in their own time and in the uniqueness of their individuality, the spiritual dimension is brought to the surface.

## Pastoral care of the family, relatives and friends

It is rare indeed that a patient has neither family, relatives nor friends. Total patient care cannot overlook the unique and intimate relationship between the patient and those accompanying him or her at the end of his or her life. With impending separation and loss, these special people have special needs at that time. Pastoral care, with its central message of salvation, should accompany the family members in their effort to cope in this highly charged emotional moment in their lives. The central message to the patient is also the message to the family and relatives. What is positive for one is positive for all.

Sometimes chaplains will find a far greater challenge coming from the family, whose helplessness and anger are placed on God. They may, therefore, encounter rebuff and even hostility. In these situations, chaplains should be able to accept such reaction, knowing that it is not meant personally. At times like this a personal encounter with a key member of the family can be greatly beneficial. Seeing the patient as a member of the family, the care of the patient and that of the family can be mutually sustaining and supportive.

The hospice, with its particular facilities for the family, can also provide the family members and all the relatives and friends with an image of the spiritual dimension that is the basis of pastoral care. The best guideline is the individual attention and appreciation of every person involved in the patient's illness and death.

## Promoting spiritual awareness in the staff

Very often members of the staff find themselves at a loss when it comes to the spiritual needs of the patient. The easy way out is to promise to call the chaplain, whose 'speciality' is in that sphere. This indicates uncertainty rather than unwillingness to become involved; it is up to the chaplain to highlight the valuable part the staff can play by simply staying with the patient as a listening and reassuring friend. After all, it was the patient who, in the first place, chose that particular member of staff with whom to share. Moreover, members of the staff need to be aware that they, and not the chaplain, may be chosen by the patient as being easier to share with in matters spiritual, than the official (and professional) minister of religion. Tradition, ignorance, prejudice, superstition and previous bad experience can create barriers that make an encounter with the chaplain appear threatening. It is essential for chaplains themselves to experience the support of the staff and to foster the staff's participation with them in the spiritual care of the patient.

## Care of the bereaved

Bereavement work is a complex and prolonged ministry. It, too, can be greatly helped by the spiritual care given before the death and after. The Christian assurances to the patient remain the spiritual background on which the pastoral care of the bereaved is based. For the bereaved, the funeral rites constitute a starting point; they should, therefore, be given careful attention by the chaplain. An intimate and deeply personal funeral service can set the tone for the recovery from grief and loss. It is, for the chaplain, a privileged moment of care for the bereaved. Because of it being a once-only and group event, it ought to be conducted with the utmost sensitivity and simplicity, so that what is said and read is easily understood at a time when understanding by those taking part can often be hindered by the emotional upheaval they are now experiencing. Much good can be achieved at funeral services. The opposite can also be true.

# SPECIFIC ROMAN CATHOLIC MINISTRY

Apart from private prayer with the individual patient (and when appropriate with the family) the Roman Catholic ministry to the sick is made up of the liturgical celebration of the sacraments: the Eucharist, the Sacrament of the Sick (the Anointing) and the Sacrament of Reconciliation (previously called the Confession). Personal prayer ought to be simple, taking into account the limited energy of the patient. Short Bible readings and traditional prayers read or recited slowly can also be very helpful. Account must be taken of those who have lost contact with any formal prayer. Above all, there ought to be no crowding of the patient with long and drawn-out prayers.

The sacraments are ideally celebrated in a community setting. At home this might be with members of the family, neighbours and friends, some perhaps from the local church. In a hospital or hospice it may be possible to gather several Roman Catholics together in a room or small ward to celebrate together. Again, any relatives, friends or staff members would ideally form the community. It has been found in a hospice setting that non-Catholic patients are sometimes very happy, and ask, to be present at a Eucharist celebration and to feel a bond with their Catholic fellow-patients. Equally, the chaplain will be happy to bring the sacraments to a single Catholic patient in privacy in whatever arrangements are suitable. Readings should be chosen with great care; sensitive topics, for example, death and dying, should be avoided since the chaplain has no control over the resulting impact on individual patients.

The Sacrament of Reconciliation is a powerful means of restoring a positive self-image and self-confidence in the patient. Extreme sensitivity is needed on the part of the chaplain whose patients may have some guilt feelings and uncertainty leading up to this sacrament. Care must also be taken to allow the patient true freedom in choosing the appropriate moment to celebrate this sacrament. It is not uncommon to find a patient burdened by family members who wish him or her to 'make their peace with God'.

The Sacrament of the Sick has recovered its original meaning and purpose: a sacrament for those who are sick. Until recently it was known as the 'Last rites' or 'Extreme unction' and was generally administered in association with imminent death. There may still be some patients whose image of the sacrament remains the same as that of their parents' or grandparents' time. Extra care is needed in this case. The sacrament is best celebrated during the celebration of the Eucharist – again, if possible, in the company of family or staff members.

## THE ANGLICAN MINISTRY

The Church of England offers a variety of ministry to the dying person, which is marked by a flexibility of application according to the needs of the patient, the family and the circumstances involved. The most comprehensive collection of rites and prayers is contained in the booklet, *Ministry to the Sick*, published in 1983 and widely welcomed as a companion to the alternative service book of 1980. In this volume there are different shortened forms of Holy Communion, including a simple form of personal preparation.

There are also forms of 'The laying on of hands with prayer' and 'Anointing', which may or need not be a part of Holy Communion. Essentially they are part of a 'healing ministry' that is prayer for the wholeness of the dying patient and they have a totally different atmosphere from the popular conception of the 'last rites'. These are also commendatory prayers for use at the time of death and, most importantly, readings and prayers that are for the bereaved family and friends. These are brief and simple and are often most appropriately used by the nursing staff immediately after the death, particularly if the family is present. Provision is also made for confession, which can be used either formally or informally depending upon the tradition or background of the patient.

The breadth of Anglican practice means that there is a great variety of approach and options within the material provided. This enables those caring for the dying to be sensitive and flexible and, which is most important, the rites and prayers are usually appropriate for nursing and other staff to use as well as the chaplain or visiting priest.

## FREE CHURCHES

These churches comprise the third main Christian group in the UK, and they share many common beliefs with each other, and with the Anglican and Roman Catholic communities. For the purposes of this chapter the nurse will find that the members of these churches share with other Christians hope for a life after death, and that dying patients and their families will look for comfort and spiritual help from their ministers. There are no special rites practised in relation to the dying person but instead an emphasis on the mercy of God, inspiration from scripture readings and spontaneous prayers together.

All Free-church chaplains come under the umbrella of the Free Church Federal Council who, amongst their other activities, have a Hospital Chaplaincy Service, which is responsible for the appointment and training of all hospital and hospice chaplains. The Free Church Federal Council is made up of about 15 free, independent churches, the largest of which are the Methodist Church, the Baptist Church, the United Reformed Church and the Salvation Army. In addition to this organization, the free churches are also members of the Hospital

Chaplains Fellowship, which is an ecumenical group of churches incorporating the Roman Catholic Church and the Church of England, in addition to the free-church representatives. In addition to this, there is also an Association of Hospice Chaplains that, again, is an ecumenical group of chaplains working specifically in the field of hospice.

Although most of the Free churches do have a sacramental ministry, most Free-church chaplains would have a gospel-based ministry of prayer, bible reading and of practical help, both to patients and to their families.

## THE NON-CHRISTIAN RELIGIONS

Nurses caring for dying patients whose religion and customs differ from their own are often worried because they do not really know how to behave, and yet they wish to do all they can to help and to support the individual and the family. It is important to remember that even though the religious affiliation may be given as Jew, Muslim, Sikh or Hindu, for example, the degree of orthodoxy with which the individual observes the various rights and customs may vary greatly. It will be greatly appreciated, and not regarded as an intrusion, if the family are asked how best the staff can meet the patient's needs.

It is, however, helpful to know a little of the beliefs of a particular religion and the implications for physical care as well as religious observance. Some information in this respect is provided here for some of the major non-Christian religions. The reader is referred to more detailed studies in the list of references at the end of this chapter.

### Judaism

The patient may belong to either the Liberal or Orthodox category of Judaism. In the case of the former there will be few special requirements, although some Liberal Jews will observe strict rules regarding their diet, which will be either vegetarian or kosher (i.e. meat must come from animals slaughtered in a certain way, and any meat from the pig is forbidden). Food is a very important feature of Jewish life, and in the case of the very ill or dying patient, relatives may wish to bring in certain favourite dishes, particularly chicken soup, which is a panacea for all ills. Orthodox Jews follow a number of strict rules regarding daily living. They will eat only kosher food, and when near to death may wish the rabbi to be with them to help them acknowledge their sins and recite special prayers. The relatives will also appreciate the presence of the rabbi because many things have to be arranged after the death of the patient and they will wish to make arrangements.

After the funeral there is a period of mourning initially for seven days, the bereaved remaining at home and receiving relatives and friends, seated on low chairs. This ritual is very comforting to the bereaved for it encourages everyone to express their grief.

## Hinduism

Hinduism has no fixed creed and many schools of philosophical thought. Hindus practise the worship of many gods, though some would say these are only different manifestations of one god. The Hindu faith is centred on the transmigration of the soul with indefinite reincarnation. When the individual dies, that person is born again and the new body depends on what kind of life he or she has led during this present one.

Prayer is very important, as is ritual cleansing and, again, a shower is more acceptable than a bath because of the need for running water; the left hand is considered 'unclean'. Hindu women also dislike, and may refuse to be examined by, a male doctor. There are strict dietary rules. Neither beef nor pork may be eaten and, in addition, cooking utensils must not have been used for these meats or their by-products, and the food should have been prepared by someone of the same caste as the patient. This makes provision of food very difficult. A vegetarian diet is acceptable but sometimes it is better for the family to bring in food. Being able to follow their religious customs is very important for the terminally ill, as this may affect the quality of their next life.

Married women wear a nuptial thread around the neck and possibly a red mark on the forehead. These should not be removed. A male may have a sacred thread around the arm, and again this should not be removed. Hindus would prefer to die at home but even when in hospital they may try to lie on the floor so that they can die as near to 'mother earth' as possible. With the use of rugs and pillows, they should be helped to do this, especially if they are being nursed in a high bed, as falling is a great risk.

For the Hindu there is a design for living: a period of education; a period of working with the world; a period of loosening of ties and worldly attachments; and a period of freedom through death. Cremation is necessary and the ashes are usually scattered on water. It is usual for the eldest son to make all the arrangements. There is a set pattern for mourning: for ten days friends and relatives visit the bereaved bringing gifts of food, clothes and money and a service is held on the eleventh day. To open the body is considered disrespectful to the individual and the family, and great sensitivity will be needed if a post-mortem examination is required.

## Islam

Islam is the religon of the Muslims, of whom there are over 900 million in the world. Most Muslims in the UK have their origins in the Indian sub-continent. Muslims believe that the religion of Islam (meaning 'submission', i.e. to God's will) was revealed by God to the prophet Muhammad in Mecca, in what is now Saudi Arabia. Muslims revere the prophets of the Old Testament and also Jesus as another prophet.

Most Muslims adhere strictly to Islamic law, and so those nursing the terminally ill need to be sensitive to certain attitudes and practices. Every Muslim says certain prayers five times a day. Even the dying patient will try to carry out this practice as far as possible, even though some of the associated rituals may not be feasible. Washing is very important before prayers. Where possible, time should be provided for the bedfast patient to wash hands, face and arms before prayers, and of the genital areas after urinating or defecation.

Friday is the holy day for Muslims, and month of Ramadan a period of fasting. Although dying patients cannot do this totally, they may wish to make some gesture towards it. Modesty is crucial to Muslims of both sexes, who would wish to be treated by a doctor of their own sex. It is important to be aware of the dietary rules observed by Muslims. The main ones are as follows:

(1) No pork or pig products are permitted. Other meat may be eaten as long as it is '*halal*', i.e. killed according to Islamic law, or if this is not available, kosher meat may be acceptable.
(2) Fish of any kind is permitted unless it has no fins or scales.
(3) Alcohol is expressly forbidden.
(4) Some Muslims will refuse all food that has not been cooked and served separately. Obviously, it is important when dying Muslims are admitted to hospital or hospice that their dietary needs are carefully discussed with their families. It may be most helpful to allow the family to bring in special food (if they live near enough) or

to ask for the help of the religious leader (Iman) of the nearest mosque.

Muslims believe in life after death and that death is God's will. However, it is likely that grief will be displayed openly. Details are given in Chapter 6 on the rituals surrounding the last hours of life, and the performance of Last Offices.

After the death, all friends and relatives are duty-bound to visit and to comfort the bereaved. Mourning usually lasts for about a month, and the widow is expected to stay indoors, as far as possible, for 130 days.

## Buddhism

Buddhist teaching is based on non-violence and brotherhood, and on a doctrine of rebirth. Buddha is revered, not as a god but as an example, and Buddhism is more a way of life than a religion. There is great emphasis on meditation to relax the mind and body in order to see life in its true perspective – this will also include meditating on one's own death. Because of this it is important that quietness and privacy are provided for the terminally ill.

Diets vary, but Buddhists are mostly vegetarian because of their reluctance to kill any creature. Certain fast days are observed that may require the individual to eat before noon and not after and, depending on the country of origin, there may or may not be strict rules of hygiene. As the administration of drugs may sometimes cloud the mind, these may be refused by the patient and may make the relief of pain difficult.

Buddhists accept the ordinary human life-cycle and there are no special rites for the dying, but patients and their families may wish to be visited by a Buddhist monk. There are many schools of thought in Buddhism and it is important to know which the patient practises if a Buddhist monk or sister needs to be contacted in order to know for whom to ask. (The Buddhist Society and the London Buddhist Centre will usually know how contacts may be swiftly made.)

## Sikhism

The Sikh has one God and there is no priesthood as such. Sikhism is concerned with the individual's relationship with God and with doing good in this life as a way to salvation. It has a strong community aspect and the community runs its own temple providing services, information and hospitality for all.

The guru who founded Sikhism gave his followers five symbols of faith: *kesh*, uncut hair, which the men wear under a turban; *kangha*, a wooden or plastic comb used to hold the hair; *kara*, a steel bangle that represents the unity of God and should never be removed; and *keipan*, a symbolic dagger that indicates a Sikh's readiness to fight in self-defence or to protect the poor and oppressed. This is worn night and day. *Kaccha*, special underpants or shorts, which represent a symbol of modesty and morality, will be worn at all times even in a shower. These must never be completely removed and when washing a patient during a blanket bath and when changing them, one leg should be removed at a time, dealt with, and a fresh pair put onto that leg before removing the other leg from the old pair.

Sikhs are not allowed to eat meat that is *halal* (killed as for Muslims). Most are vegetarian. If non-vegetarian, beef is not usually eaten and, for some, pork is also forbidden. Alcohol and cigarettes are also forbidden. The family is important to the dying Sikh as is privacy for private prayer. Cremation should occur within 24 hours of death, and families may need help with convincing the undertaker that their need is urgent. As the eldest son would normally light the funeral pyre it may be possible for him to press the button that moves the body to the furnace. The widow may fast until after the cremation. The ashes are scattered in a river or the sea.

After the cremation the family returns to the temple where the members may wash, or they may return home. The whole family remains in mourning, relatives and friends providing support. After ten days a special service marks the end of mourning.

## Shinto

Shinto or 'The Way of the Gods' is the original religion of Japan and had its origins in the worship of the spirits of nature such as the sun, forests, rivers and seas. It was also influenced by ancestor-worship and Confucianism. It grew into two main groups, Sect Shinto and State Shinto, the latter promoting patriotism to the Emperor who was thought to be descended from the Sun Goddess. The Emperor Hirohito denied his divinity in 1947. Any particular wishes of the patient and family should be sought.

## Confucianism

Confucianism is one of the principal religions of China. It was founded by Confucius and is concerned with the development of a sense of responsibility towards one another. There are specific duties and responsibilities in five areas, between ruler and subject; father and son; husband and wife; elder and younger brother; and friend and friend. They also believe in some part of the individual surviving after death. Again, any particular wishes of the patient and his or her family should be sought.

It should be realized that followers of these non-Christian religions originate from countries where family ties are close, and this tendency continues if migration to another country such as the UK occurs. It is thus understandable that a number of relatives may congregate together around the dying patient's bed and that outward signs of grief will be manifested to an extent that may be disturbing to other patients in a hospital ward. In this situation, the nurse should be ready to escort the relatives to a suitable room after the death has taken place so that they may support each other and give vent to their grief in private. Because of the close-knit family circle there is usually considerable support during bereavement from within the family and close friends of the deceased.

The nurse may meet patients from many other religious faiths than those mentioned. It is helpful if clear guidelines are available in patient areas regarding telephone numbers of religious centres where appropriate ministers can be contacted, and if some notes are drawn up for nurses with details of any religious practices that are important to patients when they are gravely ill.

# REFERENCES

Akram, M. (1984) *Religions and Cultures*, Lothian Community Relations Council, Edinburgh.

Black, J. (1987) How to do it. Broaden your mind about death and bereavement in certain ethnic groups in Britain, *British Medical Journal*, Vol. 295, No. 6,597, August, pp. 536–9.

Boag, I. (1980) Disposal of the dead, English translation of four lectures given at the Eleventh Congress of Thanatology, Paris, 12 January, *Bulletin de la Societé de Thanatologie*, No. 46, 'Funeral and mourning customs according to different religious rites', Paris.

Joseph, B. and Levenstein, M. (1980) *Jewish and Muslim Teaching Concerning Death*, St Joseph's Hospice occasional paper, London.
McGilloway, O. and Myco, F. (eds) (1985) *Nursing and Spiritual Care*, Harper & Row, London.
Neuberger, J. (1987). *Caring for Dying People of Different Faiths*, Lisa Sainsbury Foundation series, Austen Cornish, London.
Walker, C. (1982) Attitudes to death and bereavement among cultural minority groups, *Nursing Times*, 15 December, pp. 2,106–9.

## Additional reading

Ainsworth-Smith, I. and Speek, P. (1982) *Letting Go – Caring for the Dying and Bereaved*, SPCK, London.
Hector, W. and Whitfield, S. (1982) *Nursing Care for the Dying Patient and the Family*, Heinemann Medical, London.
Huilton, J. (1972) *Dying*, Pelican, Harmondsworth.
Lancerton, R. (1981) *Care of the Dying*, Pelican, Harmondsworth.
Sampson, C. (1982) *The Neglected Ethic*, McGraw-Hill, Maidenhead.
Zaechner, R. C. (1971) *The Concise Encyclopedia of Living Faiths*, Hutchison, London, 2nd edn.

# 14. Ethical Aspects

Ethics is the scientific and philosophical study that seeks to determine and to provide guidance towards goodness in human actions. Ethical principles are meant to provide a basis for everyday practice and all professions establish their own ethical codes for their members to follow.

Involvement with death and dying poses many ethical problems and dilemmas. Life itself is a person's most valuable possession, and the duty to preserve human life is upheld in the ethical codes of both the nursing and medical professions. Difficulties can arise in the interpretation of principles and their application to the actual situation when the doctor or nurse often has to make decisions in a short space of time. Sometimes two professional people will come to different conclusions about an ethical dilemma even though both have given serious and sincere thought to the problem. Cultural and religious factors can influence a person deeply in coming to a decision.

The ethics of medicine are as old as the profession itself, going back to the Hippocratic tradition. Nursing, although a younger profession, can point to a number of ethical codes emanating from both the International Council of Nurses and the Royal College of Nursing. Naturally, nursing and medical ethics are closely linked, although both professions will face distinctive problems because of the different roles and responsibilities. Because of the rapid developments in medical science, more and more crucial issues are being highlighted and publicized needing urgent consideration by all health professionals as well as society at large.

Decisions that have to be made of an ethical nature are still influenced by the respect for freedom of choice due to each human being that is the basis of Western religious and philosophical ethical tradition. Where patients are not competent to make choices, those caring for them, primarily their families, must decide the following:

(1) What is in the best interests of these individuals?
(2) What would the individuals choose for themselves if they were able to do so?
(3) What, as far as the carers can judge, is the right moral choice?

# SOME ETHICAL DILEMMAS ASSOCIATED WITH DEATH AND DYING

## The patients' rights

In endeavouring to act in the best interests of patients, the caring team must be careful to include their views as far as possible. The patients' rights have also to be balanced with those of others. For instance, a patient may wish to die at home but despite all the help that could be arranged it would create an overwhelming problem for the family. In this case it would not be right to press the issue even though it means over-riding the patient's wishes. Patients have a right to know about their illness and prognosis insofar as they wish to do so. From the right to know follows a further right – to refuse active treatment. In the dying patient with advancing cancer this could arise in relation to an option of further radiotherapy being given. Occasionally a patient may refuse to take drugs being given for symptom control. These rights must be respected by the care-givers, having ensured that the patients have had the situation fully discussed with them and that they understand any consequences likely to follow their refusal. If a patient is not lucid, then such decisions must be made for him or her.

## Use of powerful opiate or sedative drugs

The principle of relieving pain and distress in the dying patient is honourable and humanitarian, and administration of drugs where a proper regime is used should be uncontroversial (see Chapter 6). An anxiety is sometimes expressed that a nurse does not wish to be the one to give 'the last injection', implying that it is this which will kill the patient. This is erroneous; the patient having pain-control management, as described in Chapter 6, dies of the disease, not from the drugs.

The opposite situation may occur where the nurse considers that a patient is receiving inadequate analgesia and is in pain, but the doctor appears to be reluctant to alter the medication. Consulting with an experienced nursing colleague and then both discussing the matter with the doctor are the appropriate steps to take to resolve the problem.

## Maintenance of fluid and nutrition in dying patients

This is not only a practical but an emotive issue. Next to the need for oxygen, the needs for water and then food are universally recognized as the fundamental drives to maintain life. If during the terminal illness a person is unable to eat or drink normally, decisions must be taken by the carers as to the proper course of action. Those most involved hitherto will have been nurses and the patient's family, particularly if the patient is at home. Once normal intake becomes impossible, the management of the situation involves others to a greater extent, especially the doctor and dietitian.

There is no single answer to the problem, each person must be assessed individually and their entire circumstances taken into account. This is again a situation in which the patient should be included in the decision-making, if possible. One of the following options will be available:

(1) If the patient is considered to be deteriorating rapidly, becoming semiconscious and likely to die within about 24 hours, no artificial feeding will be instituted but the patient's mouth will be kept moist, with frequent care.
(2) A problem may arise when it is judged that patients, although in the terminal stage of their illness, have still several weeks to live. An example is the patient with advanced carcinoma of oesophagus, who is now having difficulty even with swallowing liquids. It might be considered right to attempt to pass a fine-bore nasogastric tube and institute tube feeding, or to commence an intravenous infusion of a suitable fluid. However, the patient and the team together may decide that he or she should not have this artificial treatment as this would only be an additional burden in the process of dying. Every means would be taken to ensure the patient's comfort and tranquillity, including medication and constant mouth care.

(3) A patient may be admitted for terminal care to hospital or hospice, or transferred home from hospital, with some means of artificial feeding already in place. This might include a gastrostomy. Unless there is some problem actually being caused by the feeding apparatus itself, the decision is likely to be that the feeding should continue until circumstances change.

(4) There has been much publicity recently about attitudes towards newborn handicapped infants. Debate centres on how the rights of such children to proper care, including ordinary provision of fluid and nutrition, should be met within the particular circumstances. Such decisions involve the parents, and doctors and nurses who have accepted responsibility for doing their best in the interests of the patient and the family. Nurses cannot opt out in such decision-making, particularly as the patients are unable to speak for themselves. One of the basic principles of nursing care is to help the patient with eating and drinking. The same ethical principles should be applied to care of the infant human being as to adults, whether the child is handicapped or not. If this is not so, the question must be asked whether a mental or physical handicap renders a person subhuman. If the newborn infant is dying, any decision regarding whether or not some means of artificial feeding should be attempted must, as in the case of adults, be taken in the light of all the prevailing circumstances.

G. R. Dunstan (1981) considers that, although nurses and doctors are not under a duty to take extraordinary means to prolong the life of the grossly handicapped newborn child, there is a duty of care discharged by ordinary medical and nursing intervention.

## Euthanasia

This Greek word literally means 'a good death'. It is the modern interpretation (popularly known as 'mercy killing') that has given rise to frequent and continuing debate, at least since 1936 with the founding of the Euthanasia Society. The name was changed in 1969 to the Voluntary Euthanasia Society and is now known as EXIT. The main way in which those subscribing to the right of a person to request euthanasia propose to operate is by the administration of a lethal dose of a drug deliberately and specifically to accelerate death in order to terminate suffering. There is a tendency to use the term 'passive euthanasia' to describe the situation where it is no longer considered helpful to continue with active medical treatment appropriate to an acute illness, but to keep the patient comfortable including the use of pain-relieving drugs. Twycross (1984) thought that the two situations were not comparable. On the other hand, Rachels (1986) maintains that there is no real moral difference between killing and letting someone die. Likewise, he does not consider that traditional distinctions between ordinary and extraordinary means of preserving life are important.

In the UK, attempts have been made in 1936, 1969 and 1976 to have a bill passed in Parliament to legalize euthanasia. All these attempts failed. In 1986 the British Medical Association set up a working party to consider the matter. In the UK the majority of doctors and nurses oppose euthanasia although there is a small but increasing pressure-group in society at large who uphold the concept in certain circumstances. In Holland there is now open practice and support of voluntary euthanasia by some doctors, although it is still illegal. Hanratty (1985) warns that once a principle is abandoned ethical support for it is rapidly eroded; a permissive Act of Parliament, even if hedged around with considerable restrictions, may eventually become the norm and almost mandatory as in the case of the Abortion Act 1967.

In the event the BMA working party published its report in May 1988 and made a clear recommendation to maintain the present law forbidding euthanasia. The final conclusion reads:

> The law should not be changed and the deliberate taking of a human life should remain a crime. This rejection of a change in the law to permit doctors to intervene to end a person's life is not just a subordination of individual well-being to social policy. It is, instead, an affirmation of the supreme value of the individual, no matter how worthless and hopeless that individual may feel.
>
> (Beecham, 1988, pp. 1,408–9)

Those who oppose euthanasia will have been relieved at the outcome of the report, but would do well to ponder on the words of Hinton (1972, p. 148), which are still timely: 'It seems a terrible indictment that the main argument for euthanasia is that many suffer unduly because there is a lack of preparation and provision for the total care of the dying'. Although there have been many improvements since 1972, there is still room for more to be done, and for other groups for whom euthanasia is advocated as a solution to their sufferings.

## Resuscitation and use of life-support systems

In a general hospital it may be a student nurse who initiates resuscitation in a patient who suddenly suffers a cardiac arrest. Clear guidance is essential in the ward as to when this procedure should be carried out, and for which patients it is inappropriate. The staff should understand why particular decisions are made. Good communications will remove uncertainty and worry that the 'wrong' action has been taken – or not. Nurses will be very involved in the care of a patient whose vital functions are being maintained by a life-support system. If it is thought to be no longer reasonable to continue ventilation of the patient because brain-stem death has been confirmed, the medical staff in charge should discuss the matter with the family and with the whole caring team before the machine is switched off. This is a traumatic situation for all concerned and it should be made clear that this is not a case of killing the patient, because he or she is already dead.

# RESPONSIBILITIES AND RIGHTS OF THE NURSE

If nurses are asked to carry out or participate in some treatment that they are convinced is unethical, they have the right to refuse to do so. It is important that such a step is only taken when the nurses are sure that they have full and accurate knowledge and understanding of the situation, and that by withdrawing they do not harm the patient in another way. An example would be where a nurse is working in an operating theatre and suddenly refuses on ethical grounds to assist the surgeon who is performing an abortion. If the patient bleeds severely the nurse would be held gravely at fault if he or she did not remain during this crisis and give assistance. The law provides a disassociation clause for non-participation in abortions and the nurse should have made his or her position clear to the theatre superintendent well in advance.

The ethical dimensions of modern medicine pose many difficult problems for the nurse, and the challenge must be met by becoming as well informed as possible regarding the principles involved. In coming to the right decisions, experience, intelligent reasoning and desire to uphold the patient's interests all contribute. In disagreeing with others one should respect the individual for views sincerely held, and be aware of the personal anguish that ethical problems can bring to those involved. Some nurses may have the opportunity to make use of the facilities offered by the Society for the Study of Medical Ethics. This society is an independent, non-partisan body that promotes the multi-disciplinary study of issues raised by the practice of medicine, nursing and other health-care professions. It publishes quarterly the *Journal of Medical Ethics* and sponsors groups in many British cities through university teaching-hospitals and medical schools. It includes in its study programmes many issues concerning death and dying.

## REFERENCES AND FURTHER READING

Beecham, L. (1988) Report on BMA Council debate: the Euthanasia Report, *British Medical Journal*, May, Vol. 296, pp. 1,408–9.

Darbyshire, P. (1987) Whose decision? Euthanasia, *Nursing Times*, 11 November, Vol. 83, No. 45, pp. 27–9.

Dunstan, G. R. (1981) Abortion – general ethical considerations, *Dictionary of Medical Ethics*, Darton, Longman & Todd, London.

Hanratty, J. (1985) *Implications of Legalised Euthanasia*, St Joseph's Hospice publication, London.

Hector, W. and Whitfield, S. (1982) *Nursing Care for the Dying Patient and the Family*, Heinneman Medical, London.

Henderson, V. (1969) *Basic Principles of Nursing Care*, International Council of Nurses, Geneva.

Hinton, J. (1972) *Dying*, Pelican, Harmondsworth.

Lamerton, R. (1980) *Care of the Dying*, Pelican, Harmondsworth.

Linacre Centre (1982) *Euthanasia and Clinical Practice – Trends, Principles and Alternatives*, Linacre Centre, London.

Rachels, J. (1986) *The End of Life: Euthanasia and Morality*, Oxford University Press.

Sampson, C. (1982) *The Neglected Ethic – Religious and Cultural Factors in the Care of Patients*, McGraw-Hill, Maidenhead.

Smith, D. (ed.) (1984) *Respect and Care in Medical Ethics*, University Press of America, Eurospan, London.

Twycross, R. G. (1984) *A Time To Die*, Christian Medical Fellowship Publication, London.

United Kingdom Central Council (1983) *Code of Professional Conduct for Nurses, Midwives and Health Visitors* (based on ethical concepts), London.

Whitfield, S. (1987) Going gently into that good night, *Nursing Times*, Vol. 83, No. 45, p. 30.

# 15. The Place of Creative and Diversional Activities

In the considerable efforts being made to achieve a near-ideal situation in caring for the dying patient, symptom control in all its aspects has understandably been a prior consideration. Allowing the patient to die in the environment of choice is not always possible but excellence of care and peace of mind for the individual and the family may compensate if, for instance, the patient would prefer to die at home but circumstances make residential care essential.

An aspect of care that is now receiving increasing attention is the need of the dying person to maintain a sense of self-esteem and meaning to their life once they are symptom free or nearly so. Using the limited time of life that is left in a fulfilling and creative way can balance the helplessness and loss of purpose induced by having so much 'done' for them. The phrase 'living to the end' is a familiar one in this context and needs careful assessment by the caring team if it is to have real meaning and relevance to the dying person's individual situation.

## CHOOSING THE APPROPRIATE ACTIVITY

The first consideration is what the patients themselves wish to do in order to occupy their day. We must be careful not to try to force the pace or infringe on the patients' rights to decide. Some may be apathetic and indeed feeling too weak to make any effort on their own part for most creative activities. However, with a little gentle encouragement there is a variety of ways in which a sense of pleasure and fulfilment may be gained without painful exertion.

Those individuals who have led an actively creative life may be able to continue a lively interest in their chosen activities almost to the end, and are a source of inspiration to others. On the other hand, many dying people have had little space for recreation in their lives, apart from television. Even these individuals may find a new pleasure in a creative pursuit if the right one can be found, and in the right presentation.

Physical handicaps, increasing weakness and perhaps total bedfastness are, of course, factors that will influence what is possible or welcome. The views of family and friends will be valuable in recalling what hobbies and interests have provided stimulation and pleasure in the past. The patient's age will also be an important factor in almost every creative activity.

## USE OF A DAY CENTRE

Increasingly, health districts are planning a terminal-care service as part of the overall provisions for the community they serve. This usually includes a day centre where patients may be brought from home, or as part of a residential unit for dying patients. Independent hospices also have seen day care as an important adjunct to residential- and home-care services.

The centre will not only aim to provide material equipment for creative and diversional activity, but also such services as hair-dressing, baths and a medical treatment centre for those patients coming from home. Community nurses find it valuable to be able to come in and keep in touch with their patients who may be at a stage of their illness where frequent nursing visits are not yet needed at home.

Where the day centre is attached to a residential hospice or continuing-care unit of a hospital, it is a vital link in bringing activity to the patient who finds it difficult to leave his or her bedside. Volunteers can provide a much-appreciated service in the day centre itself, and in the link with patients who cannot or do not wish to come to the centre.

The serving of tea and other refreshments in attractive china and at a leisurely pace is, in itself, a pleasurable activity – this accompanied by some cheerful conversation is sufficient to provide a welcome break from home or ward and to make the visit to the centre a worthwhile exercise for many patients.

# COMMON TYPES OF ACTIVITY

The following examples suggest areas of activity that can be offered to patients whatever their environment, with suitable modifications. It must be stressed, however, that the dying patient may only be able to tolerate short periods of any activity, however pleasurable.

## Music

Few people are completely immune from appreciation of some sort of music—and for many dying people music provides a deep satisfaction and emotional solace (excluding loud and jarring sounds). Actual participation in playing a musical instrument, or singing, is valuable, but for many their pleasure will take the form of listening. This may be to a chosen cassette or a personal stereo or radio, by attending a short concert or the moving experience of having a professional musician softly playing a violin or harp by the bedside of a patient dying in a hospice.

Music is a powerful evoker of memories and may bring tears when a favourite melody or song recalls some joyful or sad occasion from the past. This in itself can be a relief to the patient in opening up an opportunity to talk through some of the pains and joys of his or her life with a sympathetic listener. In a different context one recalls a gallant Irish lady slowly dying at home from the deteriorating effects of many years with Huntington's chorea, hardly able to articulate the words but greatly enjoying singing the rebel songs of her youth in her native country, with her elderly parish priest.

Several professional organizations, such as the Council for Music in Hospitals and the Guildhall School of Music are providing valuable help in bringing music to dying patients, and as a by-product this is enabling many young music students as well as mature musicians to learn much from this close encounter with the realities of the ending of life.

## Gardening

This can be interpreted widely as anything involving flowers or growing plants. A day centre or hospice will often have a garden that in fine weather gives real pleasure for patients just to sit and enjoy the sunshine, fresh air and birds. For those able to do so, raised flower-beds and a small greenhouse offer opportunities for those who have been keen gardeners to continue with some activity. At home, comfortable garden chairs, foot-rests and pillows will enable patients who wish to do so to spend some of their precious hours in their gardens, if they have one. Even the flat-dweller can derive pleasure from vases of flowers and plants. Again, this is not necessarily every dying person's personal pleasure, but as one man said, 'I never realized how beautiful the blue sky was until now when I know that I shan't see it for much longer'.

## Books

Even those who have been avid readers may find that they can only read for short periods without getting tired. Being read to can be soothing and enthralling if the reader has a good quality of voice. Taped books are widely available, and usually recorded by fine actors and actresses who have volunteered their services. A lifelong love of books may continue in practical ways. A classics master dying in his prime at home painlessly but uncomfortably from carcinoma of the liver, was daily absorbed for short periods in the last weeks of his life in re-classifying the sixth-form library of Greek authors. He had decided to undertake the task at this stage, and every day two of his pupils came to help him of their own volition. He thus, so to speak, died in harness.

## Other creative activities

Painting, drawing and sculpture are other art forms that may be ideal for some patients, given the appropriate facilities and someone with the ability to help and encourage. The degree of talent shown by the patient is immaterial; the extent to which the creation of a piece of work enriches and satisfies the creator is what matters. Needlework and knitting may be the hobby of a lifetime for a woman and can be carried out anywhere, bedfast or not. There are some exciting developments in bringing ballet and opera into the lives of dying people in hospices and hospitals.

## Diversional activities

Many patients enjoy activities that may not merit the term creative, although one should not draw too arbitrary a line. Card games are the breath of life to many people and also give companionship. Reading a newspaper and attempting the crossword puzzle may continue as a source of enjoyment to the last days of life. Watching a favourite television programme or video film also has its place. Those patients who have enjoyed a regular or occasional alcoholic drink should continue to be indulged. Indeed, the 'drinks round' or gathering at the bar is part of the encouraged pattern in the life of some hospices, not least of the benefits being the sense of continuing to share in a community social life.

## Visitors

The nurse has a special role in ensuring that visiting of the dying patient is a mutually supportive time for both patients, and relatives and friends. Frequent short visits by the immediate families will have priority, and visits by friends may have to be on a selective basis as patients and families wish. People often feel awkward and strained in trying to make their visit helpful to their loved one, and benefit from guidance that if the patient tires easily it is not necessary to talk much, just sitting and holding his or her hand in peaceful silence for much of the time is appropriate.

Short visits by children or grandchildren can give great pleasure and are helpful for both patient and children. Obviously, noisy boisterous behaviour would be tiring, and in a residential setting there should be some provision for children to be able to play away from the bedside.

A dying patient in a hospice or hospital may suddenly express a longing to visit his or her home again, realizing perhaps that this will be for the last time. Every effort should be made to meet this request even though it may be considered rather a hazardous undertaking.

## Pets

A pet animal is often the mainstay of the family unit, being a friend, companion and comforter. It has been observed that the presence of a pet reduces stress and depression, particularly in the lonely and elderly person. If a person is dying at home, there need be no break in the relationship as long as there is someone able to take on the supervision and care of the pet if this was previously provided by the dying person.

Hospices and other institutions are beginning to recognize the deprivation that will be suffered by the sudden separation of the dying patient from his or her pet – perhaps the sole companion. Dogs are a particular case in point, and it should be possible to allow the contact to be resumed in a suitable way. In a ward setting, not only the patients but their fellow-patients will gain much pleasure from these canine visits.

## A SPECIAL TYPE OF CREATIVE ACTIVITY

There is a special type of creative activity that is of fairly recent development and assuming increasing importance in the care of dying patients and their families.

### Poetry writing

When disability and illness render one unable to perform familiar tasks, or inhibit long-term planning, people often see themselves as useless and 'being done unto'. Often the time is there to reflect and create, but it is more often used to worry and to fret.

From comments made and poems written, it would seem that poetry is particularly useful as a catalyst where communication is difficult and the language of everyday conversation has proved inadequate. A poem can be a bridge between the writer and the audience, whether public or private; it may form a memorial so that a 'mark' remains after death; it may speak of love for the first time in many years and thoughts and fears that are felt to be too remote or personal may be addressed. Sometimes a poem may bring comfort to others in similar circumstances by lessening the sense of isolation.

*Being cared for*

Little, in my despair,
I wait and hear
that I will die.

It is a shock, a trauma
from which you don't recover.
Nothing is ever quite the same again.

But in my homelessness
I find a place to rest,
and also find that I am lovable.

By encouraging people to communicate new perceptions, the understanding of others can sometimes by changed; and those being cared for, who are usually perceived as fulfilling a passive role, can be seen as educators.

*The official*

He just stared,
one of those stares
that deaden all feelings
that others have warmed.

I spoke, he wrote.
Never a 'Good morning'
or a 'how-do-you-do'.
If only he could have smiled . . .

just once.

Beginning to write poetry can simply be fun; a game with words; a playing with rhyme and rhythm as with doggerel and the limerick or the simple building of word pictures. If several people can be concerned in the initial writing, much of the anxiety of attempting something new is removed.

Whilst interest in writing poetry is limited to comparatively few, the effects of the poems can be quite far reaching. For, although some poems are poetically inept – interesting and precious only to those who knew and cherished the writer – others are sufficiently mature to enrich both society and literature were they to be made public. However, for both ethical and legal reasons, nothing should be published or used without the expressed permission of the author or their next-of-kin.

## HELPING BEREAVED PEOPLE IN A CREATIVE WAY

Throughout this book emphasis has been placed not only on the care of the dying patient but also of the relatives so that, when death occurs, they feel helped and supported. All that has happened to the family from the moment of the initial diagnosis will affect the grieving process after death. Grief is a very individual process and everyone reacts differently. At one hospice a leaflet is given to every relative explaining some aspects of grief such as seeing or hearing the loved one, experiencing despair and depression or even developing physical symptoms. As well as feelings of sadness there may be self-criticism, guilt and anger (even with the loved one). This explanation often helps to reassure people that it is normal to experience these feelings.

## The help available from other people

The family, good friends and neighbours are needed to give support through what may be a long period. The whole of the first year after bereavement is fraught with anniversaries of one kind or another and the way ahead is not a straightforward upward progression. Sometimes bereavement counselling may be needed for those lacking a supportive family or friends, or for those who get 'stuck in the tasks of mourning' (Warden J. William, 1983, p. 11). The bereaved person may then turn to a specialized counselling service, such as CRUSE, or if there is an association with a hospice such a service may be offered from there. Perhaps the most important part of this service is the willingness of the counsellors to give time to *listen*, to collect and to 'earth', rather like a lightning conductor, emotions of anger and guilt, and providing some relief.

## The use of the written word

Even with regular help from a counsellor, the bereaved person may experience waves of depression between visits. For those who find this unbearable and have the ability to write, putting their feelings on to paper may give enormous relief. This may take the form of verse, prose or disconnected sentences, to be shared with others – because it has been 'shed'—or kept hidden because it is still too painfully private. A few have the ability to record their thoughts and feelings for publication in the hope that others may be helped. To read *A Grief Observed* by C. S. Lewis (1961) Faber, London, may open the floodgates for those who are dry-eyed, and bring blessed relief, but it is important to find the right book to help each individual. The following are offered as a starting point: Grollman, Earl A. (1977) *Living – When a Loved One has Died*, Beacon Press, Boston, Mas.; Mannery, Doug (1984) *Don't Take my Grief Away*, Harper & Row, New York;

and Green, Wendy (1985) *The Long Road Home*, A Lion Paperback, Tring.

## REFERENCES AND FURTHER READING

### General

Frampton, D. (1986) Restoring creativity to the dying patient, *British Medical Journal*, 20 December, Vol. 293, pp. 1,593–5.
Hospice Care Service for East Hertfordshire (charity no. 288512) (1986) Our day Hospice in operation, *Newsletter*, November, p. 1, Welwyn Garden City.

### Pets

Lord, R. (1986) Paws for thought, *Journal of District Nursing*, Vol. 4, No. 7, Jan., pp. 4–5.

### Poetry

Eisenhauer, J. (1987) Is anyone out there listening? *Ageways*, HelpAge International, 14 September, pp. 23–4.
Eisenhauer, J. (1987) I'd like to write a poem but . . . , *Ageways*, HelpAge International, 15 December, pp. 25–6.
Eisenhauer, J. (1987) *Poetry within Hospice*, St Joseph's Hospice publication, London.
Moss, L. (1987) *Art for Health's Sake*, Carnegie United Kingdom Trust, Dunfermline.

### Bereavement

Worden, J. W. (1983) *Grief Counselling and Grief Therapy*, Tavistock, London.

# 16. Care in the Home

The industrialized, affluent parts of the world have, until comparatively recently, seen a gradual move towards death occurring in a hospital or other institution rather than dying people remaining in their own homes. In the UK about 68 per cent of all deaths occur in institutions, the majority being general hospitals (Spilling, 1986).

There are several reasons for this. Families are smaller than previously so that greater strain is placed on the carers. The unmarried members of the family often do not stay under the same roof but move off to a separate existence elsewhere. Many mothers now go out to work so that a dying relative would be alone much of the day anyway. Today there is much more population movement than hitherto, so that families often live in different towns or parts of the country, and may even have emigrated.

Another possible reason for people not dying at home is fear in the care givers. Over the last half century, because of dramatic reductions in likelihood of death in infancy, childhood and young adulthood, many people reach middle age and have still never seen anyone dead or dying – especially as there has not been a major war for nearly forty years. Thus, when presented with a dying person, many families will panic, feel inadequate and urge admission for their loved one.

## ADVANTAGES OF HOME CARE

What of that loved one – where does he or she want to die? Given the opportunity, most people would like to die in their own home and in their own bed. One of the most traumatic experiences in life must be to have an ambulance drawing up at the door to take a very ill person to hospital. For that individual knows – even if they haven't verbalized it – that they are seeing their home of perhaps forty years or more for the last time. The garden, so lovingly tended and the tomato plants about to flower, will not be seen again. The dog who leapt on the bed every morning to waken its master or mistress will not be seen again, as animals are not usually allowed into hospitals. Finally, the bed warmly shared with a spouse for the past forty years will never be experienced again either. So much to lose at a time of life when such things could bring the greatest comfort to the dying. So, with a determined nurse and other members of the primary-care team, the aim should be to enable the death to take place at home. Domiciliary hospice teams around the UK and the world have shown that the trend towards dying in an 'institution' is reversible. Many of these teams report 60 to 80 per cent of their patients dying at home.

Thus admission should mainly be for social reasons – for instance, an elderly or infirm spouse, or an elderly patient living alone. Most medical and nursing problems can be resolved in the home – apart from a few occasions when a patient or family finds it difficult to co-operate for whatever reason. There are many differences between caring for a dying patient at home and doing so in hospital. Noticeable are the role reversals. The patient and the family are the hosts and the nurse or doctor is the visitor.

In hospital it is usually possible to 'persuade' patients to do things they don't like, for instance, taking multifarious pleasant or unpleasant medications and treatments. At home, patients are the rulers of their domain, not frightened people in bed with labels on their wrists to distinguish them from their neighbours. They can show the nurse the door if they do not like his or her approach or what he or she is offering.

Another difference is that in a hospital setting, although relatives are treated with polite courtesy, they might be regarded as a bit of a nuisance – they clutter up and untidy the ward, they often want to be talked with and ask awkward questions, and they are always bringing flowers that have to be put in water and that get knocked over when the curtains are pulled round the bed!

At home the patient and family are considered to be one unit requiring care. Many times the relatives need as much, if not more, help than the patient.

## Assessment

With practice this should become continuous and almost subconscious. It begins before meeting the patient. What sort of area is the home in? Does the outside look cared for or neglected? What do the curtains at the windows look like: ragged and dirty or immaculate – or somewhere in between? What sounds are there before the door opens – arguing and raised voices, dogs and screaming children, or nothing? Consider the state of the person opening the door – do the eyes look away, look anxious or frightened or weary, or bright and happy and welcoming? Is the home well cared for and well loved, or is it a cold, sad, lonely home? Is the neglect long term or due to the illness of the patient? Note the arrangement of furniture – chairs in isolated positions may indicate the nature of the occupants.

The emotional state of the people in the home needs assessing: for example, is the spouse defensive or nervous or over-protective? The patient's manner of greeting and subsequent conversation should reveal whether he or she is angry, anxious, depressed, terrified, happy, dull, unintelligent, unkempt, in pain, restless, agitated or confused.

Conversation with the patient and family and examination of the patient should also reveal all that is relevant in relation to nausea, vomiting, pain, bowels, bladder, mouth, sleep, cough, pressure areas, mobility, oedema, dyspnoea, wounds, discharges, bleeding and appetite.

All of these aspects should be assessed by the nurse (and the general practitioner will make his or her own assessment). The findings need to be accurately recorded. Nursing notes in the patient's home should, however, contain only information that would not alarm or upset the patient or family if read by them. Such matters as the degree of acceptance or denial of the diagnosis would have to be recorded at the health centre or wherever the more formal notes are stored. The patient's insight should be assessed but without probing too deeply. Asking patients what they had radiotherapy for will often give a pointer to their degree of insight. On a first meeting, that is probably as far as the questioning should go in relation to diagnosis and prognosis – unless the patient is obviously wanting to discuss these matters further. At the first meeting it is also useful to enquire discreetly about the patient's religious faith, and how meaningful it is to him or her. The nurse will then have an idea as to whether or how the clergy should be involved later on. Throughout the patient's illness, communication is a vital aspect of care. This has been developed in Chapter 2.

## CARE OF THE FAMILY

The degree of effective help and support given to the family can make the difference between their coping or not coping. If they cannot cope, then the patient will usually have to leave home and be admitted to hospital. This may mean that a spouse will feel guilty and the subsequent bereavement will perhaps be more painful. The family have the rest of their lives to live after the death, and a distressing death and difficult bereavement period could drastically affect those lives, especially that of the spouse.

In families there is often sibling rivalry, or one child may do most of the caring while the others feel guilty and become even less supportive. Thus, when the patient's needs have been met, the nurse often finds him- or herself having a fifteen-minute 'doorstep chat' or else is spirited into the kitchen. He or she can then start to pick at and unravel some of the knots in the family, and allay some of their fears.

As mentioned earlier, fear of death is often why families do not cope. It is necessary to ascertain the nature of the fears. It can be difficult for a nurse to appreciate the incredible ideas held by the public about death. It is often thought to be explosive at the end, with 'guts' spilling out and 'things' coming from the mouth. There is an idea that cancer creeps up in the throat – especially if the patient has a bronchial carcinoma – and strangles the patient so that he or she will choke. Simple explanations, for example, about the 'death-rattle', and relaxation of sphincters at death, will allay these fears. Another idea is that the patient will die in agony. With inadequate control of pain and other symptoms this can, unfortunately, happen.

Reassure the family that someone will always be available, even if only to answer a question on the telephone. Reassure them that the patient will be given the best possible care and will probably die peacefully in sleep – so peacefully that they may not realize immediately that he or she has died.

Check on the amount of sleep, food and recreation that the main care-giver is having. Often there are many visitors and the spouse spends all day making tea and sandwiches. Offer to answer any questions they have. Reassure them that the patient will not be 'told' anything he or she does not wish to hear. Teach the family whatever nursing techniques they want to do or are capable of doing. It is imperative not to increase their anxiety by asking them to perform tasks such as giving suppositories if such things frighten them. It is important to remember to praise the efforts of the family and to encourage them.

Some spouses will deny the impending death – their bereavement is likely to be difficult. Others will feel guilty about many things. If it relates to the care, the spouse should be reassured that the best nurse possible is the one who has known the patient for forty years and knows exactly how he or she likes their tea made, and that without him or her the patient would have to be in hospital.

Relatives often ask for a prognosis because of taking time off from work. Although very tempting it is usually unwise to predict such matters. Very few babies (unless induced) are born on the expected day and few of us die when expected. A time limit can, in fact, cause more problems and anxiety for the family when death is quicker or slower than anticipated. It would be more useful, with the relative's agreement, to write a note to his or her employers, for example, thanking them for being so helpful and understanding in allowing Mrs X time off to care for her very ill mother!

Another way to make life easier for the relatives is occasionally to deliver some of the medication so they do not have to keep queuing up at the doctor's surgery or the chemist. If the patient is still paying for prescriptions, he or she may be eligible for an exemption on the grounds of 'a continuing physical disability which prevents me leaving home without the help of another person'. The forms can usually be obtained in the doctor's surgery or post office, etc., and once completed by the patient and doctor, and posted to the family practitioner committee, the patient can then obtain free prescriptions. If there is time, allow them to go to the shops while nursing care is being given to the patient. Encouraging the relatives to cope when they feel they cannot is a decision that needs to be skilfully assessed. At the time the family may feel too much has been asked of them, but after death they are usually pleased and delighted to find that they could manage. However, such pressure does require careful evaluation before being applied – some people cannot cope and should not be pushed too far.

## The needs of children

Children in the family need care and often it is necessary to talk about it with the adults first. There is a tendency to hide children away from death in case it has some bad effect on them. The opposite is true. If, when someone has died, people behave as though there is something in the room so awful that a child cannot see it, he or she will grow up believing that death is too terrifying to behold. Children acquire attitudes from adults. It is easy to ask children if they would like to say goodbye to Grandma. They can be taken into the room and asked if they would like to kiss her goodbye. It is important to remember that an explanation of the death in adult terms may be misinterpreted by a child and produce undue anxiety. Obviously each child will have individual needs, and should not be forced into any situation where he or she is uncomfortable.

Children should be included in the grieving and not made to feel outsiders. There is usually no reason why they should not attend the funeral. There may be particular problems for the children when a parent dies. Can the other parent cope? This needs to be anticipated well before the death. The help of a social worker is likely to be necessary.

## CARE OF THE PATIENT

The room or environment is of paramount importance. The situation is often improved if the living-room is used as a bedroom. The advantages are that the patient remains in the circle of the family and is not isolated upstairs. It also saves the care-giver from constantly going up and down stairs to attend to the patient's needs and makes supervision much easier with less anxiety. Such a rearrangement should only be effected if all parties agree. Even if they are not going to move the patient's room it may, with permission, be useful to move some of the furniture in the room to allow easier access to the patient.

The nurse needs to have frequent contact with the family by phone or visit. The aim is to anticipate needs rather than deal with a problem once it has arisen. The latter simply increases the family's anxiety, reducing the likelihood of keeping the patient at home. As the illness progresses new symptoms can and do present fairly frequently. The nurse needs to be aware of them in order to alert the doctor. The general practitioner should be given regular information and he or she can be kept on his or her toes by the nurse, for example, diagnosing oral thrush (very common) and suggesting nystatin drops for it! The number of visits by the nurse should increase as the patient deteriorates.

Medication, if prescribed confusingly at different times, will either be taken randomly or not at all. It is a good idea to request the doctor to prescribe so that drugs can be fitted easily into a 4-, 8- or 12-hourly regime. Writing the medication out clearly will also increase the likelihood of accurate administration.

# Equipment

Equipment for the dying patient needs to be provided sooner rather than later – later is likely to be too late. Ripple mattresses of the large cell or Pulsair type can be very helpful in the prevention of pressure sores. If obtainable, a Spenco or Roho mattress can also be excellent. Bed cradle, bed, commode, urinal, feeding cup, bedpan, incontinence pad and sheeting, Zimmer frame and wheelchair may be needed and are usually available through local authorities, or Red Cross organization.

Remember that in a patient's home there is no hospital linen-cupboard with an inexhaustible supply – only a tired family frantically borrowing from neighbours. Therefore, incontinence needs to be anticipated so that a mattress is not ruined. An ideal draw mackintosh is made by cutting a black polythene-bag (which most homes now have) down one long side and across the bottom. This can be put under the bottom sheet or draw sheet. Draw sheets can be manufactured by dissecting an old sheet. Families will often urge the nurse to cut up their best linen – this should be resisted!

When a patient is dying, much of the management of the urinary tract can be initiated and carried out by the nurse (with prior agreement of the doctor). Thus, if a semiconscious patient is incontinent or has an obvious retention with overflow, the natural thing will be to catheterize the patient without having to waste the precious time and comfort of the patient by obtaining equipment or trying to contact the doctor who may be out on his or her rounds. Condom drainage for male patients may be helpful if there is no retention.

Similarly, management of the bowel should be readily available. To have to wait another day or so in order to obtain suppositories simply prolongs the patient's discomfort while constipation turns into a faecal impaction. Should there be circumstances where a nurse could not catheterize or give immediate bowel care to a dying patient, then a plan should be made before the need arises. For example, a patient with carcinoma of the bladder may need to be hospitalized if a catheter is required, in case of acute haemorrhage.

The provision of equipment such as a commode may need tact and understanding. It is hard to recognize that the body one has taken for granted for so many years now no longer works properly. Patients may need to find out for themselves that they are unable to get to the toilet, before accepting a commode or urinal.

When patients are dying at home, the week or so before unconsciousness develops can be difficult for them and their families. Patients get cross at their weakness and inability, and may displace their anger on to their families. This may increase their anguish. However, as patients lose consciousness and begin to let go, the families' anxieties may become easier. This may also be because the nursing visits will have increased. A wife may be able to wash her conscious husband, but once he is unable to move himself the sensitive skill of a nurse may be needed to make the patient refreshed and comfortable. The frequency of 'turning' a patient at home may depend on how much the family can do, or the amount of domiciliary nursing available. The patient will need to be turned even in his or her own soft bed not less than 8-hourly. Relatives can be taught how to use foamstick applicators for cleaning the mouth, and also how to give sips of water or medicine from them. A male patient, by this time, does not care if, for example, he is not shaved, but the family's morale is lifted if his appearance is as normal as possible. A battery-operated razor is a useful piece of equipment in the nurse's bag.

An unconscious patient's medication needs to continue. Usually an 8-hourly regime can be organized in the home. Oxycodone suppositories (available only from Boots the Chemist) are usually preferable to injections. One oxycodone suppository is equivalent to approximately 30 mg morphine by mouth. The advantages are as follows:

(1) It is effective for 6–8 hours.
(2) It causes less discomfort for the patient.
(3) A relative may be able to insert it, thus reducing the number of nursing visits required, and helping them to feel in control of the situation.

If sedation is needed for restless patients, chlorpromazine (Largactil) suppositories 100 mg may be used. Rectal diazepam 10 mg is likewise often very effective. If injecting diamorphine, then methotrimeprazine 25–50 mg (as Nozinan) may be given in the same syringe. (Methotrimeprazine has greater strength and is in less volume than chlorpromazine in equivalent injection.)

Continuous medication is increasingly being given via a subcutaneous needle and syringe driver. Again, various combinations of drugs can be given simultaneously and the syringe renewed daily.

Nurses often sit patients up to prevent chest infections. Many patients dying of carcinomatosis and pneumonia are much more comfortable on their side with pillows giving plenty of support in the back, between neck and shoulder and between the knees. Nothing looks more distressing to a family than a semi-conscious patient lolling around either upright or semi-upright in bed.

## AFTER THE DEATH

After the patient has died and the family have been comforted, the body needs to be attended to. The nurse should be guided by the family, but in most instances it is not appropriate to do the full Last Offices as the funeral director can do these much more professionally. However, it is necessary in a home situation to remove catheters, straighten and tidy the body, insert dentures and support the jaw. The last is very simply done by wedging an appropriate-sized article between the chin and claviculosternal notch. A small perfume bottle or new bar of soap is often just right. The head should be on one or two pillows so that the sheet can be pulled just over the chin. The family can then be escorted in to say goodbye if they so wish. They often appreciate it if the nurse offers to contact the funeral director for them, who will collect the body after a doctor has certified the death. The nurse should ensure that a doctor has seen the patient not less than two weeks before the death in order to avoid unnecessary complications with legal requirements. Thus, for a patient dying at home, anticipation is the key to care. The other aim is maximum effectiveness with minimum fuss!

## LIAISON ROLE OF THE NURSE

Efficient communication with other district nurses is essential, including full and useful notes. 'GNC given' is totally inadequate and is unfortunately seen too frequently. Night nurses staying with the patient for the last few nights can often make the difference between death at home and a moribund patient being transported to hospital. This service may be provided by a nurse funded partly by the local authority and partly by the Marie Curie Memorial Foundation. Some districts will have direct access to Marie Curie nurses, others have a 24-hour nursing service and provide their own night sitters. This latter can have disadvantages. If the district is unduly busy, the night sitter may only spend a very few hours with the patient or there may be more patients requiring a night nurse than the number of nurses available. This leads to uncertainty for the family and increases anxiety. Again, communication between day and night nurses needs to be carefully co-ordinated.

Recreational therapy is vital in the home as much as in hospital. Patients feel frustrated by their weakness and a burden to their family. It is important to encourage a useful activity so that they feel that they are contributing to society. A recreational therapist can usually decide what is appropriate for each patient. 'Live until you die' is a useful expression in these circumstances.

Many patients benefit from visits by the clergy and this should be arranged if required. It is important not to pressurize the patient with religion that may not be welcome. Social workers are an integral part of the team (see Chapter 8). Briefly, they are invaluable for making sense of complicated financial tangles in which some families find themselves. They can produce relatively rapid miracles by bringing forward a telephone installation or discovering a grant of money for a family in debt.

Their principal function before and after death is to unravel some of the psychosocial problems; to anticipate and plan to prevent further distress, for example, where children are about to lose a parent. The social worker's shoulder is often also invaluable for other professionals caring for the patient! The fresh view or insight a social worker can bring to a situation is often very different from that of a nurse or doctor. The intrepid home-help service can also make the difference between a patient coping at home or not. If the patient lives alone the home help may be the main carer.

Physiotherapists can be very helpful for gentle rehabilitation, exercises and massage. Gentle chest physiotherapy and postural drainage may be the treatment of choice for a dying patient with a chest infection. The ingenuity of the physiotherapist is often stretched to produce interesting-looking pieces of equipment out of foam rubber or polystyrene – whatever necessary to improve patient comfort. An occupational therapist may be involved to make minor home adaptations such as improved stair bannisters or bath rails. Complicated expensive and lengthy alterations are usually not appropriate.

The nurse must liaise with the general practitioner, who may have known the patient and family for many years. Sometimes, however, the doctor may believe there is nothing he or she can do and so feels awkward visiting the patient. The nurse may tactfully indicate that the patient would be pleased to see the doctor anyway – and this is indeed so. It may also be necessary for the nurse to apply persistent persuasion if the patient's pain and other symptoms are not adequately controlled. Any hospice would be happy to give telephone advice to a general practitioner, and may be available for domiciliary visiting.

If a patient needs a paracentesis, this can be done very simply by the doctor in the patient's home, using for example, peritoneal dialysis cannula plus receptacle for the drainage. This is done very successfully by some domiciliary hospice teams already. It saves an unnecessary trip to hospital or even admission for the procedure.

Local volunteer agencies may provide extra company to sit with the patient, thereby enabling the spouse to go shopping or to the dentist, or simply to have a break from the house. Meals-on-wheels service may be needed occasionally for patients living alone. The special local laundry service, if available, is not often needed because by the time the patient becomes incontinent he or she usually has only a few days to live. If the patient is admitted to hospital or hospice it is always helpful to send an explanatory note, however brief, with the patient. It is important to provide enough information about the patient's condition to make the transition less traumatic. If a relative is able to accompany the patient this should be encouraged.

## SPECIALIST DOMICILIARY CARE

Increasing expertise within in-patient hospices resulted in some patients returning home, with their pain and other problems under control. To try to preserve the improvement, hospice staff began to visit patients at home, and specialist domiciliary teams emerged. Today the majority of in-patient hospices and hospital support teams will provide a team to visit the patient and his or her family at home. Most will have an interdisciplinary approach – and as well as nurses will comprise doctors, social workers and perhaps clergy and physiotherapists. They often provide a seven-days-a-week service, as well as round-the-clock availability.

Macmillan nursing or nurses were the other main system to develop. This was due to generous financial assistance from the Cancer Relief Macmillan Fund. Thus Cancer Relief provides an initial three-year funding of a nurse or nurses with district training, on the understanding that the National Health Service will undertake subsequent funding. These nurses (around 400 in the British Isles) are based with, and work alongside, the community nurses – the latter continuing to be the primary nurse. Macmillan nurses may share some of the regular nursing care of the patient. It is envisaged that community nurses will acquire some of the specialist knowledge more effectively, by working and 'living' so closely with the Macmillan nurses.

Neither Macmillan nurses nor domiciliary hospice teams seek to 'take over' the patient from the general practitioner or district nurse. The aim is to enable additional knowledge to be available, where appropriate, to enhance the care of the patient as he or she reaches the end of their life.

## REFERENCES AND FURTHER READING

National Association of Health Authorities (1987) *Care of the Dying – A Guide for Health Authorities*, King Edward Hospital Fund for London, London.

Spilling, R. (1986) *Terminal Care at Home*, Oxford University Press.

# 17. Care of the Dying Patient in Hospital: Special Aspects

Why should this type of care be any different from caring for a patient in a hospice? The answer is, of course, that it need not be different but there are important aspects in teaching and changing of attitudes that can make all the difference between a patient dying peacefully and one whose death is disturbed.

This chapter describes, using St Thomas's Hospital Support Team as a model, how staff can be taught to care for dying patients amongst the everyday happenings of a busy ward; how nurses and doctors can come to terms with death and dying and go on to teach others; and how relatives can be encouraged to take on the caring of the patient at home, so long as they are able. Finally, this chapter comments on the needs of dying patients in specialist areas and the staff who care for them.

## TEACHING STAFF TO CARE FOR DYING PATIENTS IN A BUSY WARD

In December 1977, a team – consisting of a consultant and her registrar, both radiotherapists working in their spare time, a full-time sister, a part-time social worker and the hospital chaplain – was formed, to advise nurses and doctors at St Thomas' Hospital in London (Bates *et al.*, 1981; Saunders, 1980) how to control the symptoms of patients suffering from terminal malignant disease.

The hospice movement had been in operation locally for about ten years and a considerable number of nurses, doctors and medical students had visited and been taught at St Christopher's Hospice. Despite this education, it was observed in the hospital and in the community that patients were still suffering pain and other distressing symptoms from their cancers.

Whilst nurses and doctors did care and agreed with the basic principles of keeping their patients symptom free and alert, they found it difficult to put them into practice without careful guidance. Many were apprehensive about the use of strong analgesia. They had seen evidence of the misuse of drugs amongst patients coming to casualty, and had read about it in the press.

These staff needed to be taught how symptoms could be controlled, as well as keeping their patients alert, with the added satisfaction of seeing most patients go home. They needed to understand addiction and whether it would affect these particular patients.

The World Health Organization (1979) defines addiction as

> A state, psychic and sometimes also physical, resulting from the interaction between a living organism and a drug, characterized by behavioural and other responses that always included a compulsion to take the drug on a continuous or periodic basis in order to experience its psychic effects, and sometimes to avoid the discomfort of its absence. Tolerance may or may not be present.

Dying patients require their pain to be controlled and do not require the drugs for their psychic effects. In fact, if pain is stopped by other means, then analgesia can be reduced and sometimes discontinued without ill effect.

Nurses and doctors were interested in knowing how analgesia could be most effectively used. They needed to understand how long drugs lasted, and the importance of titrating drugs to the patients' needs. They also needed to know about the side-effects of these drugs and how they could be avoided. Another important aspect of their education was to know that some drugs were inappropriate for the care of patients with chronic pain of cancer.

As a team, their mode of action is to visit patients, at the request of their consultant, on the day of referral, if possible. It is important to start by discussing the patient with the nurse in charge, and the ward doctor if available, and to read the patient's medical history. Armed with this information the team doctor and sister introduce themselves to the patient. With the patient's permission they sit down and encourage him or her to talk about his or her problems as he or she sees them, to recount the illness and his or her social situation and to ask questions, if the patient so desires. It is important that on this occasion the patient is given time so that a sense of trust begins to be built. At the end of the interview it is explained to the patient what the team are going to suggest to the doctors and nurses, that they are only giving an opinion, not taking over the care and that they, or perhaps just the sister, will return the next day.

The next stage is to write the problems, as the patient sees them, in his or her case-notes and to suggest solutions. A note is also made of the patient's insight into his or her illness.

Discussion with the ward staff is again important. Sometimes suggestions about the nursing care of the patient, tactfully given, are important. For instance, a lemon mouthwash may be more refreshing for somebody who can hardly swallow. Crushed ice-cubes to suck may be easier to manage than a drink. Salt and soda mouthwash is excellent for cleaning a dirty mouth.

Salt and soda mouthwash:

Sodium bicarbonate 2.5 qm
Sodium chloride 2.5 qm
Purified water to 1 l
(2 weeks' expiry time)

The dietitian's help may be sought when eating or drinking is difficult. The loan of an angle pillow, Spenco mattress, heel or elbow pads, may make the patient more comfortable. The question of why temperatures are being taken and fluid balance charts maintained can also be discussed. The assistance of the diversional therapist or librarian could be sought, or an appointment made with the hairdresser.

At the same time it is important for the nurse in charge to know that the team sister, who might be seen as a threat to his or her authority, only wants to help the patient to be free of symptoms and to be given the best quality of life for the time he or she has left. The team sister also wants the nurse to understand that caring for the terminally ill can be satisfying but that it is stressful, and that the team sister is there to give any support or advice if it is needed.

When staff are frantically busy it is appropriate for the team sister to offer practical help for a dying patient: perhaps by sitting and holding the dying patient's hand or by feeding another in a leisurely fashion;

helping to make a bed; taking a prescription to pharmacy; collecting a book from the library; or just sitting and listening or chatting. These small actions may help the patient, but they will also teach the nurses how care is put into practice.

The patient is revisited daily during his or her hospital stay. Following visits need not be so long, but if a patient trusts the team and wants to ask questions, then the visit may be longer. Gradually the team may learn what the patient knows about the illness and what else he or she wants to understand.

The team need to interpret patients' gestures, pick up clues and cues, verbal or non-verbal, and be ready with honest answers in language they can understand, sometimes illustrated by a simple drawing. This information must be written in patients' notes and explained to the nurse in charge, often encouraging him or her to learn how to give further information if questions are asked. By observing a patient whose symptoms are gradually being controlled, nurses and doctors begin to see how they can do this themselves, first with assistance and then alone.

One of the first results of the team's work at St Thomas' Hospital was to alter the attitude of prescribing the old Brompton Cocktail. Previously the implication of prescribing Bromptons implied that no more could be done for the patient. It was prescribed mostly with little imagination and usually had the same ingredients, diamorphine 10 mg, cocaine 5 mg, chlorpromazine 25 mg, alcohol, honey or syrup to 10 ml, irrespective of need. If this mixture did not control pain, injections were given and if they did not keep the patient and nurses quiet, then increasing doses of sedation were added. This was given not because the doctors and nurses did not care, but because they had not been better informed. The team tried to teach nurses and doctors a better way of prescribing a simple morphine mixture in chloroform water, to add an anti-emetic if required, to give it regularly, 4-hourly, and to titrate the strength of the analgesia against the patient's pain. They also taught that there was no virtue in pain, as some might have thought; that the patients had chronic pain, not the type of acute or post-operative pain that staff, particularly on surgical wards, were familiar with.

We also needed to explain that the pain of bony secondaries, apart from the treatment by radiotherapy, was best controlled by the antiprostaglandin-type drug, such as aspirin, indomethacin, ibuprofen, etc., and that this could be given as well as morphine.

Pain in its various types needed to be explained. As well as physical pain, the patient may have social or mental pain. Nurses are in a unique position to ferret out particular problems and to try to solve them, sometimes with the help of the chaplain or social worker.

At a later stage the team began to introduce other analgesic drugs in to their teaching, such as MST Continus (slow-release morphine sulphate). These different drugs caused other teaching problems in that staff needed to have explained the different ways they worked, that a 4-hourly regime was not appropriate; that other regular analgesia could not be used with buprenorphine (as it is a partial opiate antagonist) and it does not seem to be a useful drug for patients with cancer. It is important, however, in hospital to use new drugs and not be complacent about just using the well-tried 'friend'. By using them we may find better ways of making our patients' lives more tolerable.

It is also important for nurses to know that drugs can be given by other routes apart from the mouth. Suppositories are extremely useful if a patient cannot swallow, or is vomiting. Analgesic drugs, such as oxycodone, morphine and diamorphine, and non-steroidal anti-inflammatory drugs, like aspirin and indomethacin come in suppository form, as do some anti-emetics, chlorpromazine, prochlorperazine, cyclizine and domperidone. Another drug that has been produced in this form is diazepam that seems, from the team's experience, to be more effective rectally than by injection. When regular analgesia can only be given by injection, the Greaseby syringe driver is very helpful, delivering a steady subcutaneous infusion over 24 hours (Regnard and Newbury, 1983).

When a dying patient's symptoms are well controlled, nurses do not seem to be so concerned about nursing him or her in a separate room. Some patients prefer to stay in the ward. It is sometimes beneficial for other patients to observe a patient dying peacefully and to know that the nurses are watching him or her carefully and that relatives are encouraged to stay. It is equally good for other patients to be nursed in a single room, particularly when relatives want to stay all the time, and to be involved with the care. This is especially relevant when a patient has been nursed at home but has had to be re-admitted for the last few days of his or her life. To encourage a family to continue to help at this stage can be very beneficial in their bereavement.

Apart from teaching in a practical way, day by day, it is essential to have the opportunity for classroom teaching, because not all nurses work on wards where the team are invited to advise. Classroom teaching was originally given to trained staff so they could understand why the team was involved with only some patients. They were taught how symptoms could be controlled and the importance of the team advising rather than taking over, in order to teach other nurses and doctors to care in the future and to avoid confusion amongst patients.

The next group to be taught were nurses in introductory block. It is important for them to discuss the fact that patients do die – everybody does one day; and that dying is not a failure and, although it is sometimes sad, it does not need to be depressing so long as patients die peacefully, with symptoms well controlled. It is helpful for them to suggest the nursing problems that may be encountered in the care of this group of patients and how they will be able to alleviate them. Often this is the first time these young people have discussed death.

At a later stage nurses are taught about symptoms and how they can be controlled and the team discusses whether in fact this is happening in the hospital. It would be useful if medical students could join nurses during this lecture; they are going to work together in the future and to discuss such an important topic together could be very advantageous.

During their community secondment, students are taught by one of the team's community sisters about the care of patients dying at home. Before they take their state finals they are given some problem-solving exercises involving hospital care and planning for home care. This is an opportunity for revision and for looking ahead to a charge-nurses' role.

It is important that all newly-appointed nurses and doctors learn that a team exists in the hospital, and how they can be contacted and their mode of action. New staff nurses have a two-hour teaching session on 'Communicating bad news'. This takes the form of role play and many examples of difficult situations can be played out with helpful discussion between scenarios.

Teaching also takes place in seminars on the wards. On these occasions particular patients can be discussed; the team talk about problems and whether they were overcome or not. It is an opportunity for nurses to voice their feelings, anger, frustrations, sadness or satisfaction. The team can also discuss other patients who have gone home and who are enjoying a relatively good quality of life, and others who have died peacefully with their families, at home.

Although not every acute general hospital will have introduced a support team to assist staff in the manner described, many ward sisters have found that the practice of allocating nurses to care for individual patients as far as possible, rather than task allocation, does help to ensure positive attitudes towards the needs of the dying patient and the sorting out of priorities, even in a ward with many different competing pressures on the staff. Some nurses find that when the principles of the nursing process are being applied in their ward it is also a help towards providing emotional as well as physical care to a dying patient and the family.

But whichever process is adopted, it remains of paramount importance to ensure that the patient's symptoms are controlled. The sister needs to have knowledge of how this can be achieved, so is able to advise the doctor if the need arises.

## COMING TO TERMS WITH DEATH AND DYING AND TEACHING OTHERS

When symptoms are controlled, nurses feel much more at ease with their patients. When the patient has a symptom that the nurse is powerless to control, the temptation is to ignore the patient, or to spend little time with him or her. Nurses and doctors do not feel unhappy at using strong analgesia if they see patients alert and mobile, with their pain controlled, able to return home and sometimes resume employment.

Staff do not fear dying if they see patients die peacefully, knowing that if an unpleasant symptom does arise there is a team within the hospital whose advice can always be sought. Being honest with patients when they ask questions about the nature of their illnesses and passing this information on to other members of staff, can only make for a more relaxed atmosphere in which to work. If staff are content that patients are really comfortable, they are able to discuss with relatives in a more straightforward way what is going on and why. They are also able to encourage them to continue this caring at home, with help from community staff.

Nurses and doctors who have learnt good terminal care can teach their juniors, by example, in the wards. They can also take this knowledge to other wards, where perhaps these skills are not so widely practised. Finally, when they leave the hospital, they can take this expertise to other hospitals, knowing that if they look after patients with symptoms that are not easily controlled, they can always refer back to the team for further advice.

Some nurses and doctors will still find it difficult to come to terms with dying, and perhaps this is because they cannot contemplate their own deaths, but they may be able to share their feelings individually with a member of the team, which may be a means of support during a period of stress.

## TEACHING RELATIVES HOW TO CONTINUE WITH CARE AT HOME

Relatives will usually only consider taking a patient home to die if most symptoms are controlled. They are often very apprehensive and need to be approached gently. Very few families these days have observed a person dying, except dramatically or violently on television. They, therefore, have no reason to think dying will be any different in reality.

Nurses in charge need to explain about the advantages of going home, if that is what the patient wants; how drugs are given and that a clearly written instruction card will often be a great help. The nurses need to enquire whether help will be required at home, and whether the patient will have to use stairs. They may suggest bringing the patient's bed into the living-room. They should know the height of the bed at home, and practising getting in and out of one of similar height in hospital will ensure that it can be done safely. They should ask where the toilet is: the loan of a commode may be helpful; whether the patient is going to require a community nurse to assist in his or her care or, if the family want to do the nursing themselves, whether they are capable of it; whether a home help or meals-on-wheels would be needed and if financial assistance can be obtained. Questions such as these can be answered with the help of a social worker.

When a patient known to the St Thomas's Support Team is going home, a doctor from the referring team contacts the patient's general practitioner, to see whether he or she is agreeable to one of the support team's community nurses continuing to support the patient and family at home. (These nurses are attached to the district service but work similarly to the hospital sister, in an advisory capacity with the district nurses and general practitioners.) If permission is given the team is able to give the patient and relative telephone numbers and explains that if advice is needed, somebody is always on call. This is a great reassurance to relatives, who perhaps have had difficulty in the past in obtaining help. Many are reluctant to ask the advice of a doctor, fearing the question may be regarded as stupid but feeling more able to ask a nurse.

It is also important to let the family know that, should they be unable to continue the care, the patient will be able to be re-admitted to hospital, or perhaps it would be more appropriate for referral to be made for admission to a hospice. At times it is useful to send a patient home for a trial day, or weekend to find snags that can then be solved before a final discharge. When a patient is going home to be alone, an occupational-therapy assessment and home visit before discharge are very useful. Nurses and relatives need to make careful plans before a terminally ill patient is discharged home. Experience has shown that a hastily discharged ill patient soon returns to hospital.

## CARING FOR THE OLD PERSON WHO IS DYING IN HOSPITAL

For these patients we need to consider a longer time span, generally speaking, and to discuss quality of life and how that can be maintained (British Geriatric Society and Royal College of Nursing, 1975). If the geriatric patient is dying from malignant disease then the same principles should be followed as already mentioned. Of the patients cared for at St Thomas's, 60 per cent are over 65 years of age.

Many geriatric patients die from arteriosclerotic disease, perhaps the terminal stage being a sudden coronary thrombosis. Usually it is inappropriate to resuscitate such patients but rather to ensure that they are pain free, not left alone and that relatives are fully informed of the situation. Others have a series of cerebrovascular accidents, perhaps none very severe but each leaving the patient in a weaker state. It is important that the patients' dignity is maintained, that they are dressed in their own clothes, that attention is given to hair, teeth and nails, that they are encouraged to be as independent as possible. Pneumonia may be the final illness, which should not usually be treated with antibiotics, but by 'tender loving care'. They should be turned frequently, their mouths kept clean, and sips of iced water given. They may become hot and sweaty, when cotton nightclothes will be cooler – their own, rather than the hospital variety, will look more pleasant. The use of a fan will make them more comfortable. If they become 'bubbly', then an injection of hyoscine 0.4–0.6 mg given 4–6 hourly will dry the secretions and quieten them. If they are anxious, diazepam or chlorpromazine given by suppository will relieve this symptom.

When geriatric patients are dying in hospital, or old people's homes, it is important to explain to their friends what is happening. They may have known the patient for a long while and may want to sit with him or her and say goodbye. They will be realizing that their own deaths may not be far away and observing a friend die peacefully, with good care, can serve to make them less afraid.

Many old people have been brought up with far more respect for, and interest in, Christianity than the present generation and it is important that they are offered a visit by the minister or priest.

Some of the nurses will have become very fond of their patients, whom they may have looked after for a long time. These nurses should be given opportunities to talk about their sadness. They and some of the other patients may wish to attend the funeral. This should be encouraged as a useful outlet for grief. Perhaps flowers from the funeral will be sent to the home or ward, so that they can be enjoyed by the remaining patients and staff.

## CARING FOR THE DYING PATIENT IN INTENSIVE CARE UNITS

Nurses caring for these patients are often under additional strain because of the following:

(1) The patients are often young.
(2) The nurses and doctors have been working under extreme pressure to cure the patient and death will feel like utter failure.
(3) The death is sometimes very soon after admission and the family will be extremely shocked and distressed.
(4) The medical team will be caring for other patients who are similarly acutely ill, possibly in the same area.

How do nurses care in this very clinical atmosphere, electric with anticipation? They have to remember that they are looking after a human being, albeit attached to many pieces of equipment, who can usually hear what they say, and the way that they say it, although the patient may not be able to answer. He or she can probably feel the nurses' caring hands, although he or she may not be able to move. A patient, who may be in pain or have other needs and be unable to shout, requires the nurses' senses to anticipate his or her needs and to alleviate them. All this is stressful and requires nurses to have special qualities.

The nursing team needs to be headed by a person with great sensitivity to the feelings of the staff. He or she needs to comfort, explain, encourage and show concern for the staff and the relatives, as much as care for the patients.

It is important for doctors and nurses working in intensive care to have opportunities to discuss patients in team meetings, with other specialists to help them, such as a psychologist, chaplain or social worker.

## CARING FOR THE TERMINALLY ILL PATIENT WITH RENAL DISEASE

Staff must cope with the problem of deciding not to treat renal patients or abandoning dialysis treatment. Another problem is the disappointment of patient, relatives and staff following kidney-transplant rejection. The patient will probably have been known in the renal department for many years; he or she and the family may have become friends of the staff. The same principles apply in end-stage renal failure as in terminal cancer. The symptoms must be controlled in the best way possible and patients and families given clear information and support in a kind and understanding fashion.

Patients will be lethargic and drowsy, so the nurse, or perhaps a relative, will need to give help with general care, allowing the patients to keep as much independence as they are able to cope with. If their appetites are poor, it is important that meals should be small and attractively presented. Keeping to a rigid diet is inappropriate; rather they should be allowed to eat and drink what they fancy. They will often be nauseated, which may be relieved by cyclizine 50 mg given twice daily. If they also have hiccups, then chlorpromazine will relieve this symptom as well as the nausea. It can conveniently be given by suppository, if this route is acceptable to the patient.

If patients have pain then this should be relieved in the most appropriate way; there is no point at this stage in withholding potent analgesia, if it relieves symptoms. Their skin may be dry and itching: arachis oil will relieve dryness; crotamiton (Eurax) cream may relieve the itching.

Mouth care is extremely important, because their mouths will be very dry and their gums may bleed. They may also develop *Monilia*, which will be relieved by nystatin suspension or miconazole (Daktarin) gel. Another problem that may be very distressing to patients and families is realizing there is no drainage from a catheter, in which case removal should be considered.

Patients may also have fits, or muscle twitching, which can be controlled by diazepam 5–10 mg given 8 hourly. Relatives, patients and staff need to be kept fully informed as to why medicines are given and how they will help, and if they do not relieve a symptom, they should be stopped.

Staff will sometimes be very distressed after such a patient dies and should be given the opportunity to talk about their sadness as well as successes, and to discuss the preventive side of the illness.

In conclusion, dying patients can be cared for in hospital just as well as in a hospice, so long as nurses pay attention to the details of basic care in a sensitive way and doctors prescribe appropriately. These combined efforts will lead to better care, improved patient and family support and enhanced job fulfilment.

## REFERENCES

Bates, T. *et al*. (1981) A new concept of hospital care, *The Lancet*, Vol. I, pp. 1,201–3.

British Geriatric Society and Royal College of Nursing (1975) *Improving Geriatric Care in Hospital*, London.

Regnard, C. and Newbury, A. (1983) Pain and the portable syringe pump, *Nursing Times*, 29 June, pp. 25–8.

Saunders, B. (1980) Terminal care support team, *Nursing*, July, p. 657.

WHO (1979) *Expert Committee on Drug Dependency*, 16th Report, Technical Report Series No. 407, World Health Organization, Geneva.

# 18. Care in a Hospice: Special Aspects

A current definition of hospice is a community of people devoting their time exclusively to the care of dying patients, and sometimes the frail elderly and chronic sick or disabled as well. The term is not synonymous with a special building; hospice type of care may be given in a patient's home or in a ward set apart for the purpose in a general hospital.

Hospice care of dying patients, for whom the goal of cure is now inappropriate, aims to offer a complete service in which the emphasis is on freeing the person from distressing symptoms and ensuring that those caring for him or her have the time, skills and compassion to support the patient effectively until death, and the family throughout this time and in their bereavement.

It has been pointed out that the dying patient and family can also be given excellent care in an acute hospital ward. This, of course, is true but because of many conflicting needs staff can find it difficult to achieve what they wish to provide. Time may be lacking, personnel in short supply and the physical environment deficient in various ways. Doctors and nurses working in the community may also be frustrated in their desire to give a high-quality service to dying patients for similar reasons.

Those who have worked in hospices for a number of years have been able to build up a fund of knowledge and understanding, backed up by research, precisely because the resources are available for them to devote all their time to this field of care. Their expertise is being increasingly shared with other professional health workers; thus hospices can act as resource centres for improving the care of dying patients over a wider sphere.

# SPECIAL FEATURES OF RESIDENTIAL HOSPICE CARE

The wards should be bright and cheerful in colour and design; the ideal basic size seems to be a four-bedded unit, with some single rooms for those whose condition makes this more suitable, with their agreement. Large windows where patients can see people and traffic moving, if they are used to an urban environment, give a feeling of unity with the living world. Country dwellers, on the other hand, will appreciate being surrounded by beautiful natural scenery.

Unrestricted visiting is encouraged, since the patient and family need frequent contact with each other. Relatives and friends should feel welcomed, and their physical and emotional comfort considered.

## Reception and admission

When patients, sometimes accompanied by relatives, arrive at a hospice, it is the custom for the trained nurse in charge to greet the patients at the entrance and escort them to their own ward where he or she will be responsible for their care. In this way, patients are treated as true guests with courtesy and a warm welcome. It is common for the nurse to be with the relatives while the doctor is taking a history from patients, and examining them. This can be an opportunity for anxious and sad relatives to unburden themselves to a sympathetic listener. If they have been looking after the patient at home, there may be an expression of guilt at not being able to continue, and a feeling of failure. They are likely to be very tired, and apprehensive as to how the patient will come to terms with the new environment. The nurse should ensure privacy whilst interviewing the relatives, and provide comfortable chairs for them. The atmosphere should be unhurried to enable the nurse to obtain the necessary details about the patient (these can be added to later). Some type of nursing history sheet should be used, which will also be of value to doctor, social worker and other professional members of the caring team, for instance the physiotherapist.

The doctor will also wish to meet the relatives to ensure that they have an accurate understanding of the situation, and there may be a pressing reason why the social worker should be involved at an early stage. Unless the patient is near to death on admission, which can be the case, the relatives will want to see the patient settled before they go home, and should be offered a cup of tea, sitting with the patient. The usual precaution of obtaining a telephone number should be taken, and assurance given that the relatives are welcome to telephone or call whenever they wish.

A significant feature of hospice care, and one that has already been mentioned, is that time is made available to spend with patients not only when some physical procedure needs to be carried out, but at other times, simply providing companionship and a willingness to listen. This means that an adequate ratio of staff to patients is essential. Follow-up care of bereaved families is an important service, developed mainly by social workers, often with a team of trained volunteers. However, nurses have a part to play here because they will often have built up a close relationship with the family of a dying patient and may attend the funeral. They can help with the follow-up care by inviting the family to feel welcome to call into the ward from time to time to maintain contact.

Finally, the fact that hospices are relatively small in comparison with general hospitals helps to foster a sense of close community among staff, which will be sensed by patients and relatives. Rigid hierarchical barriers are out of place, and consultation and sharing of problems is beneficial to patients and staff.

It is essential for a hospice to be situated near a general hospital where facilities such as an X-ray department (and radiotherapy), clinical laboratories and dentistry are available. The need for such technical assistance will not occur frequently, but can bring considerable relief on occasion to individual patients. For instance, a single dose of radiation therapy can bring dramatic reduction of pain for a patient with malignancy of bone.

The pace of life in a hospice is much more relaxed than in the large general hospital. Staff will try to go at the patient's pace rather than follow their own inclination, and to aim at an informal and homely style of ward management. There should be opportunities for patients to go home for a day or a weekend if they wish, provided the family can cope and no extra strain or burden will be put upon them. This requires consultation between doctor, nurse and social worker before finalizing the matter with the patient and family.

The homely quality of a hospice is enhanced by the absence of a multiplicity of charts hanging on beds, by little or no evidence of intravenous infusions, and by the freedom from the inevitable bustle and noise of trolleys taking patients to and from operating theatre or other departments. All this activity is necessary and justifiable in institutions devoted to cure as well as care, but it is an inappropriate intrusion into the peaceful surroundings of dying patients in a hospice.

Because of the considerable interest being shown at present in hospice work, both by professionals and the lay public, there are many requests to be 'shown round'. This commendable interest must be channelled in a suitable way, as too many groups or individual visitors walking through the wards can be an excessive invasion of the privacy due to dying patients and their families, and a strain for staff. It is usually preferable to arrange talks illustrated with slides or a film showing the work of the hospice, and keep tours to a minimum. This is usually accepted with understanding, particularly when it is explained that it is not customary to isolate the patient and family behind screens during the last hours of life.

The in-patient care of a hospice is usually combined with a home-care service. The latter is often known as a Macmillan service, being supported by Cancer Relief Macmillan Fund. This requires close co-operation and efficient communication between all staff so that if and when a patient is admitted for residential care, the home-care team are able to keep in touch with the situation. The main reason for admission is to give the caring family a temporary respite from their responsibilities, or there may be other reasons. Sometimes, the patient naturally deteriorates and dies in the hospice.

The qualities that go into the making of a hospice are not exactly definable. Klagsbrun (1981) states that although a hospice need not be a religious organization, it would seem essential that there is a spiritual dimension to its structure – to the rational human being, suffering and death have to make sense ultimately in order for the person to remain human.

## HISTORY OF THE HOSPICE MOVEMENT

The word 'hospice' has its origin in the Roman word '*hospes*' – meaning both a host and a guest. From this tradition of hospitality, both hospitals for treatment of the sick, and hospices for giving temporary help and accommodation to travellers and care to the dying developed. Hospitals can be traced back to the ancient world, but the dominant influence in the growth of hospices was Christianity (although the two concepts were interchangeable for several centuries).

Most of the credit for early hospices must be attributed to the Knights Hospitallers of the Order of St John of Jerusalem. These were founded in Malta in 1065, primarily for the task of caring for the sick and dying on pilgrimage to and from the Holy Land.

At the peak of their flowering, records show an attitude of great consideration and respect for the needs of the individual – what would be called today a holistic approach to care. The same was true of the medieval hospices operating throughout Europe; 750 were in existence in England alone.

Following the suppression of the monasteries and the dispersal of religious men and women, the sick, poor and dying were left without help and medicine and nursing remained at a low ebb for a considerable time, hospitals at that period being a place to be dreaded and avoided at all costs.

## The modern hospice

It was not until the middle of the nineteenth century that the old idea of the hospice began to revive. The Sisters of Charity, founded by Vincent de Paul in 1600, had worked quietly for three centuries among the poorest and most despised members of French society, and during the nineteenth century influenced such pioneers as the Protestant pastor Fliedner (who founded Kaiserswerth), Florence Nightingale and Elizabeth Fry.

In 1840 an Irishwoman, Mary Aikenhead, opened in Dublin a place of shelter and care for the incurably ill and dying and called it by the old medieval name of 'hospice'. She founded a new order of nuns, the Irish Sisters of Charity, who in 1906 opened a similar house in London – St Joseph's Hospice, which has continued until the present day in caring for dying patients and those with chronic illnesses. Just before the opening of St Joseph's Hospice, two other hospices had opened in London—St Luke's, founded in 1894 by a Methodist minister, Mr Barrett, has been rebuilt and is known as Hereford Lodge. The other hospice, the Hostel of God, was started by a community of Anglican sisters. This closed for some years but is now operating under lay management and has been renamed Trinity Hospice.

While this development was proceeding in Europe, a parallel revival of the old hospice ideal was taking place in America, through the work of a Dominican order of nuns founded by Rose Hawthorne. Their first hospice opened in New York in 1899, and was followed by others. In the 1950s an important development was the establishment of the Marie Curie Foundation, which aimed to relieve the distress of patients dying with cancer, and the strain on their families. Homes were set up to provide hospice care. The highest point of the hospice movement in this century so far was reached through the work of Cicely Saunders. In revolutionizing the approach to control of pain and other distressing symptoms in dying patients and in re-emphasizing the right of the patient to a peaceful and dignified death, she has led the way and inspired others to introduce hospice care all over this country and in North America.

At St Joseph's Hospice, where she was appointed as the first full-time medical officer, and began her special work for dying patients, she was able to build on the tradition and practice of loving care carried out for more than half a century by this Christian community, whose original priority had been relieving the distress caused by wide-spread tuberculosis in East London. Many of the victims died at home or in the hospice, tended by the sisters. In then founding St Christopher's Hospice in 1967, Cicely Saunders drew together the threads of care traced back over nearly 2,000 years, and enriched the work with a new emphasis on scientific research and teaching.

## PRESENT AND FUTURE TRENDS

In the UK there are now (1988) 124 hospices for residential care, 176 Macmillan teams and 400 Macmillan nurses. Much financial help and guidance continues to be given by Cancer Relief Macmillan Fund with particular emphasis on home care. Most hospices are largely independent, although increasingly some State help is forthcoming. Some hospices have been built through voluntary subscription and have subsequently become the responsibility of the NHS health authority. Other charitable bodies helping to build and maintain hospices are the Marie Curie Foundation and 'Help the Hospices'. There are other types of home-care organizations, for instance, 'Hospice at Home', examples of this one being in Tunbridge Wells and Peterborough.

Hospices now tend to be relatively small in size, say between 12 and 25 beds, in comparison with the older hospices such as St Joseph's and St Christopher's.

With the much greater interest in the needs of dying people and their families, both by the health-care professions and the general public, the whole subject has been opened up for research and debate. As the basic concepts of hospice care become more widely understood and applied in hospitals (where about 60 per cent of people in the UK die), some believe that hospices should 'plan for [their] own obsolescence', linked with the provision of counselling, support and good symptom control for patients and relatives, upgrading of community terminal care, and a vigorous teaching programme for young doctors and nurses. This will result in a hospice having only a few beds, and not necessarily functioning in a special unit on its own, but as a centre associated with schools of medicine and nursing (Wilkes, 1981). A detailed and well-documented analysis of the effectiveness of hospice care, including cost-benefit, is needed to justify separate hospice care (Torrens, 1981). Finally, there is a challenge to be met in the application of hospice concepts to a broader section of care: since it has been widely accepted as having achieved much for dying patients, other groups such as the chronic sick, the mentally handicapped and the frail elderly deserve the same efforts to be made on their behalf.

Many countries throughout the world are giving much thought to the most appropriate way in which hospice-type care can be developed. In some countries, rather than building free-standing hospices, existing institutions are used in which an improved care service for dying people can be based. In others, particularly in the USA, there has been a great proliferation in home-care programmes.

An increasing number of well-established hospices have education departments catering not only for their own staff but also in providing education in terminal care for colleagues in surrounding health districts and beyond. This includes medical students and student nurses.

Although home is the ideal place in which to die, this is not always possible. A hospice can be a haven of peace for the patient and family, particularly because of the lack of hurry and tension inevitable to some extent in an acute hospital ward.

## Acceptance of death

Those of us whose privilege it often is to sit by the bedside of a dying patient know well that the moment of death need be neither frightening nor painful, but a peaceful end to the functioning of the body. This was brought home to me as I sat at the bedside of an only child – Ronnie – who was dying of cancer. His father and mother sat beside him praying silently. We seemed to be enveloped in an atmosphere of great peace. Ronnie was just 9 years old. Suddenly the silence was broken when his father said, 'Sister, we have had Ronnie for 9 wonderful years. We realize that he is only a loan from God; now we give him back. We shall be very lonely, but he is going to a better home and one day, please God, we shall join him'. This remarkable acceptance came after months of suffering – both parents rebelled at first and could not accept this cruel cross, but gradually they found peace.

## Overcoming fear

For many people the thought of death and dying is fearful. The fear may relate to death itself – how it may come and what may be found after death. The practice in a hospice of not hiding the dying patient behind curtains during his or her last hours can have a calming and reassuring effect, as can be seen by the following incident.

Mrs X was a frail, worried little lady of 50 years. She knew that she was dying and was very frightened. A few days after admission to the hospice she said one morning, 'I am not afraid of dying now since I saw Dora slip away. [Dora was a patient in the opposite bed and they had become friends.] It was so beautiful – Dora had just had her hair done and she looked so pretty when suddenly she cried out that she felt queer and wanted Sister. Sister and doctor came, then the chaplain. They all knelt down and prayed. Sister held Dora's hand and she went so quietly and peacefully. I hope I go that way too'. Mrs X did 'go that way' a few days later.

This gentle passage from life to death can only be achieved if we have succeeded in a large measure in relieving any distressing symptoms of mind, body and spirit. Some patients will have lived their lives according to particular religious beliefs and will find comfort in the confidence of eternal life to which death is the awakening. The person with no belief in an after-life may also die calmly and peacefully since to him or her when death comes all is over. The constant presence of a caring staff eager to give comfort and support to all without discrimination of race or creed must be the hallmark of a hospice.

## Some views expressed by patients and relatives in a particular hospice

The following are answers given by some patients when asked how they would describe a hospice:

- 'A home from home.'
- 'Not like a hospital – just like a beautiful big drawing-room. Full of loving people!'

- 'A place where I know I am wanted.'
- 'A place where people have time to listen.'

## Bereavement

Terminal care does not end with the death of the patient whose sufferings are over – those of the family continue, sometimes for a long time. Professional support and help may be needed, and social workers in particular will visit the bereaved family or single relative when it is thought to be helpful. Some hospices have set up a bereavement service using trained counsellors or visitors. The custom that some of the hospice staff attend the funeral is much appreciated by the family. A card sent by the hospice to the spouse or close relative on the first anniversary of the death – simply saying 'We are remembering you' – is described by many as a great solace.

## A wider view of hospice care

Patients in the terminal stage of malignant disease form the main group of patients admitted for residential care in a hospice. Many hospices also care for a small number of patients with severe neurological disease when they are terminally ill. There is already one hospice for dying patients with AIDS (the London Lighthouse) and several others will be opened. Some hospices, such as St Joseph's, include units for the care of people with severe chronic conditions who, although they may have many years still to live, are not candidates for a regime aimed at 'cure'. Instead, the hospice principle of living life to the full whatever the remaining span is applied. Residents live in comfort and dignity in a homely atmosphere using their talents and interests in a fulfilling way. Not all institutions giving care to dying patients, or in the wider sense of support for frail and handicapped people, are necessarily called hospices. One thinks of the homes run by the Marie Curie Foundation, Sue Ryder Homes and Cheshire Homes. None the less, all are imbued with the philosophy of the ancient medieval foundations and in the continuing hospice traditions of today.

## REFERENCES AND FURTHER READING

Hanratty, J. (1988) *Care of the Dying – A Philosophy of the Care of Terminal Illness*, St Joseph's Hospice, London.

King Edward's Hospital Fund for London (1987) *Care of the Dying: A Guide for Health Authorities*, National Association of Health Authorities, London.

Klagsbrun, S. C. (1981) Hospice – a developing role, in C. M. Saunders *et al.* (eds) *Hospice: The Living Idea*, Edward Arnold, London.

Lamerton, R. (1980) *Care of the Dying*, Pelican, Harmondsworth.

Manning, M. (1984) *The Hospice Alternative: Living with Dying*, Souvenir Press, London.

Saunders, C. M. *et al.* (1981) *Hospice: The Living Idea*, Edward Arnold, London.

Stoddard, S. (1978 and 1979) *The Hospice Movement*, Vintage Books and Jonathan Cape, London.

Torrens, P. (1981) Achievement, failure and the future, in C. M. Saunders *et al.* (eds) *Hospice: The Living Idea*, Edward Arnold, London.

Wilkes, E. (1981) Great Britain: the hospice in Britain, in C. M. Saunders *et al.* (eds) *Hospice: The Living Idea*, Edward Arnold, London.

## ACKNOWLEDGEMENT

We would like to acknowledge the help of Anne Eve, Cancer Relief Macmillan Fund, for providing some statistics.

# Appendix 1: Patient Care Study

It seems right to finish this book with an account of a patient and her family, because many of the facets of care described in the various chapters were drawn together during the last weeks of the patient's life. The contribution has been written by a nurse who was closely involved in the caring process.

## CARE STUDY: ROSE AND JAMES

### Patient and family

Rose was a 69-year-old woman living with her husband, James, in a self-contained maisonette in East London. They had been married for three years. For both of them it was a second marriage, their first partners having died. Rose had a son and daughter by her first husband, both were married with children. Before her illness Rose had seen her children regularly and greatly looked forward to the visits. While Rose was in the hospice both her children managed to visit her each week, but it was not possible for any other members of the family to visit. Rose's favourite hobby had been ballroom dancing, she and James had met dancing. When she talked about dancing Rose's face would light up.

James had had one operation to replace a hip joint and was waiting for the other hip to be done.

## Past medical history

Rose had suffered with the usual childhood illnesses. She had also had rheumatic fever as a child. She had a long-standing history of claustrophobia. Over the years Rose had learnt to avoid claustrophobic situations and the condition did not interfere with her enjoyment of life.

More recently Rose had suffered with occasional facial neuralgia, which was very painful. Her general practitioner (GP) had prescribed carbamazepine 200 mg to be taken four times a day, which worked well.

## Present illness

Rose went to see her GP in March 1987 with a two-month history of a persistent cough. Her doctor referred her to the local hospital. She was admitted for investigations that led to a diagnosis of oat-cell carcinoma of the bronchus with superior vena cava obstruction.

## Treatment

Rose was treated with a course of six treatments of chemotherapy. Re-assessment showed no improvement in her condition so she commenced on a course of radiotherapy treatment. Rose became much weaker and found the radiotherapy treatment very stressful, so it was discontinued. Rose was referred to the hospice home-care team for assessment and support.

## Home care

The home-care doctor visited Rose on 10 November. He found an ill lady with advanced carcinoma of the bronchus and metastatic spread. Rose appeared to be aware of her diagnosis and prognosis but unwilling to talk about it.

Rose had developed large, painful swellings on her skull about a month previously. She had gradually become weaker with increasing dyspnoea, malaise, dysphagia and a feeling of choking. These had become worse over the last couple of weeks. Rose's main problems seemed to be weakness, constipation, pain – particularly over her skull, shortness of breath, frontal headaches and a potential sacral pressure sore.

At this time Rose was sitting up in a chair. She was caring for her own hygiene needs and able to climb the stairs. She struggled to maintain her independence but found it increasingly difficult due to weakness. She refused offers of help from the district nurse but occasionally allowed James to help her.

Her husband was finding the situation very difficult. He said Rose made constant demands and his efforts to help her were belittled, nothing he did was right. James was worried about coping and talked about his painful hip.

Over the next few days a sheepskin was delivered so that Rose could lie more comfortably in bed. She said her sleep was disturbed by coughing. She complained of frontal headaches and of aching all over. She had had her bowels open with a loose stool, which she said was due to the laxatives. James said that Rose was vomiting several times a day, but when asked Rose would not admit it.

The social worker was asked to visit because of the deteriorating emotional situation. She talked to Rose and James together and formed the opinion that Rose had been the dominant partner. Her illness had forced a role reversal and James felt unsupported. James mentioned Rose's restless and confused behaviour, such as cutting off buttons and unpicking the sheet, which he found very frightening.

The Macmillan nurse visited on 16 November and noted that Rose was weaker. She was now ready to accept help with washing and needed assistance to transfer from bed to commode. The skin over her sacral area was red but intact.

## Assessment of the situation

During the next few days James was becoming increasingly anxious and agitated about coping with his wife. He said that Rose was very demanding and could not be left. Although medication had been prescribed and was available, Rose refused to take it although she complained of pain. The Macmillan nurse mentioned the possibility of admission to the hospice for a period of respite care but at this stage Rose refused to consider this. On 22 November James telephoned the nurse and demanded that Rose should be admitted to the hospice as neither he nor his wife were sleeping and he could no longer cope. He was very angry and could not understand why Rose should be consulted in the matter.

The Macmillan nurse and the social worker visited the home together.

It was explained to Rose and James together that a hospice bed was available. Rose refused to comment, but while the nurse washed her and attended to her needs, she gently talked about the hospice and that James was at present too exhausted to care for her. Towards the end of the visit Rose was asked directly if she would agree to admission and she nodded her consent. A night sitter was arranged for that night so that James could, it was hoped, obtain some rest, and admission and transport to the hospice were arranged for the next day. The social worker gained the impression that both husband and wife were frightened by the deteriorating situation and James was becoming so angry about everything that he was hardly able to listen to what was being said.

## Admission to the hospice

Rose and James arrived at the hospice on 24 November and I went to meet them at the entrance and welcome them. I accompanied them to the ward (Rose was in a wheelchair). I helped Rose into bed and observed how thin she was and frail, with a wary but determined expression. She remained silent when I asked her a few simple questions to try to break the ice. She and James were left sitting together quietly drinking a cup of tea while awaiting the doctor's arrival.

## Medical assessment

The doctor who examined Rose on admission had some difficulty because she refused to speak to him; she appeared to have withdrawn into herself, and James spoke for her. The doctor noted that Rose had an enlarged liver and that the right lower lobe of her right lung had consolidated. She had three very tender lumps on her scalp, candidiasis (thrush) at the back of her mouth and a superficial pressure sore. Although according to the home-care notes, Rose had been prescribed morphine 5 mg every four hours for pain, there was some doubt that she was taking the medication. In view of her pain, nausea and dysphagia the doctor decided to commence the use of a syringe driver containing diamorphine 20 mg and cyclizine 100 mg. He also prescribed Nystan suspension 2 ml four times a day for the thrush and Benoral suspension 10 ml twice a day to help in controlling her bone pain. He explained the purpose of the medication to Rose and advised her to try to drink as much as she could. The doctor saw James and explained the seriousness of Rose's condition and her poor prognosis.

## Nursing assessment

I talked to James to discover how he felt. He seemed to accept Rose's diagnosis and that the radiotherapy treatment had been unsuccessful. He was still resentful and angry, talking at length about how hard he had tried; how nothing he did seemed to be right; and how his arthritis made everything more difficult. He had tried to change Rose's position but on his own he seemed to hurt her more than help her. He thought that Rose should have been admitted sooner to the hospice. Once he had 'let off steam' James calmed down and said that it had helped to talk things over. He supplied personal details for Rose and their telephone number. I asked him whether Rose was a member of a particular religious faith; he said that she believed in God but did not attend a church. After assuring him that he could telephone and visit his wife whenever he wished, James said goodbye to Rose and went home.

Having been with the doctor when he examined Rose, I had been able to make certain observations about her general condition, and present and potential problems. Because of her present reluctance to talk, it was inappropriate to subject her to much questioning at the moment, and the nursing history sheet could be finally completed later in the day.

## Nursing care plan

Rose's main problems were identified and a care plan drawn up as in Figure 1 (see p. 250).

## Implementation of care plan

As the afternoon progressed Rose appeared to relax a little more. She answered questions about her immediate needs, but did not volunteer any comments. She seemed less withdrawn and watched the ward around her with interest. That evening Rose had a *grand mal* fit. Diazepam 10 mg was given *per rectum* with good effect. Rose slept for the evening and all that night.

The following morning Rose was still drowsy. She was able to understand what was being said but too sleepy to answer. The doctor decided to commence a trial of steroids and prescribed dexamethasone 2 mg three times a day; this was to relieve the headache and reduce the possibility of further fits. By mid-morning Rose had not passed urine since admission. She said she did not feel uncomfortable. A catheter was suggested to Rose, who agreed. A size 14 Foley catheter was passed and left *in situ*, 100 ml of urine drained immediately.

Rose's days on the ward settled into a pattern. She slept for long periods at night. Between position changes and drinks, Rose was most comfortable lying on her side. She had porridge or milk for breakfast, according to how she felt. Each morning, after a wash or a bath, she sat in a chair on a Roho cushion, which she found comfortable. Rose was very frail and needed supporting with pillows but she appreciated the change of view. Drinks were offered and she particularly liked vanilla ice-lollies.

If Rose wanted some lunch James or one of the staff would help her. For the first few days she tended to have soup and a soft pudding. She generally refused any supper, but might have ice-cream and a cup of tea. In the afternoon Rose liked to return to bed to doze. She would sit up in bed for supper and drinks but was more comfortable lying on her side because of her painful scalp lesions.

Rose could manage liquid medication fairly well with help, as long as she wasn't rushed. At times Rose brought up moderate amounts of saliva, and she liked to have a paper tissue in her hand to clear it from her mouth. The amount of saliva varied from day to day, some days there was none.

## Progress notes

The morning was Rose's best time of day, when she tended to be brighter and more alert; quite ready to respond and occasionally to initiate conversation. Rose had a lovely smile, her eyes would sparkle and her face light up. Generally Rose became less alert as the day progressed, becoming tired and sleeping or dozing for much of the time.

James visited regularly; he came every morning about 11.00 and would stay for a couple of hours, talking to Rose and helping her with her lunch. He would return again in the evening and stay for an hour or so. Sometimes when he visited, James seemed to be particularly anxious, hovering over Rose as though not sure what to do. When one of the staff spoke to him he would sit down and seem to relax.

*Figure 1 Nursing Care Plan, 24 November, 1987*

| Problem | Goal | Action |
|---|---|---|
| Pain | To be comfortable and pain free | Ensure efficient working of syringe driver<br>Give oral analgesia as prescribed<br>Monitor effectiveness<br>Change position with care – painful scalp lesions |
| Nausea | Free of nausea and vomiting | Give anti-emetics as prescribed |
| Immobility | Assist with functions of daily living<br>Comfortable position | Change position two hourly<br>Sheepskin under feet and heels<br>Observe skin for potential pressure sores |
| Loss of power in left arm | Assist with functions of daily living | Give assistance with eating and drinking |
| Sacral pressure sore | Promote healing, prevent further deterioration | Keep sacral area clean and dry<br>Change position two hourly<br>Use Spenco mattress/Roho cushion<br>Clean sore daily with Betadine and protect with a dry dressing |
| Dehydration | Comfortable mouth | Rose likes ice lollies<br>Offer frequent drinks $\frac{1}{2}$–1 hourly when awake<br>Moisten and clean mouth using sponge sticks with water or glycerine and Thymol |

| | | |
|---|---|---|
| | Adequate urine output | Offer commodes when changing position<br>Ensure catheter able to drain freely<br>Empty urine bag at 06:00 and 18:00, chart output in Kardex<br>Keep vulval area free of talc |
| Dry mouth/thrush | Moist mouth, infection free | Encourage frequent drinks<br>Clean dentures night and morning<br>Offer glycerine and Thymol mouthwashes after meal<br>Give Nystan suspension as prescribed |
| Constipation | Bowel action every 2–3 days | Give oral laxatives as prescribed |
| Difficulty with personal hygiene | Clean and comfortable at all times | Daily bath/bed bath<br>Observe skin for potential pressure sores<br>Do not use talc around catheter |
| Rose appears anxious/withdrawn | Relaxed atmosphere, Rose able to talk | Establish a good relationship<br>Be friendly even if response is minimal<br>Allow Rose time to talk |
| Loss of appetite | Encourage eating, don't let it become a problem | Encourage soft diet<br>Give assistance as required<br>Don't let Rose feel she has to eat if she doesn't want to |
| Headaches | Comfortable/pain free | Give dexamethasone as prescribed<br>Position head with care |

The night of 26–27 November Rose slept for only short periods. She was coughing up large amounts of thick sputum and became very frightened. One of the night staff sat with her, Rose talked about death and her fears of dying. Talking about her fears seemed to settle Rose and she eventually fell asleep.

Rose had not had her bowels opened since coming to the hospice, she said it was several days since her bowels had worked. The previous day a rectal examination had shown her lower rectum to be empty. I suggested she should have an enema, Rose said she did not mind, as long as it worked! The foot of Rose's bed was raised slightly and a disposable phosphate enema given. Rose was worried about making a mess but I assured her that any mess would be my fault. After 30 minutes we helped Rose onto a commode and she had a good bowel action. We helped Rose to have a full bath before she sat in her chair. For the rest of her stay Rose's bowels were opened every 2–3 days with oral laxatives and suppositories.

When Rose had been with us for a few days James remarked how much better she seemed. He asked if she might be able to go home. I explained that Rose seemed to feel better because her pain was controlled so she felt brighter and more relaxed; but she was still very frail. I said that although it was possible she might improve enough to go home again, I thought in her present condition he would have difficulty looking after her. He seemed satisfied with the explanation and even slightly relieved; I wondered if James thought we might want to discharge Rose home now she seemed a little brighter.

## The last few days of life

On the afternoon of 29 November Rose had an episode of diarrhoea. She did not seem to be aware of it. Laxatives were omitted from her drug regime for two days and no further episodes occurred. By 30 November Rose was noticeably weaker. She tended to become slightly muddled about the time of day or whether she had had lunch. Rose did not appear to be upset by the muddles and they did not last long. Rose was sleeping more of the time. On 2 December Rose seemed to feel pain when she was moved. The dose of diamorphine in her syringe driver was increased to 30 mg over 24 hours.

Rose became progressively weaker over the next few days. She was sleeping more and more but was still alert when she was awake. She sat up in a chair for the last time on 4 December. She ate only ice-cream for lunch and had frequent sips of water. That day when we saw James coming into the hospice and told Rose he was coming her face lit up in anticipation.

That evening, Rose was much weaker; she slept, only waking when her position was changed. The staff nurse spoke to James about her increasing weakness; he seemed to be aware that she would die soon. That night Rose slept for long periods. The night staff noted that she seemed to have pain when she was moved, but settled very quickly afterwards. During the night she was incontinent of a large amount of faeces; she did not appear to be aware of either the incontinence or being washed afterwards.

On the morning of 5 December Rose was extremely weak. When her eyes were open she appeared to understand what was said to her, but she was unable to respond. As she appeared to be experiencing some pain, the medication in her syringe driver was increased to diamorphine 40 mg with cyclizine 100 mg.

James visited in the morning and sat with Rose until about 4.30 p.m., when he left saying he would be back in an hour or so. One of the staff sat with Rose holding her hand. She died very peacefully at 5.15 p.m. The staff nurse on duty rang James and told him Rose had died. James asked what happened next. He was asked to return to the ward in the morning. The staff nurse thought that James sounded in control of himself, but persuaded him that he should telephone his stepson and daughter and ask them to come round to the house so that he was not alone that evening. He agreed to do so.

James came to the ward the next morning. He was seen by the ward Sister who encouraged him to talk about how he felt. He seemed calm, and slightly relieved that Rose's illness was over; sad that she was dead, but glad she was no longer in pain. Sister explained how to register the death and that this should be done before he approached an undertaker. James appeared to think that Rose's cremation could take place at the hospice and seemed slightly daunted by the thought of an undertaker. Sister suggested that he should see the social worker who had visited Rose and James at home. James agreed and he was taken to her office.

The doctor looking after Rose wrote to her GP and hospital consultant, telling them about her stay in the hospice and that she had died.

## Evaluation

Rose and James were assessed as very anxious and unable to cope with Rose's illness at home, and Rose was reputed to be frightened of hospitals. Like many patients, Rose was anxious at first, but she soon began to relax. The ability of the hospice team to make her more comfortable enabled Rose and James to enjoy each other's company for the time that was left. I think the support of the staff helped James to cope with the knowledge that Rose was dying and with her death.

James was a rather lonely, elderly man, and although Rose's son and daughter did visit her each week there seemed to be little communication with James and they appeared to be content to leave him to maintain contact with the hospice staff and not to be involved in this. Neither James nor Rose wished to have any religious ministration, although they appreciated a friendly word with the chaplain each day. In fact, with the help of the social worker, the family came together to arrange the funeral and the stepdaughter volunteered to keep in touch with James as she lives fairly near.

This care study was written by Christine Fox, RGN, while undertaking ENB course 931, 'Continuing care of the dying patient and the family'.

## FURTHER READING

British Medical Association and Pharmaceutical Society of Great Britain, *British National Formulary* (1985) No. 10 and (1987) No. 13.
Capra, L. G. (1986) *Care of the Cancer Patient*, Macmillan, London.
Gould, D. (1985) Pressure for change, *Nursing Mirror*, Vol. 161, p. 16.
Gould, D. (1987) 'Patients and pressure sores', *Nursing Times*, Vol. 83, p. 47.
Regnard, C. F. B. and Davies, A. (1986) *A Guide to Symptom Relief in Advanced Cancer*, Haigh & Hochland, Manchester.

## NOTE

No detailed drug glossary has been included in this care study as such information is available elsewhere in the book. Likewise, a description of the use of a syringe driver is given in Chapter 5.

# Appendix 2: Useful Addresses

CRUSE, National Organization for the widowed and their children
CRUSE House
126 Sheen Road
Richmond
Surrey TW9 1UR
01-940 4818/9047

Marie Curie Memorial Foundation
28 Belgrave Square
London SW1X 8QG
01-235 3325

Cancer Relief Macmillan Fund
Anchor House
15–19 Britten Street
London SW3 3TY
01-351 7811

The Society of Compassionate Friends (for bereaved parents)
6 Denmark Street
Bristol BS1 5DQ
0272 292778

Stillbirth and Neonatal Death Society
28 Portland Place
London
W1N 4DE
01-436 5881

BACUP (Information and support service for cancer sufferers)
121–3 Charterhouse Street
London EC1M 6AA
01-608 1661

The Terence Higgins Trust – BM/AIDS
London WC1N 3XX
01-242 1010

Health Education Authority
Hamilton House
Mabledon Place
London WC1H 9TX

Hospice Information Service
St Christopher's Hospice
51–9 Laurie Park Road
London SE26 6DZ
01-778 9252

National Association of Funeral Directors
57 Doughty Street
London WC1
01-242 9388

# ADDRESSES OF SOME RELIGIOUS BODIES

The Islamic Cultural Centre
146 Park Road
London NW8 7RG
01-724 3363

The Buddhist Society
58 Eccleston Square
London SW1V 1PH
01-834 5858

Jewish Joint Burial Society
North-Western Reform Synagogue
Alyth Gardens
London NW11 7EN
01-455 8579

United Synagogue (Orthodox)
Woburn House
Upper Woburn Place
London WC1H 0E7
01-387 4300

The Hospital Chaplains' Fellowship
c/o Reverend David H. Robinson
Wallsgrave Hospital
Clifford Bridge Road
Wallsgrave
Coventry
West Midlands CV 2DX
0203 613232

The Association of Hospice Chaplains
c/o Reverend Colin Kassell
St Catherine's Hospice
Malt House Road
Crawley
Sussex RH1O 6BH
0293 515224

# Index

"Growing up in church and Christian schools, I was taught that Jesus's parables were basically about how we should live. To be sure, many of the parables do show us God's standard for our lives, but they also reveal how we have failed to live up to that standard, and how God in his infinite mercy has done for us what we could never do for ourselves. My friend Jared Wilson shows how Jesus used parables to illustrate the upside-down and counterintuitive ways of God compared to our ways. We see how the parables are not a witness to the best people making it up to God, but rather a witness to God making it down to the worst people—meeting our rebellion with his rescue, our sin with his salvation, our guilt with his grace, our badness with his goodness. Thanks for the reminder, Jared. I keep forgetting that this whole thing is about Jesus, not me."

**Tullian Tchividjian,** Pastor, Coral Ridge Presbyterian Church, Fort Lauderdale, Florida; author, *One-Way Love: Inexhaustible Grace for an Exhausted World*

"Jared Wilson's new book is a punch in the gut. Gone are the tame, bedtime-story versions of the parables we've been told in the past. Instead, Wilson invites us to see them afresh with all of their explosive, imaginative power."

**Mike Cosper**, Pastor of Worship and Arts, Sojourn Community Church, Louisville, Kentucky

"In showing us the parables of Jesus for what they are (and are not), Jared Wilson invites us into a deeper understanding of their author and the kingdom he came to establish. *The Storytelling God* teaches us to read and reflect upon the parables with great care, and rightly so. The parables, and this book, point the way to life abundant."

**Scott McClellan,** Communications Pastor, Irving Bible Church, Irving, Texas; author, *Tell Me a Story: Finding God (and Ourselves) through Narrative*

"My own bookshelf has precious few commentaries on the parables and this will definitely fit nicely into that gap. In fact, this book is actually two books for the price of one. Part devotional commentary and also doubling as a solid gospel tract. This book serves the gospel straight up on a plate. His chapter commenting on the gospel and the poor is worth the price of the book alone. Clear, straightforward, biblical, gospel-centered writing. Definitely recommended reading."

**Mez McConnell,** Senior Pastor, Niddrie Community Church, Edinburgh; Director, 20schemes

"With a characteristic combination of wit and wisdom—humor and sobriety—Wilson grabs your attention, fixes it upon Christ, and keeps it there for the duration of the book. Readers in search of a pastoral introduction to biblical parables that is rich with real-life applicability can gladly make room for this volume on their bookshelf."

**Stephen T. Um,** Senior Minister, Citylife Presbyterian Church, Boston, Massachusetts; author, *Why Cities Matter*

# THE STORYTELLING GOD

# THE STORYTELLING GOD

## Seeing the Glory of Jesus in His Parables

**Jared C. Wilson**

CROSSWAY
WHEATON, ILLINOIS

*The Storytelling God: Seeing the Glory of Jesus in His Parables*



Published by Crossway
1300 Crescent Street
Wheaton, Illinois 60187



Cover design: Faceout Studio, www.faceoutstudio.com

First printing 2014

Printed in the United States of America



Trade paperback ISBN: 978-1-4335-3668-7
ePub ISBN: 978-1-4335-3671-7
PDF ISBN: 978-1-4335-3669-4
Mobipocket ISBN: 978-1-4335-3670-0

**Library of Congress Cataloging-in-Publication Data**

Wilson, Jared C., 1975–
The storytelling God : seeing the glory of Jesus in his Parables / Jared C. Wilson.
pages cm.
Includes bibliographical references and index.
ISBN 978-1-4335-3668-7
1. Jesus Christ—Parables. I. Title.
BT375.3.W55 2014
226.8'06—dc23 2013026734

Crossway is a publishing ministry of Good News Publishers.

VP 24 23 22 21 20 19 18 17 16 15 14
15 14 13 12 11 10 9 8 7 6 5 4 3 2 1

To David McLemore,
who has helped me love Jesus
more deeply

"Christianity is the story of how the rightful king has landed, you might say landed in disguise, and is calling us all to take part in a great campaign of sabotage."

—C. S. Lewis, *Mere Christianity*

# Contents

# Introduction

Throw away your Flannelgraphs. They are flat and soft, and the story of Jesus is neither.

I don't remember the day I sat down to read the Sermon on the Mount for the umpteenth time (it was about ten years ago), but I do remember the distinct feeling that I was really reading it for the first time. I felt gut-punched and mind-blown. The text had not changed, but certainly *something* had. The words I'd been reading since I was old enough to read were finally familiar. And they scared me. I felt disturbed, interrupted. If the point of gospel ministry is to comfort the afflicted and afflict the comfortable, I counted myself at that time in the latter camp.

Matthew 5:8, the sixth of the Beatitudes, is a good example: "Blessed are the pure in heart, for they shall see God." Jesus isn't saying anything new, really, since this promise of blessing echoes King David's statement in Psalm 24:3–4. I don't know if it really had registered with me before that day what having a pure heart entailed, but it most certainly struck me that my heart was not pure. It is frustratingly difficult to keep it pure. I don't even have to think about thinking impurely—I just do. So when I read that the pure in heart are the ones who get to see God, I freak out a little. Okay, I freak out *a lot*. If purity of heart is the standard, how will I ever get to see God? And is there any passage of Scripture scarier than Matthew 7:21–23?

> Not everyone who says to me, "Lord, Lord," will enter the kingdom of heaven, but the one who does the will of my

> Father who is in heaven. On that day many will say to me, "Lord, Lord, did we not prophesy in your name, and cast out demons in your name, and do many mighty works in your name?" And then will I declare to them, "I never knew you; depart from me, you workers of lawlessness."

These words push me to the end of myself, driving me back to the first word, the first beatitude in Matthew 5:3: "Blessed are the poor in spirit, for theirs is the kingdom of heaven." Matthew 5:8 shows me the depths of my poverty; Matthew 5:3 shows me the riches that await me upon this realization, upon my owning of it as the truth about myself. The afflicted receives comfort.

The rest of the Sermon on the Mount is like that, too, constantly revealing God's standard of living—the blueprint for what his kingdom on earth looks like lived out—and constantly driving us back to Jesus in desperation for this kingdom in spite of ourselves.

Actually, all of Jesus's teaching is like this, including the parables. When these oft-repeated stories from Jesus strike us as sweet, heartwarming, or inspiring in the sentimental sense rather than the Spiritual sense, we can be sure we've misread them. A generation of churchgoers grew up hearing the parables taught more along the lines of moralistic fables—illustrations of how to do the right things God would have us do. And they are that. But they are more than that. Some of these narratives are only a few lines long, but every parable, long or short, is fathoms deep and designed to drive us to Jesus in awe, need, faith, and worship. When we treat them as "inspiring tales," we make superficially insipid what ought to be Spiritually incisive.

In Matthew 13, after a barrage of parables, we are told that Jesus "said nothing to them without a parable" (v. 34) and that this approach fulfilled the prophecy of Psalm 78:2: "I will open my mouth in parables; I will utter what has been hidden since the foundation of the world" (Matt. 13:35). When Jesus teaches a parable, he is not opening up "Chicken Soup for the Soul" or a fortune cookie but a window to the hidden heavenlies. He is revealing a glimpse of eternity crashing into time, a flash photo of his own wisdom brought to bear. The parables give us a direct portal to the kingdom of God being done on earth as it is in heaven. "Indeed," Edward Armstrong writes, "they are sparks from that fire which our Lord brought to the earth."[1]

The parables are in some sense the truer and better editions of Ransom of *Perelandra*'s appraisal of the ancient myths: "gleams of celestial strength and beauty falling on a jungle of filth and imbecility."[2] And just as the ancient myths point in their falsehoods to the Myth that is fact, the parables in all their earthiness and everydayness point in their truisms to him who is called True (Rev. 19:11). In other words, the parables don't just tell us about the true ways of life but shine into darkened hearts the way, the truth, and the life (see John 14:6).

The word *parable* from the Greek means "to cast alongside," and like the seeds cast in one of the few parables for which Jesus offered an interpretation, the parables may land on rocky soil. It is there that they are often softened for duller spiritual senses, when it is the senses that ought to be softened instead. I'll say more about that in the first chapter. For now, though, it is enough to say that the parables are designed to stir those whose antennae are tuned to their frequencies, and to confound those whose antennae are not.

Because the real-life and common scenarios of the parables belie their otherworldly power, it is imperative that we continue to click "refresh" on our familiarity with them. I hope this book will help with that. It's possible for familiarity to breed apathy or numbness if we come to Jesus's stories in lackadaisical, unexpectant, unsubmissive ways. Instead, let us come again and again to the "old, old story" of Jesus and his love and behold his power freshly, ever-newly.

[1] Edward A. Armstrong, *The Gospel Parables* (London: Hodder & Stoughton, 1967), 11; quoted in Vernon D. Doerksen, "The Interpretation of Parables" in *Grace Theological Journal* 11.2 (1970): 3–20.
[2] C. S. Lewis, *Perelandra* (New York: Macmillan, 1965), 201.

No, the parables are not flat felt. They are white-hot sparks. And if the parables are sparks, let us scatter them far and wide. May they set our vision for Christ's kingdom afire, and may our teaching of these stories be torch-wielding, our sharing of their gospel nucleus be an illumination of the light of the world, that he who is the radiance of God's glory might cover the very earth the parables put in their crosshairs, like the waters cover the sea.

1

# Postcards from the Revolution

The Gospel of Luke shows us that Jesus began his public ministry in an instance of brilliant audacity. He went to church on the Sabbath like a good Jew, proclaimed the coming of the Lord's favor according to the prophet Isaiah like a good preacher, and then, stunningly, in essence said, "This prophecy is about me" like a good instigator. The congregation was stirred, pleased. Who wouldn't want to hear that the prophecy of Isaiah 61 was being fulfilled? They "all spoke well of him" and found his proclamation "gracious" (Luke 4:22).

But the tide turns. As so often is the case throughout the Gospels, the crowd attracted to Jesus becomes the crowd crying for his blood. What happened? Jesus finished his self-centered sermon and sat down among them. Maybe that's what did it. He should have drawn a sword or issued an altar call. Instead he took a seat.

"Wait a minute. Isn't this Joseph's kid?" someone says.

Hearing their murmuring, Jesus adds a coda from the pews:

> "Doubtless you will quote to me this proverb, 'Physician, heal yourself.' What we have heard you did at Capernaum, do here in your hometown as well." And he said, "Truly, I say to you, no prophet is acceptable in his hometown. But in truth, I tell

> you, there were many widows in Israel in the days of Elijah, when the heavens were shut up three years and six months, and a great famine came over all the land, and Elijah was sent to none of them but only to Zarephath, in the land of Sidon, to a woman who was a widow. And there were many lepers in Israel in the time of the prophet Elisha, and none of them was cleansed, but only Naaman the Syrian." (Luke 4:23–27)

What happens next is one of the quickest mood shifts in the history of mood shifts. The crowd that had been marveling, that had been struck with the impression of grace, "were filled with wrath" (v. 28). Instead of shaking his hand at the narthex door, they drive him out of it. Right out to a cliff, ready to throw him off.

Now, I have preached some bad sermons in my day (and have plenty of bad sermons yet to preach), but none of my sermons—as far as I know—ever drove anyone to want me dead, still less to physically attack me. But if we are reading the text correctly, we will see it wasn't a bad sermon that stirred up wrath, but a good one. A very good one. It was the inauguration of the public ministry of the climactic good news itself, actually. But something in that addendum drove the point home in such a way that it drove its hearers to murderousness.

Jesus recalls the way God has preserved his people in the past by passing over the likely to minister in the nooks and crannies to the unlikely. In a nutshell, he is saying to his congregation, "You probably won't accept me. So this message is not for you. It's for widows and Syrians." This is what we might call a public dis-invitation. They don't teach this model in preaching classes at seminary. Some pastors work for years to perfect the art of the altar call. No one practices an altar refusal.

From the very beginning, Jesus insists that the kingdom is not for the healthy but the sick (Matt. 9:12). The prophecy itself makes this clear! Who is the gospel for, according to Luke 4 and Isaiah 61, but the poor, the brokenhearted, the captive, the mourner, and the faint? And if we may add in the preamble to Jesus's epic kingdom announcement, the Beatitudes introducing the Sermon on the Mount, we include the meek, the hungry, the thirsty, the pure, the merciful, and the peacemaking.

Jesus is turning something upside down, and for that the angry crowd wanted to turn *him* upside down.

But really Jesus is turning something right side up. And when we read the parables he employed to teach the crowds throughout his ministry, we could do a lot worse than to see them as narrative portraits of rebellion against rebellion. The rightful king has landed, and he is leading an insurrection against the pretenders to his throne.

As the crowd in Nazareth has Jesus between rocks and a high place, he calmly passes through them and walks away. Jesus, like the stories he told, didn't look like much, but the power of the eternal God was in there.

This story in Luke 4 illustrates something central about the illustrations we call the parables, namely, that they are not for everyone. Jesus's message of the day of the Lord's favor sounds wonderful . . . until he says it's only for certain people. He says a similar thing about the parables. On the one hand, this is counterintuitive because we think of the parables as "sermon illustrations" of a sort, stories designed to make Jesus's teaching plain and clear and easy to understand. But on the other hand, the way the parables actually function is *entirely* intuitive—which is to say, you either get them or you don't. More on that in a bit, but for now, let's pan out to see the larger context of Jesus's ministry. The parables can't be understood without it.

## The Gospel of the Kingdom

When Jesus, and John the Baptist before him, went about preaching that the kingdom of God (or "heaven," to use Matthew's circumlocution) was "at hand," they were clearly not saying the kingdom was coming thousands of years from then. They had no illustrated charts or infographics chronicling an eschatological timeline involving

Israeli statehood, Russian tanks, American Blackhawk helicopters, Swiss supercomputers with ominous nicknames, and UPC tattoos. They said, "It's here. It's arriving now." In Mark 1:15, Jesus seems as unequivocal as you can get: "The time is fulfilled, and the kingdom of God is at hand; repent and believe in the gospel."

This makes sense when we read back in Luke 4 that Jesus says, "Today this Scripture has been fulfilled in your hearing" (v. 21). Matthew summarizes the message of Jesus as "the gospel of the kingdom" (Matt. 4:23; 9:35).

The gospel of the kingdom is the announcement that Jesus the Messiah has arrived and has begun restoring God's will on earth in and through himself. The fulcrum upon which this restoration turns is Christ's substitutionary work in his sinless temptation, suffering, death on the cross, and resurrection from the grave.

Through Adam's disobedience, sin entered the human race, affecting human dominion and the environment. Look at all that is cursed in Genesis 3:14–19. If we cannot tell from the world itself that the whole place is messed up and we along with it, the truth is plain enough throughout all the narratives that make up the Bible. From the fall of mankind onward, the Scriptures show us the breakdown between man and God, man and man, and man and the created world. When Adam and Eve, deceived by the Serpent and driven by their prideful lusts, ate the forbidden fruit in the hopes of greater peace, the result was the diminishing of it. So the Old Testament portrays a broken world groaning under the weight of the consequences of its sin. But it also portrays the loving faithfulness of a holy God who will not let sin and the Serpent have the last word. Every new day the patriarchs are breaking covenant, and every new day God is keeping it.

The promise of vindication may come as early as Genesis 3:15, which casts a long shadow to the foot of the Messiah in the New Testament, pierced in crucifixion yet victorious *in the crucifixion* over the Serpent. After the four hundred years of silence that began at the closed door at the end of Malachi, God's people are ripe for redemption. Jesus's preaching ministry from top to bottom proclaims this inevitability and the purpose and effects thereof. In his incarnation he is the second Adam (Rom. 5:12–14), redeeming the human experience from the first Adam's failure. In his teaching he is Wisdom made manifest, fulfilling the Law and the Prophets and actually embodying what they foretold. In his miracles he is signaling the in-breaking of God's restorative kingdom. In his suffering and crucifixion he willingly submits to the wrath of God owed to true sinners and thereby satisfies the wages of sin and conquers its power. In his bodily, glorified resurrection he conquers the power of death and becomes the firstfruits (1 Cor. 15:22–24) of the promises like those in Psalm 16:9–10 and Job 19:26. Everything rad is coming true.

The kingdom is at hand because it is at Jesus's hands. In his ministry, from that first explosive sermon on that Sabbath day in Luke 4, it comes violently (Matt. 11:12).

But if the gospel Jesus and his disciples preached was the gospel of the kingdom, what *is* the kingdom, exactly?

Some may say that the kingdom is heaven, and in some sense it is, but too many who say this have in mind a celestial place of disembodied bliss, the place the Scriptures sometimes refer to as paradise. Matthew, as we have noted, speaks of "the kingdom of heaven" rather than "kingdom of God," but what is in view here is not some extraterrestrial, spiritual locale. Matthew's intended audience is Jewish, and because the name of God is unutterably sacred, he substitutes "heaven" where the other Gospels use "God." Therefore, Jesus was not really preaching that the location of paradise is "at hand," at least not in any material way. In any event, since God is omnipresent and the locale of paradise, whatever that locale *is*, is best thought of as the place where God is, heaven has in some sense always been at hand. For instance, heaven broke into earth in the temple religion of the Old Testament Israel. Heaven was "at hand" in the Most Holy Place. No, when Jesus preached the kingdom, he was not specifically talking about the place we often think of when we hear the word "heaven."

Some will say that the kingdom of God/heaven is the church. There is an element of truth in this as well, but it still will not do.

The church indeed cannot be prevailed against by the gates of hell (Matt. 16:18), which sounds a lot like the forecast of the kingdom in Daniel 2:44 (among other texts). But the kingdom and the church are distinguished in numerous places. In Luke 17:21, Jesus says that the kingdom is "in the midst of you," which makes little sense if the kingdom *is* you. It could be that Jesus is saying the kingdom is in the midst of you *plural*, you together, as in the body of believers. But when we read the descriptions of Jesus and his disciples preaching the gospel of the kingdom and hear the commands to the church to preach the kingdom, it ought to be clear that Jesus is not preaching "the church," still less that the church ought to be preaching itself. "For what we proclaim is not ourselves, but Jesus Christ as Lord" (2 Cor. 4:5).

The place heaven is not the kingdom, and the people called the church is not the kingdom, but the gospel of the kingdom of God tells us something about heaven and calls the church to do the telling. The kingdom is the manifest presence of God's reign. George Eldon Ladd puts it like this:

> When the word refers to God's Kingdom, it always refers to His reign, His rule, His sovereignty, and not to the realm in which it is exercised. Psalm 103:19, "The Lord has established his throne in the heavens, and his kingdom rules over all." God's kingdom, his *malkuth*, is His universal rule, His sovereignty over all the earth. . . . The Kingdom of God is His kingship, His rule, His authority. When this once is realized, we can go through the New Testament and find passage after passage where this meaning is evident, where the Kingdom is not a realm or a people but God's reign. Jesus said that we must "receive the kingdom of God" as little children (Mark 10:15). What is received? The Church? Heaven? What is received is God's rule. In order to enter the future realm of the Kingdom, one must submit himself in perfect trust to God's rule here and now.[1]

[1] George Eldon Ladd, *The Gospel of the Kingdom: Scriptural Studies in the Kingdom of God* (Grand Rapids, MI: Eerdmans, 1998), 20–21.

Again, there is some sense in which those who receive the kingdom "receive" the church and heaven, but those are the benefits of embracing the yoke of God's sovereignty, the implications of the gospel. What the gospel announces is that the God-man Jesus of Nazareth is doing the Messiah's work of tearing the veil between heaven and earth through his sinless life, sacrificial death, and glorious resurrection. He brings the manifest presence of God's reign into fallen mankind and broken creation. And since he is bringing this reign in and through himself as king, he is preaching himself.

The parables, then, serve this end: they proclaim, in their unique way, the gospel of the kingdom of God and Jesus as king of that kingdom. The glory of Christ is to be had in the parables, provided the parables are had at all.

But while the glory of God has been brought to bear in the reign of Christ in and through Jesus's ministry and atoning work, the effects of sin continue and the brokenness is still to be endured for the time being. Habakkuk 2:14 holds out a vision for the world's end that has God's glory covering the entire earth like the waters cover the sea—itself a parallel to the Revelation forecast of Jesus as the illuminating sun of the new heavens and the new earth. In the teachings of Paul and Peter, in the prophecies of John in Revelation, and in the teachings of Jesus himself, we understand that while God's kingdom is "at hand," it is also not fully here. We may say that Jesus Christ inaugurated the kingdom, but he has not yet consummated it. He will do this at his second coming. Therefore, a biblical understanding of the nature of the kingdom of God keeps in tension the reality that the kingdom is both "already" and "not yet." As we will see, the parables capture this tension as well.

## The Kingdom Story

God is the greatest storyteller ever. Our most brilliant, most captivating, most spellbinding authors have nothing on him. All good stories are but pale reflections and imitations of the great story of God's glory brought to bear in the world. The Bible is a book of books, a combination of stories that tell one larger story, and in the Bible we have the overarching and thoroughgoing added element that the story is true. Only God can write a myth that is at the same time historical, factual. Only God can write a biography that is at the same time a history of biographies to come, because God is the only creative person who is also omniscient. Only God can write a story that resonates not just in the power of the imagination or the heart or the mind, but in the very soul; only God can write a story that brings dead things to life. Only the word of God quickens, divides, heals, resurrects. The poetry, the history, the laws, the lists, the genealogies, the proverbs, and the prophecies together make up the mosaic of God's vision for the universe with himself at its center.

What is the grand story that God is telling? It begins with his triune self as the only eternal good and holy, and then moves to his creation of the world and the men and women in it, creatures specifically designed to glorify him and enjoy him forever. But as in every good story, there is a conflict, a crisis. Mankind seeks his own glory, his own enjoyment apart from the Creator, and the result is death. Wretched men that we are! Who will rescue us from this body of death? (see Rom. 7:24).

Every good story has a hero, and God himself is the unparalleled hero of his story. Since the story is about his glory, this only makes sense. So throughout the Old Testament narratives, we will see just how frail and stupid the "heroes of the faith" really are. Only a few escape their narratives without blemish, but even an upstanding man like Boaz has a prostitute for a mother. Abraham lies and finagles, Isaac capitulates and spoils, Jacob schemes and wrestles, Joseph is a gullible braggart, Moses stutters and stumbles, David lusts and backstabs, and the list goes on and on. Why? Because they're sinners. But also so that we will see the one who is true and faithful, the hero of the story, the real dragon-slayer between the lines, hidden in the shadows, biding his time until the moment he is pleased to come and instigate the story's eucatastrophe, the moment at which all heaven breaks loose.

While the Old Testament heroes fail and fumble forward, God promises judgment and vindication, the former to the unrepentant workers of wickedness and the latter to his covenant children. These are the two primary things we want in a good story when our hearts are right: justice and a happy ending (or at least the hint of one to come later). This double-edged dynamic recurs throughout many of Jesus's parables.

The Old Testament is fraught with warnings and brimming with promises. If you read it right, you will feel the anticipatory tension building all the way into the last chapter of the Old Testament, where we see these ominous and ecstatic words of prophecy:

> For behold, the day is coming, burning like an oven, when all the arrogant and all evildoers will be stubble. The day that is coming shall set them ablaze, says the LORD of hosts, so that it will leave them neither root nor branch. But for you who fear my name, the sun of righteousness shall rise with healing in its wings. You shall go out leaping like calves from the stall. And you shall tread down the wicked, for they will be ashes under the soles of your feet, on the day when I act, says the LORD of hosts. (Mal. 4:1–3)

There is the warning of justice and the promise of a happy ending wrapped into one teaser. And when this story closes, we can almost picture a "To Be Continued" title card appearing on the screen.

Every good story has a twist. In the true story that God tells about his glory brought to bear in the world, there are twists within twists. The really big twist is that God himself becomes the man who is the prophesied Messiah, rather than just anointing one more joker to add to the long line of jokers he's used throughout history. God is aiming at concluding the story and beginning a new one, and since only the pure in heart will see God (Ps. 24:3–4; Matt. 5:8) and there is no pure heart to be found under heaven (Rom. 3:12, 23), he does the job himself. This has been his plan from the beginning, hidden but evident in the ancient stories. When Jesus, beginning with Moses and all the Prophets, interpreted in all the Scriptures the things concerning himself to the disciples on the road to Emmaus (Luke 24:27), I like to think the burning they felt in their hearts was a magnified version of what I felt when Bruce Willis realized at the end of *The Sixth Sense* that he was dead. The movie flashes back to scene after scene leading up to this revelation, showing that the attentive viewer might have picked up on it at one of many points before the end. That's good storytelling.

The twist of the incarnation gives way to other surprises that should not be surprises at all. The Messiah does not immediately take up arms against the occupiers. He does not come riding in on a white horse. Instead, common, ordinary people take up palm branches and welcome him on a donkey (Matt. 21:1–11). This is his triumphal entry, and it was prophesied (Zech. 9:9). This is just one telegraphed surprise. Psalm 22 and Isaiah 53 project the crucifixion, but this part takes the disciples by surprise too. The resurrection is deepest in the shadows of the Old Testament, so it is the biggest surprise.

Paul later writes this about Jesus's victory over death:

> But in fact Christ has been raised from the dead, the firstfruits of those who have fallen asleep. For as by a man came death, by a man has come also the resurrection of the dead. For as in Adam all die, so also in Christ shall all be made alive. But each in his own order: Christ the firstfruits, then at his coming those who belong to Christ. Then comes the end, when he delivers the kingdom to God the Father after destroying every rule and every authority and power. For he must reign until he has put all his enemies under his feet. The last enemy to be destroyed is death. (1 Cor. 15:20–26)

This is just an excerpt from an epic chapter about the gospel (see vv. 3–4) and its beautiful fallout, but it declares the veracity of Jesus's resurrection, reveals that its power is the ongoing power to do the same for the dead in Christ someday, and captures all of this wonderfulness within the proclamation of Jesus's kingship. The passage also shows us the "already" and the "not yet" of the kingdom of God, affirming Christ's present reign and yet confirming that there is an all-encompassing revelation of this reign still to come.

In the story that God is telling the world, the resurrection was the turning point in his plan to execute justice and work a happy ending, but the resolution remains to be watched for. Let us sit on the edge of our seats. The historical work of Christ's resurrection tells death that its days are numbered. The resurrection activates the Christian's power over death. And someday death will be totally destroyed.

Then the next story will begin. The Scripture's vision of the second coming of Christ, upon which occasion mankind will be judged, the spiritually dead consigned to eternal condemnation and the dead in Christ raised to resurrection life, and when the new heavens and new earth will subsume the cursed land, is glorious.

It is this epic kingdom story that Jesus's little puzzle-stories distill.

## What Are the Parables?

There are two errors readers of the Bible make most often about the parables of Jesus, each a pendulum swing away from the other. The first error is to believe that the parables are simplistic religious illustrations, almost spiritual folktales. In this erroneous reading, the parables are read superficially, as moral lessons. The parables are of course fairly simple up there at the surface—some of them simpler than others—and there are clear moral lessons in the stories. But the parables are more complex than that. On the other hand, there is another school of thought, equally erroneous, that would have readers poring over the parables as if they were some kind of Magic Eye hidden-picture painting. It is definitely possible to *over*think the parables, by which I mean to read them with too much speculative scrutiny, ransacking every point and detail for every possible meaning it may have locked up, squeezing symbols out of symbols, bypassing the primary intent of the story for some imaginative concoction of biblical connections.

The way some people read the parables reminds me of Aesop's Fables. And the way others read them reminds me of the way some discern clue after perplexing clue in their Beatles albums as evidence for a cover-up of Paul's having died in a car accident.

The parables are simple and complex, but they are not simple and complex *like that*.

The parables are also not allegories—at least not in the normal literary sense. Allegory is a form of literature in which material figures represent immaterial virtues or vices. So in Bunyan's *Pilgrim's Progress*, the character Timorous represents fear and Mr. Worldly Wiseman represents worldly wisdom. In our day, distinction of genres has been muddled a bit, so we tend to regard any story with symbolic elements in it as allegorical, but it was not always this way. C. S. Lewis's *Chronicles of Narnia*, for instance, are not allegories, even though they often are referred to as such, and Lewis himself said as much. If Aslan was symbolic for the virtue of sacrifice or some such thing, he would be allegorical, but Aslan is a material figure (a lion, in this case) who represents another material figure (Jesus), and in fact, Aslan in the stories isn't meant to symbolize Jesus so much as to *be* Jesus, except manifested in a different form in that alternate world.

The parables of Jesus could be said to contain allegorical elements, some more than others, but they are not themselves allegories, strictly speaking. While we could say the characters in the parables represent certain virtues or vices—the good Samaritan could represent compassion or mercy, for instance, or the older brother in the prodigal son story could represent legalism or pride—they more directly represent certain kinds of people. Jesus definitely deals in the world of virtues and vices, but he is most immediately interested in the world of human beings, their hearts, their words, and their deeds.

It is common also for people to refer to the parables as "sermon illustrations." I have heard this explanation employed in the defense of using creative elements in a worship service, of using spectacles and production to attract people to church, and even in defense of abandoning the ministry of proclamational preaching. Jesus told stories, so the reasoning goes, in order to illustrate, to explain, and to clarify.

As in the allegorical approach, there is some truth to this understanding of the parables. There are real senses in which the parables illustrate, explain, and clarify. But if the parables are really analogous to what we today call "sermon illustrations," then Jesus was a terrible teacher, because the disciples kept saying they didn't understand them. If you have to explain your illustration—to decode it, as it were—it's not a very good illustration. Or at least, it's not functioning the way a sermon illustration is typically supposed to function. As we will soon see, the parables are designed to obscure as much as to clarify. This is not what preachers and teachers aim to do with illustrations.

Now we know some of the things the parables *aren't*. So what are they?

Robert Stein says it's nearly impossible to define *parable*.[2] That Jesus tells a variety of parables—some involving characters and others not, some offering positive examples and others negative, some sounding more like proverbs or similes than stories with a narrative—makes it somewhat difficult to nail down precisely what a parable is. One common definition is that a parable is "an earthly story with a heavenly meaning," and that is true as far as it goes, but it doesn't go far enough, since the parable of the rich man and Lazarus appears to be a "heavenly story with a hellish meaning."

If we uncover the Greek tradition behind the word *parable*, we could say that a parable is a short story, allowing that some of these stories are unconventional, more like vignettes or sketches. But if we go to the Hebrew tradition, from which Jesus would have been drawing more deeply in his ministry anyway, we learn that the Hebrew word for parable is rooted in *mashal*, which essentially

[2] Robert H. Stein, *The Method and Message of Jesus' Teaching* (Philadelphia: Westminster, 1978), 39.

means "proverb." This root grounds a more versatile definition for *parable* and appears to best fit the multifaceted approach of Jesus to parable-telling. In the Old Testament we find that proverbs, stories, riddles, and similes are all identified with the word *mashal*. A *mashal* is an illustration of wisdom.

With this background in mind, Jesus's parables, briefly put, are wisdom scenes. But despite their common settings and scenarios, these aren't scenes of common wisdom. Jesus was not just throwing out some homespun tales of cleverness and ingenuity. The parables function in Jesus's ministry as representative stories about the kingdom of God.

Overthinking the parables can take us far afield of the immediate impact they mean to make. I know a fellow whose meticulously constructed parable interpretation code locks in leaven/yeast as always referring to sin, which reveals he has not been meticulous enough, considering that Matthew 13:33's parable tells us that the kingdom of heaven is like leaven. Overthinking has also caused many a headache with regard to the parable of the persistent widow (Luke 18:1–8) and the parable of the dishonest manager (Luke 16:1–10).

Parables are illustrations meant to run alongside their points and reveal them in rather immediate ways. In other words, if you are deciphering in the parable of the prodigal son that the pigs symbolize one thing, the feast another, the table the feast is served on still another, the robe placed on the son yet another, and so on, you have likely gone too deep to see the immediate point—that Jesus has come for sinners. There are other points the prodigal son story makes, but that is the main one.

Nearly every one of Jesus's parables has one primary point. Some have only one point. Others have one main point with one or two secondary points. Some have one or two equally primary points. Craig Blomberg has argued fairly convincingly that most of the parables feature one point per character.[3]

In any event, the parables aren't literary scavenger hunts. Med-

[3] Craig L. Blomberg, *Interpreting the Parables* (Downer's Grove, IL: InterVarsity Press, 1990).

itation on them will reveal previously unnoticed nuances, but they are designed to showcase their central truth right away to those ready to hear it.

We have had a framed print of Rembrandt's masterpiece *The Return of the Prodigal Son* in our home for about ten years now. It hung over our mantel in our house in Nashville and now hangs prominently over my writing desk in our house in Vermont. I never get tired of looking at this work of art because I always notice something new. At first glance, it doesn't seem to contain much detail. At first glance, the focal point seems to be the only point. There in the foreground, illuminated by some mysteriously focused light, is the repentant son on his knees before his compassionate father, his face pressed into the paternal bosom. This is the main point of the painting and the main point of the parable. To the returned son's right stands his older brother, arms crossed. He is also illuminated, since in the story his role is prominent. In the darkness of the background are other figures. Who are they? Over the years I have discovered new things about the painting. I never noticed, for instance, that one of the father's hands looks more feminine than the other. I didn't notice for a long time that the prodigal son had what appears to be a scabbard on his belt. Is there a dagger in it or not? In the upper left of the painting there appears to be a feminine figure standing in a doorway. Is this the mother, not mentioned in Jesus's parable? A sister? Just a servant? These are all interesting details, just as there are interesting details of varying significance in the biblical parable, but the main point is right there in the light—the father welcomes his "sinful" son with the same love as he has for his "righteous" son, and in fact this story (and painting) turns the assumed perspective of the sinful and the righteous inside out, as does the parable of the good Samaritan.

## What Do the Parables Do?

The parables are wisdom scenes. But what wisdom are they picturing, and what are they revealing in this picturing?

Jesus is the embodiment of the wisdom of God—he is the Word of God—so at their center, the wisdom scenes of the parables picture the centrality and supremacy of Christ. But they come at this central proclamation in a variety of ways, revealing different applications and implications of Christ's lordship. The parables, in fact, give us peeks behind the veil between earth and the place where God's will is most manifest; they show us glimpses of the day when that veil is torn and that world conquers and integrates with this one.

Blomberg writes,

> The central theme uniting all of the lessons of the parables is the kingdom of God. It is both present and future. It includes both a reign and a realm. It involves both personal transformation and social reform. It is not to be equated either with Israel or the church, but is the dynamic power of God's personal revelation of himself in creating a human community of those who serve Jesus in every area of their lives.[4]

The parables show us that the kingdom of the "gospel of the kingdom" is God's reign over all creation, not just part of it. So in the parables we see the effect of God's reign and the expanse of it too. These gospel stories provide glimpses of what God's reign will look like.

Basically, the parables show us what "your kingdom come, your will be done, on earth as it is in heaven" (Matt. 6:10) *looks like*. Jesus did the same thing with his teaching in the Sermon on the Mount. Those aren't stories, of course, but direct proclamations, but the aim is the same—to reveal what the kingdom of God, brought to bear in creation, is and does. Since the fall, the way of the world has been to destruction. We all like sheep have gone astray, obeying the lusts of the flesh and worshiping the god of our bellies, following the prince of the power of the air, and dutifully slouching toward hell along with the conveyor-belt system

[4] Ibid., 326.

of "the world." Our hearts are idol factories, and we spend every moment apart from Christ on the assembly line exceeding quota. The parables, though, show us how Christ-centeredness rebukes, subverts, and sabotages the sinful kingdoms of the world.

This revolutionary work begins with the Spirit's quickening of dead hearts to receive the treasure of Christ through the open hand of faith. Until that point, the kingdom of God is a puzzling thing, a ridiculous thing, a repulsive thing. In Luke 8:10, Jesus says that the parables confound those who are not privy to "the secrets of the kingdom of God." There we see a vital connection between the parables and that mysterious, Spiritual wisdom they represent. But we also see a vital truth about how these stories of Jesus work, or don't work, in the hearts of those who hear them.

### How Do the Parables Work?

Someone once wrote film critic Roger Ebert and asked him why critics loved Sofia Coppola's film *Lost in Translation* so much while audiences in general didn't appreciate it. Ebert responded that the film transmitted on a different frequency than audiences are accustomed to receiving. I was reminded of this tidbit from Ebert's "Movie Answer Man" column only a couple of days later while overhearing a conversation in a restaurant in which two men discussing the movie revealed no hints of even knowing what it was about.

Is it true that some works of art are broadcasting on frequencies of understanding and appreciation that only certain readers, hearers, and viewers are tuned to receive? I think so. And I think this hypothesis about the subjective reception of and appreciation for creative works reveals a deeper truth about how the parables of Jesus function.

On the level of direct readership, any person of average intelligence can interpret the parables. The disciples appeared to fumble with the meaning while on the immediate scene, but with the benefit of centuries of hindsight and the completion of the biblical canon, it doesn't take a J. I. Packer to make heads or tails of basic parabolic interpretation.

We can start by looking at the context. Some of the parables come as responses to specific questions asked of Jesus. So the questions help us decipher the answer. To whom is Jesus talking? What predicament are those people in? Some parables conclude with an explanatory note, a "then" to the parable's "if." Jesus often helps his hearers out by connecting the dots for them, as in the parable of the man who built his house on the rock, for instance (Matt. 7:24–27). But when he doesn't make the meaning explicit, we can look for other contextual clues.

How does the parable end? Most of the parables have a climax or "end stress." What is stressed at the end? That is usually the central point of the parable, whatever else may precede it.

With what teaching content or narrative scenes does the Gospel writer surround the parable? Is there a connection there?

These are all basic principles for understanding the immediate point(s) of a parable of Jesus. But the immediacy of the parables is something more potent than mere cognitive understanding. The parables, as the wisdom of God, are aimed not only at the mind but also at the heart. And since the parables preach the gospel of the kingdom—like the gospel itself—they are not taken to heart by everyone who hears them. Paul writes,

> The natural person does not accept the things of the Spirit of God, for they are folly to him, and he is not able to understand them because they are spiritually discerned. (1 Cor. 2:14)

This difficult truth is in full effect when it comes to the parables, and Jesus illustrates this truth about parables (and the gospel of the kingdom in general) *with* a parable!

> And when a great crowd was gathering and people from town after town came to him, he said in a parable, "A sower went out to sow his seed. And as he sowed, some fell along the

> path and was trampled underfoot, and the birds of the air devoured it. And some fell on the rock, and as it grew up, it withered away, because it had no moisture. And some fell among thorns, and the thorns grew up with it and choked it. And some fell into good soil and grew and yielded a hundredfold." As he said these things, he called out, "He who has ears to hear, let him hear." (Luke 8:4–8)

That concluding admonition is another clue to how the parable works. Those who have the ears to hear will hear the story. In other words, the "natural man" won't be able to understand the power of the parable, but the Spiritually abled person will. He has been given the ears to hear it.

Simon Kistemaker puts its simply:

> When we hear a parable, we nod in agreement because the story is true to life and readily understood. Although the application of the parable may be heard, it is not always grasped. We see the story unfold before our eyes, but we do not perceive the significance of it. The truth remains hidden until our eyes are opened and we see clearly. Then the new lesson of the parable becomes meaningful.[5]

The parable of the sower is one of the few parables that Jesus took the time to interpret for his disciples:

> Now the parable is this: The seed is the word of God. The ones along the path are those who have heard; then the devil comes and takes away the word from their hearts, so that they may not believe and be saved. And the ones on the rock are those who, when they hear the word, receive it with joy. But these have no root; they believe for a while, and in time of testing fall away. And as for what fell among the thorns, they are those who hear, but as they go on their way they are choked by the cares and riches and pleasures of life, and their fruit

[5] Simon J. Kistemaker, *The Parables: Understanding the Stories Jesus Told* (Grand Rapids, MI: Baker, 2002), 9.

> does not mature. As for that in the good soil, they are those who, hearing the word, hold it fast in an honest and good heart, and bear fruit with patience. (Luke 8:11–15)

We will come back to this parable for a closer look later on, but for now what we see in Jesus's interpretation of the story is that the message gets shared everywhere without distinction, but only good soil receives the seed in such a way as to bear fruit. In the same way, the parables need the good soil of a Spiritually enlightened heart to take root.

Since the parables themselves come from the mouth of Christ, they contain the power to open eyes and ears to behold what they reveal. "Faith comes from hearing, and hearing through the word of Christ" (Rom. 10:17), and this Spiritual truth is no less in effect in Jesus's telling of stories. The parables in their power enlighten the elect to understand the parables in their content.

At the same time, the parables that illuminate themselves to the effectually called obscure themselves to those spiritually darkened. The same sun that melts the ice, as they say, hardens the clay. Jesus says as much himself:

> Then the disciples came and said to him, "Why do you speak to them in parables?" And he answered them, "To you it has been given to know the secrets of the kingdom of heaven, but to them it has not been given. . . . This is why I speak to them in parables, because seeing they do not see, and hearing they do not hear, nor do they understand. Indeed, in their case the prophecy of Isaiah is fulfilled that says:
>
> > "'"You will indeed hear but never understand,
> > and you will indeed see but never perceive."
> > For this people's heart has grown dull,
> > and with their ears they can barely hear,
> > and their eyes they have closed,
> > lest they should see with their eyes
> > and hear with their ears

> and understand with their heart
> and turn, and I would heal them.'
>
> But blessed are your eyes, for they see, and your ears, for they hear. (Matt. 13:10–11, 13–16)

Is Jesus actually saying he speaks in parables to make sure that people won't hear or see the truth of the kingdom? Yes.

Again, if the parables are meant to be one-to-one analogous to sermon illustrations, they make a terrible job of it, since they are designed to simultaneously bless the Spiritually sensitive and confound the dull. This should not shock us, as we see it played out constantly in the life of the church today. The beauty of Christ and his gospel continues to captivate millions of believers all over the world and drive them to passionate worship while it simultaneously disgusts, angers, or bores millions of others.

I continue to remind myself of the Spiritual prerogative behind a sinner's response to the gospel every time I share it with someone. Sometimes a man's response to the gospel of the kingdom looks like when Tom Hanks "discovers" fire in *Cast Away*. Other times it looks like the guy in *Office Space* when his supervisor asks him about the TPS reports. "For the word of the cross is folly to those who are perishing, but to us who are being saved it is the power of God" (1 Cor. 1:18). The day of the Lord's favor is a new dawn to widows and lepers, but to the self-centered, self-righteous rabble, it's just any old day. The parables are just any old stories to some, but they are smart bombs of glory to others.

The parables are postcards from heaven. "Wish you were here," they say. Supernaturally, however, they can transport us exactly to the place they depict, the place where God's kingdom is coming and his will is being done on earth as it is in heaven. As Jesus conducts his kingdom ministry, he lays these stories on thick, seeding the alien nation of God with rumors of that other world, casting shadows of the realer reality like the flickering images on the walls of Plato's cave.

As we survey the parables of Jesus in this book, I hope you will be praying along with me that God would open the eyes of our hearts to behold the one who is the radiance of his glory. These earthy stories are awash in Christ's glory. Let us steep in them, meditate on them, lay them to heart.

Once upon a time, a king came to earth to tell stories, and the stories contained the mystery of eternal life.

2

# A Radical Refocus

Over the first three years of my pastorate at our church in Vermont, I had undertaken the task of ensuring the accuracy of our membership rolls. The existing membership list had not been updated in many years. There were many people on the list who had moved or died, or had simply stopped attending the church, in some cases decades ago. I sent out letters to the inactive members I could reach, encouraging them to revisit with me their interest in membership so that we could discuss their long absence, as well as the church's statement of faith and membership covenant. I was not surprised, honestly, that the nature of this contact irritated a few recipients of the letter. What I found both funny and sad at the same time were those who said in response that they would now withhold money they had planned to give the church in the event of their death. If they couldn't be a member, they reasoned, they weren't going to support the church.

I found it odd that these folks could not see the logic at work in saying that someone who hadn't participated in church life in years, who had shown no interest in supporting the church in any other way, and who had been grumbling about the church's very existence probably wasn't an ideal candidate for membership. Further, I don't suppose it occurred to any of these people that the church doesn't really care about their money. In their minds, withholding some (dubious) financial endowment was thought to be a great punishment. What they didn't understand is that we don't care about their money. We don't want their money. We want them to have our Jesus!

The ex-members picking up their piggy banks and going home were spitefully attempting a sort of blackmail; it is the way of the world to assume that justification is bought by the leveraging of worldly treasures. But it is the way of the kingdom to stay tuned to eternity.

In turning everything right side up, Jesus is putting a great many things upside down. As we survey his message and ministry in the four Gospels, we learn that he is constantly subverting values and expectations, and yet he is simultaneously fulfilling the essence of the desires at the root of these values and expectations.

The Jews of Jesus's day expected Messiah to storm the castle, so to speak, and cast out the oppressors. Jesus's eschewing of a militaristic messianism was most assuredly a continual head-scratcher for such people. And yet he was in fact overthrowing the government. He was in fact subverting the powers and principalities. As he cast out demons and put the authorities to shame (even on the cross, an alleged defeat), he was proving that the government was on his shoulders (see Isa. 9:6). So-called spiritual meanings and fulfillments are not less real than literal meanings and fulfillments; they are more real. When the Son sets a man free, he is really free. Even if he's in prison. The apostle Paul certainly thought so, which was why he sang praises while in shackles and said beautifully frustrating things like, "To live is Christ, and to die is gain" (Phil. 1:21).

Paul was a spiritually free man, which meant the powers oppressing him likely could not figure out what to do with him. What do you make of a guy who believes living or dying means the same thing—union with Christ? If he lived, he had Christ. If he died, he had Christ. Indeed, Paul reckoned himself already dead to the world and alive to Christ (Gal. 6:14), so he had put all his eggs in the basket of John 11:25. He had totally abandoned himself to the sovereignty of God, having found Christ of surpassing worth compared to anything and everything else.

## What Is Supremely Valuable?

Like Paul, if we have found Christ's work reframing our understanding of life and death, certainly everything else must be reevaluated as well. And one of these important areas of reevaluation is the concept of treasure. What is it that we really value? What is of supreme worth? What is the currency of the kingdom? Using the language of the world's values, Jesus helps us see what is supremely valuable:

> The kingdom of heaven is like treasure hidden in a field, which a man found and covered up. Then in his joy he goes and sells all that he has and buys that field. Again, the kingdom of heaven is like a merchant in search of fine pearls, who, on finding one pearl of great value, went and sold all that he had and bought it. (Matt. 13:44–46)

How do we know that the treasure and the pearl in these short companion parables are of supreme value? Because in the first, the man sells everything else he owns in order to buy the whole field. Don't get bogged down in the detail about his covering up the treasure. This does not correspond to anything we ought to do in terms of obscuring or hiding the kingdom but is just an indication of how precious the treasure was for him. He was so zealous for ownership that he was trying to make sure it would still be there when he came back. I do this in a store when I want the last of a certain item but can't buy it at the moment. Ever stick a shirt on a different rack so it won't be snatched up before you can come back and claim it? Similar concept. Jesus isn't telling us we need to cover up the kingdom. He's just showing us that our behavior should reflect how valuable it is to us. "For where your treasure is, there your heart will be also" (Matt. 6:21).

The merchant also shows how valuable this particular pearl is by selling everything he has in order to purchase it. In the first parable, we do not know if the man was searching for treasure or not. It may be that he simply stumbled upon it while working the field or walking across it. In the second parable, we see that the merchant's job was looking for valuable pearls. Finding that one pearl of supreme value put an end to all his searching. He sold all in his inventory in order to buy it.

This is like the kingdom, Jesus says. You may not be looking for Jesus and his kingdom at all. Or you may be a seeker of some kind, constantly trying out new philosophies and religions. My friend Jeff was like the merchant. In his youth he was always on the lookout for the meaning to the universe. He tried out various spiritualities, all in a sincere attempt to find fulfillment for his aching heart and a reason to live. From LSD to Buddhism to homegrown religious cults, he invested in a lot of searching—until he heard the words of Jesus in the Sermon on the Mount and was compelled to sell everything he had in order to gain Christ. He gave his heart to the Lord and never looked back. His searching was done.

But whether you're looking for it or not, it is the kingdom that really does the finding. And once we've been found by it, we're willing to lose all for it. That is how valuable it is. If we have Christ and his kingdom, we have all that matters.

The logic of this upending of values is not plain to many. No doubt the fellow selling all his pearls looked a little foolish to those who did not understand the value of the one pearl he'd found. Similarly, the man selling all his stuff to buy a field might have looked silly to those who had no idea a treasure was hidden there. And so in the two thousand years since the kingdom's inauguration, those who have given up worldly treasures left and right to walk the narrow path after Jesus have been viewed as crazy or stupid or both. Nonbelievers cannot see the value; therefore, they cannot see the logic. They do not realize that what looks foolish is actually very, very wise! R. T. Kendall writes,

> The interesting thing is, it is possible to lose your head and keep it at the same time! You lose your head in your joy in knowing God and don't care if people think you are crazy. Yet you are probably at your sanest when you come to the place

> where you abandon all else but your desire for God. Once you have truly experienced the anointing of the Spirit, your money, reputation, love for the world, fear of what people will say and so on all pale into insignificance.[1]

## The Contrast of Glory

It is not possible that the Bible is against wealth per se, since it speaks favorably of it in numerous places.[2] What the Bible is against is greed, materialism, injustice, and miserliness—thus all the reminders that wealth is fleeting, that trusting in it is vanity, and thus all the dire warnings to the wealthy, including the difficult command to the rich young ruler to sell everything he had and give it to the poor. What the Bible is against is treating wealth—or any other temporal thing—as our treasure.

When Zacchaeus gives half of his stuff to the poor and repays fourfold what he has defrauded others of, he is not showing that money is bad but that salvation in Christ is infinitely better. He shows us the truth many don't see until they really see: when you see the kingdom as precious, you see lesser treasures as dingy. The sheen is off. "Do not lay up for yourselves treasures on earth," Jesus says (Matt. 6:19). This is easier to do when you can see the moths and oxidation in the sunlight of Christ's glory.

The pearl merchant did not sell all his inventory because he found one more pearl, but because he found the "be-all and end-all" of pearls. When Christ becomes our be-all and end-all, this sort of trade-off makes total sense. It is the contrast provided by captivation in Christ's glory, which is eternally rich and incomparably beautiful. When we really see Christ as our saving security, the loss of all else seems a worthy risk. Jairus was willing to risk his position in the synagogue to ask for Jesus's help with his dying daughter because he had been pushed, by his position of desperation, to consider what was truly valuable. The Philippian jailer took his prisoners to dinner, risking his position, because he had

[1] R. T. Kendall, *The Parables of Jesus* (Grand Rapids, MI: Chosen, 2006), 53.
[2] E.g., Deuteronomy 8:18; Proverbs 12:27; 13:11.

witnessed the liberating glory of Christ. Over and over again in the Old Testament, we see the patriarchs and the prophets leaving places of comfort and familiarity to risk life and limb out of faith in God's promises. Why? Because they had tasted and seen that the Lord is good. And a taste of God's goodness ruins you for worldly delicacies.

The apostle Paul had ample wealth stored up in success and achievements. He had all the merit badges and first place trophies. But once he'd seen the light of Christ, they looked like garbage:

> If anyone else thinks he has reason for confidence in the flesh, I have more: circumcised on the eighth day, of the people of Israel, of the tribe of Benjamin, a Hebrew of Hebrews; as to the law, a Pharisee; as to zeal, a persecutor of the church; as to righteousness under the law, blameless. But whatever gain I had, I counted as loss for the sake of Christ. Indeed, I count everything as loss because of the surpassing worth of knowing Christ Jesus my Lord. For his sake I have suffered the loss of all things and count them as rubbish, in order that I may gain Christ and be found in him . . . (Phil. 3:4–9)

The gospel of Jesus Christ solves the innate problem we have of "glory greed." We are, every one of us from birth, incompetent thieves of the glory that belongs only to God. We know in our insidest insides that we fall short of his glory, and so we are constantly clawing and scratching to make up that difference in some way. This is how all sin is fundamentally idolatry and how all accumulations of worldly treasures—be they material goods or religious merit—are fundamentally acts of self-worship. Then in the gospel of Christ, God forgives our petty theft, sets us free from the bondage of our idols, and unites us Spiritually, irrevocably, and satisfyingly to himself. Now the glory we tried to steal is shared with us freely, and it is real glory this time, not these pathetic knockoffs we think will do the trick. We tried to cover ourselves with fig leaves or with mud from the pigsty. Filthy rags, they are.

But Jesus knows we are starving for glory, knows we need covering, and rather than expose our shame, he clothes us with the finest coat there is—himself.

## The Glory of Christ in the Hidden Treasure and the Pearl of Great Price

"The kingdom of heaven is like treasure hidden in a field."

"The kingdom of heaven is like a merchant in search of fine pearls."

As we have seen, Matthew's "kingdom of heaven" is a circumlocution for "kingdom of God," seeking to avoid offense with his Jewish audience. The phrasing tells us something else important, however. It is not personal fulfillment or individual salvation that is like a treasure or a pearl of great price—it is "the kingdom." The kingdom is certainly not less than personal fulfillment and individual salvation, but it is most definitely more. And understanding this is essential to understanding what makes the treasure of Christ so surpassingly valuable. It is not simply forgiveness of sins and assurance of heaven that trusting in Christ brings—as wonderful and generous as those gifts are! It is so much more. "He who did not spare his own Son but gave him up for us all, how will he not also with him graciously give us all things?" (Rom. 8:32).

What we receive in receiving Christ is his kingdom. The manifest reign of God takes dominion in our hearts as it goes about subduing the entire earth. "I am making all things new," Jesus declares in Revelation 21:5. The richness of Christ's salvation for sinners in justification and sanctification and glorification is shaping them for the richness of the world to come. When we "get saved," we aren't just receiving the redemptive thing God is doing in our lives; we are also embracing the redemptive thing God is doing in the world. Having the eyes to see salvation in this way helps us to see worldly treasures as pitiful. It is the kingdom of heaven that is a treasure worth selling everything to own, because the kingdom of heaven covers everything and becomes our everything.

In these parables we find a vision of the gospel itself, and thus of Christ's glory. The Word of God, the second person of the Trinity, sharing the substance of the Father and the Spirit, set aside the glories of the riches of his heavenly throne to inhabit the flesh and blood of his creation. He did not regard his deity as something to be leveraged. He emptied himself. Jesus set his golden crown aside to take the thorns. And in releasing his grasp of his heavenly glory for a time, he takes our hand and delivers us with him back into his glory for all time. It is Jesus who has treasured the kingdom above all else. It is Jesus who has sold all he had to gain a greater greatness. It is Jesus who has bought the treasure of salvation by buying the whole field of creation. The parables reveal Jesus's glory because they are pictures of his denying himself and taking up the cross, which are the grounds of his exaltation by the Father (Phil. 2:9–11). It is by being named among the transgressors that Jesus is given the name that is above every name. He considered all things loss compared to the surpassing worth of the glory to be had when the mission was accomplished.

## Rich toward God

Again, the parables of the hidden treasure and the pearl of great price show us that the kingdom of God operates on a completely different currency than any other kingdom in the world. We see this truth prefaced by Jesus as he unfolds the great blueprint of the kingdom in his Sermon on the Mount. He instructs us to hold stuff loosely. If someone asks for your shirt, give him your coat too. Give and lend to whoever asks. These are clearly not ways to become rich . . . unless the reward we have in mind is not monetary.

Consider a complementary parable, that of the rich fool:

> Someone in the crowd said to him, "Teacher, tell my brother to divide the inheritance with me." But he said to him, "Man, who made me a judge or arbitrator over you?" And he said to them, "Take care, and be on your guard against all covetousness, for one's life does not consist in the abundance of his

> possessions." And he told them a parable, saying, "The land of a rich man produced plentifully, and he thought to himself, 'What shall I do, for I have nowhere to store my crops?' And he said, 'I will do this: I will tear down my barns and build larger ones, and there I will store all my grain and my goods. And I will say to my soul, "Soul, you have ample goods laid up for many years; relax, eat, drink, be merry."' But God said to him, 'Fool! This night your soul is required of you, and the things you have prepared, whose will they be?' So is the one who lays up treasure for himself and is not rich toward God." (Luke 12:13–21)

In this parable we find a perfect example of a man so caught up in the pursuit of bigger and better, he neglected to invest in things that ultimately matter. All of the foolish rich man's energy was tied up in improving his property, and when he felt that was accomplished, he became lazy and gluttonous. The problem isn't really in improving one's financial state or even in resting and enjoying oneself. The problem is in doing only those things and not preparing for eternity. He stored up treasure for himself but was not rich toward God.

John Piper drives this point home with a real-life parable of his own:

> I will tell you what a tragedy is. I will show you how to waste your life. Consider a story from the February 1998 edition of *Reader's Digest*, which tells about a couple who "took early retirement from their jobs in the Northeast five years ago when he was 59 and she was 51. Now they live in Punta Gorda, Florida, where they cruise on their 30 foot trawler, play softball and collect shells." At first, when I read it I thought it might be a joke. A spoof on the American Dream. But it wasn't. Tragically, this was the dream: Come to the end of your life—your one and only precious, God-given life—and let the last great work of your life, before you give an account to your Creator, be this: playing softball and collecting shells. Picture

> them before Christ at the great day of judgment: "Look, Lord. See my shells." *That* is a tragedy. And people today are spending billions of dollars to persuade you to embrace that tragic dream. Over against that, I put my protest: Don't buy it. Don't waste your life.[3]

What has happened? This couple is earth-rich but God-poor. When the day of accounting comes, when the kingdom's currency is requested for entrance into paradise, wealthy, fun-loving, permanent-vacation-taking souls come up totally empty-handed.

Some may read this parable of the foolish rich man or John Piper's tale of the retired couple and think to themselves, "Ah, they should have cared more for others. If they had given more money away, they'd have the treasure of having done good." And it is imperative that we do good to others, but that kind of saving is a poverty all its own. When we reach the gates of paradise and are asked for the currency of the kingdom to prove our right to enter, we had best not try to hand in our own righteousness. The Bible says "all our righteous deeds are like a polluted garment" (Isa. 64:6), and "For by works of the law no human being will be justified" (Rom. 3:20a).

No, when the opportunity to present your justification for entry into everlasting rest presents itself, you need only present an empty hand, saying, "I have nothing of my own to offer. I have sold it all for the pearl of great price, the righteousness of Christ, and that I have received through faith, which makes me totally vested in his unsearchable riches. My Savior in the great grace of God has purchased my entrance for me." Now, *that* would be rich.

You may have accomplishments galore, religious and otherwise. You may be good enough, smart enough, and "doggone it, people like you!" You may be brimming with excellence! But don't try to buy grace with any of that. Grace is free, but it is not so cheap.

The deal is *all of Christ* for all of your nothing. Don't cheapen the treasure with your currency. Come and buy the unsearchable riches of grace with your poverty of spirit. That is all he will accept.

---

[3] John Piper, *Don't Waste Your Life* (Wheaton, IL: Crossway, 2007), 46.

# 3

# Uncommon Knowledge

Jesus was the smartest man who ever lived. We have to get that through our thick skulls if we want to make a hill of beans' difference for the kingdom in this world. So often we think of Jesus as spiritual in a way disconnected from reality. Jesus is religiously idealistic, we reason, but not "street smart." Jesus knows how things ought to be, but he's not so incisive on how things *really* are. Jesus is a good teacher, but in the popular imagination pretty much a naïve one. Dallas Willard explains:

> The world has succeeded in opposing intelligence to goodness. . . . And today any attempt to combine spirituality or moral purity with great intelligence causes widespread pangs of "cognitive dissonance." [As with Jesus,] Mother Teresa . . . is thought of as . . . nice, of course, but not really smart. "Smart" means good at managing how life "really" is.[1]

But as we've already argued, to say the kingdom is advancing Spiritually is not to say that it is advancing in a non-real way; quite to the contrary, it is advancing in a more real way. (This, incidentally, is why I often prefer capitalizing the word *Spiritual*

[1] Dallas Willard, *The Divine Conspiracy* (San Francisco: HarperCollins, 1998), 135.

when referring to the work of God or his children. It reminds us that our work is derived from and empowered by the third person of the Trinity, the Holy Spirit. This keeps our Christian Spirituality from being a vague spirituality, simply a Christian-flavored variation of what we find equally fuzzy in other religions and lower-case spiritualities.)

The reality is that Jesus knows exactly how things really are, and in fact he knows how things really are better than anyone else. We may look over the ethos of the Sermon on the Mount and find the whole thing utterly impractical toward getting ahead in the world, but one of the underlying points of the Sermon is that getting ahead in the world is a losing gambit to begin with. We come to Jesus's teaching looking for tips on playing checkers, when all along he is playing chess.

There is good reason for this. As God, Jesus is omniscient. He knows everything. In Mark 1:22 we read, "And they were astonished at his teaching, for he taught them as one who had authority, and not as the scribes." The sort of authority Jesus is wowing them with here is not the kind simply accumulated through years of study. Jesus taught, with the kind of authority that suggested he had mastered the material, that he was in fact the material world's very master. His authority comes not from education but from authorship. "He told me all that I ever did," the Samaritan woman declared (John 4:39). Yes, sister, because he foreknew it all, declared it all, and saw it all.

It makes total sense, then—real, actual, logical sense—to believe Jesus. He is no fool who believes the man who knows everything.

## Building Wisely

"Work smarter, not harder."

"Measure twice, cut once."

These handyman proverbs are principally aimed at those of us who like to assemble furniture without consulting the instruction manual and figure out how to get un-lost without the bother of stopping to ask for directions. But sometimes working smarter *is* working harder. The reason people avoid reading instructions and asking people for directions is that they are stubborn know-it-alls, and properly preparing for the task at hand is extra work. We are looking for shortcuts. We'd rather get something done than get it done right.

This principle certainly plays into the way most people live their lives. Life is short; best not waste it. So we try to pack in as much fun and as little work as possible. But eternity is long. No one seems to be planning for it. They are so scared of wasting a few short decades that they'll blindly trade in eternity for a mix of fleeting pleasures, like trading a birthright for some bean soup.

There is no bean soup worth the birthright. And there is nothing in the world worth losing the soul. But we'll take the shortcut when the appetite strikes us right.

My wife and I sometimes watch a show on HGTV called "Holmes on Homes," in which gruff, straight-talking host Mike Holmes visits families who have endured remodel nightmares at the hands of sketchy contractors. Holmes finds that his predecessors have used unsuitable materials, have improperly installed those materials, have disregarded quality and safety inspections, and often have absconded with the customer's money, leaving their jobs partially and poorly done. What Holmes does is essentially fix a multitude of cut corners. He works smarter and therefore harder.

People are the same everywhere and in every time. Using the familiar language of construction, Jesus addressed the takers of shortcuts in one of his more famous parables:

> Everyone then who hears these words of mine and does them will be like a wise man who built his house on the rock. And the rain fell, and the floods came, and the winds blew and beat on that house, but it did not fall, because it had been founded on the rock. And everyone who hears these words of mine and does not do them will be like a foolish man who

> built his house on the sand. And the rain fell, and the floods came, and the winds blew and beat against that house, and it fell, and great was the fall of it. (Matt. 7:24–27)

When I was a child, we sang a song about this parable in Sunday school. I've forgotten the tune, but I remember the gist: be smart or you'll get wiped out. In the context of Jesus's original audience, the washing out of one's home was a real danger, especially in the land of dry wadis. Rainfall is not too common in the desert regions of Israel, so you could hardly blame someone for building without thinking too much about flooding. But when a good hard rain does come, the gulches may overflow with flash floods. Devoid of long-term planning, poorly built homes can be washed away.

"These words of mine." Jesus wants us to know that long-term life-planning is wise when it revolves around his teaching. And since his teaching was self-referential and self-centered, real wisdom is Christ-referenced and Christ-centered. If you only live once, it might make sense to live by bread alone, but if life goes on even after the death of the perishable body, it makes more sense to live by every word that proceeds from the mouth of God.

"If you will live according to my words," Jesus says, "as if I am the one who knows the way life *really* is, as if in fact I am the center of the universe, you will be prepared when devastation comes."

How?

In the short term, on this side of the veil, we will know where to turn when suffering comes. We will grieve, but not like the hopeless. We know how life really is. We will hurt, but we will not despair. We know how life really is. We will cry out, but we will not shake our fist. We know how life really is. Because we know *who* life really is (John 14:6). Paul elucidates the Spiritual logic this way: "We are afflicted in every way, but not crushed; perplexed, but not driven to despair; persecuted, but not forsaken; struck down, but not destroyed" (2 Cor. 4:8–9).

The storm comes, and the wise are not utterly destroyed because they know that the one who controls the storms has secured their souls for all eternity. And even if he requires their lives for the moment, he will return their lives to them in glorious abundance. There is nothing God will take from the Christian that he will not give back in some way, infinityfold.

That is the long-term wisdom. Jesus wants to know who we believe he is. Just a good teacher? An idealistic sage? One more entry in the pantheon of prophets? A pretty smart guy but not really clued-in to the way things work?

> Simon Peter replied, "You are the Christ, the Son of the living God." And Jesus answered him, "Blessed are you, Simon Bar-Jonah! For flesh and blood has not revealed this to you, but my Father who is in heaven. And I tell you, you are Peter, and on this rock I will build my church, and the gates of hell shall not prevail against it." (Matt. 16:16–18)

As we believe in Christ, we become more like Christ. United with him in faith, we are as secure as he is. Thus, Peter becomes a rock, and so do all confessing Christians. The church is built upon the confession of Christ as God and King. When the storm of hell comes to condemn, the persecuted church stands secure.

This brings up a rather important point: Notice that no amount of building on the rock kept the storm away. The strongest rock did not ward off the rain. The rain falls on the just and the unjust alike (Matt. 5:45). This is a promise of Jesus: "In the world you will have tribulation" (John 16:33). When he tells us that the gates of hell will not prevail against the church, he is emphatically not saying that there will be an absence of violence. Similarly, Paul tells us to take up a shield (Eph. 6:16). We are told over and over to stand firm (1 Cor. 16:13; Gal. 5:1; Eph. 6:13; Phil. 4:1). We are told to hold fast to the word (Rom. 12:9; 1 Cor. 15:2; 1 Thess. 5:21; Heb. 4:14; 10:23). We are told to mature so that we will not be "carried about by every wind of doctrine" (Eph. 4:11–14). We are told to be wise as serpents (Matt. 10:16). Why? Because confessing Christ is not a force field against trouble.

The way some pitch Christianity, I do not see how they make room for the disciples being scared out of their minds in the storm-rocked boat while Jesus slept. The life of faith seems less Galilean and more Disney World, perhaps like one of those slow-moving boat rides through artificial happy-fun-lands, Christians merely passing through, safely observing, detached spectators to the world but not participants. But Christianity emphatically does not make every day a Friday. Unless we mean the biblical Friday, the historical church's Friday, the Friday of the cross.

No, becoming a Christian does not ward off trouble. In fact, biblically speaking, it seems to entail the promise of more trouble. No one by becoming a Christian becomes exempt from the suffering common to every human being in this fallen world—we still get sick, we still get hurt, we still die. And on top of that, the Christian embraces the cross of Christ, opening himself up to scorn, mockery, and persecutions of various kinds.

But having built on the rock of the Word, we know that even if the storm kills us, we will live. Cheer up, then, Christian! Should heaven and earth pass away around you, it's not the end of the world.

None of this building on the rock is simply about intellectual assent, however. It is about faith. And faith is not works, but it certainly gets to work: "Everyone who then hears these words of mine and does them . . ." (Matt. 7:24). So to build on the rock is just that—to *build*. Belief in Jesus means rolling up the sleeves and activating the elbow grease. "The kingdom of heaven has suffered violence, and the violent take it by force" (Matt. 11:12).

## Serving Wisely

Jesus's Olivet Discourse—Mark 13 and Luke 21, but the longest version is in Matthew 24—is Jesus's most detailed prophetic announcement in the Gospels, and it is perhaps the most complicated in all the Bible. What exactly is Jesus referring to? A time of tribulation within the lifetime of his audience? The end of the church age at some point still future to us? Both, and several points in between? Complicating matters is Jesus's own admission of not being privy himself to the timing of these end-time events (Matt. 24:36). And at the end of Matthew's presentation of the discourse, he records Jesus delivering a barrage of parables—five in a row—each in growing complexity:

The fig tree (Matt. 24:32–35)
The thief in the night (vv. 43–44)
The wise and wicked servants (vv. 45–51)
The ten virgins (25:1–13)
The talents (vv. 14–30)

The parable of the talents is followed by the matter of the sheep and the goats, which is rather parable-like itself.

Capping off one of the most difficult passages in Scripture is this set of illustrations which themselves require interpretation. The Olivet Discourse in all its unwieldy glory is fairly obfuscating. Smart, godly students of the Scriptures have disagreed on the finer points of this material for centuries, but there appears to be one common thread running through the discourse proper and the concluding parables. We see it in the parable in our immediate focus, the tale of the wise and wicked servants. Jesus warns,

> Who then is the faithful and wise servant, whom his master has set over his household, to give them their food at the proper time? Blessed is that servant whom his master will find so doing when he comes. Truly, I say to you, he will set him over all his possessions. But if that wicked servant says to himself, "My master is delayed," and begins to beat his fellow servants and eats and drinks with drunkards, the master of that servant will come on a day when he does not expect him and at an hour he does not know and will cut him in pieces and put him with the hypocrites. In that place there will be weeping and gnashing of teeth. (Matt. 24:45–51)

On the surface, the parable resembles the satirical bumper sticker poking fun at evangelical expectation: JESUS IS COMING. LOOK BUSY. This is not far off from the point, although Jesus is of course not some ignorant boss fooled by busywork.

No, but it is just like Jesus to tell us to stay alert for things we don't understand. And that appears to be the primary point: alertness; and as part of alertness, diligence. Indeed, diligence in serving is alertness. The wise servant operates as if the absent master is actually there, managing the household. He does not exploit the master's apparent delay. He wants to be found faithful, so he stays faithful. The wicked servant, on the other hand, has on his car the bumper sticker WHEN THE CAT'S AWAY, THE MICE WILL PLAY. He lacks discipline, care, allegiance. Wickedness has become normative for him, and he is drunk, not just on wine but on his own foolishness. The wicked servant is spiritually slobby: "Eat, drink, and be merry, because, you know, *whatever*."

When the master returns, it is not as if he's happened upon the wicked servant at some exceptional time. It's not like the moments at work where the manager only happens to walk by the office when you're on your coffee break. The wicked servant is ruled by neglect.

The connection between this parable and the larger Olivet Discourse, and the way Jesus concludes this parable, show us that the stakes are very high. The parable gives us a glimpse into eternity. We're not talking about merit badges and reprimands; we're talking about eternal prosperity and eternal condemnation. The wicked servant no doubt knew he had a master, but he certainly didn't live as though he did. He did not hear the master's words and do them. When the storm of judgment came, he was utterly devastated. Dismembered, actually, is the imagery Jesus uses to convey the seriousness of the message. He is consigned to the place of eternal conscious torment. He is given over to eternal death because he didn't look alive in the meantime.

Alertness and diligence. These are the marks of the wise servant. He knows, first, that he has a master. He then acts like it.

Every day he denies himself, takes up his cross, and follows Jesus. He is not saved by his works, but he works because he knows that saved people work. He knows working smarter is working harder. He won't take shortcuts, because he knows that a lifetime of diligence is not to be compared to the eternal rest to come. "Blessed is that servant whom his master will find so doing when he comes. Truly, I say to you, he will set him over all his possessions" (Matt. 24:46–47).

So the servant will keep plugging away, building up the calluses on his hands, knowing that as he's building on the rock for his master, his master is in heaven preparing a mansion for him, too.

## Jesus, the Embodiment of Wisdom

The scariest part of these parables to me is found in their larger context. In the parable about the steward, the faithlessness that results in dismemberment and eternal condemnation comes from a lack of expectation. You could almost say that the fool didn't know any better. In a real sense, he didn't. The master came at a time when he was not expected. The implication is that one should stay vigilant, alert. The admonition is that one should turn off the autopilot. This is a heavy admonition, especially to a sleepwalking evangelical church living as if the master's delay in returning is just "how things really are."

In the parable of the two builders, the context makes the implications even more frightening. When Jesus says, "Everyone then who hears these words of mine and does them" (Matt. 7:24), the word "them" connects the parable to the Sermon on the Mount in general, but to the immediately preceding passage in particular (Matt. 7:21–23), which involves the condemnation of some who prophesied in Jesus's name, cast out demons in Jesus's name, and did mighty works in Jesus's name.

What gives? If they could do such things in the name of Jesus, which, as Jesus appears to be saying in 7:24, is the important thing, how could they be sent to eternal destruction? "I never knew you," Jesus says (v. 23). And there is the difficult truth to sort out in the midst of hard work: it is not our hard works that save, but Jesus's hard work. It is apparently possible to do a whole bunch of stuff "in Jesus's name" that has no real connection to him whatsoever.

It is possible to be good without knowing God. Many church people have a hard time understanding this. They rightly understand that loving God means loving our neighbors in sacrificial service, but they struggle to see how our good works testify to the gospel without being the gospel itself. This is easier to see in places where good works aren't hard to come by. I live and minister in a small rural town in Vermont. The people here are generally very nice. They are kind to each other and extremely helpful.

Whenever tragedy strikes a neighbor, our church of course steps in to assist in any way we can. In the last couple of years our town has seen at least two families lose everything they own to house fires. The church has been instrumental in raising money and collecting clothes and providing whatever else might be needed, from food to help with housing. But so has the larger community. The church does not distinguish itself very easily in such situations, because people here—Christian and non-Christian alike—genuinely care about each other and are interested in helping the less fortunate. This is not a complaint. It's a great thing to live in such a community! But at the same time it is a reality the church of Jesus Christ must sort through. "Being good" does not always help us stand out. As it always is, the difference between the Christian and the moralist is the gospel. The difference is Jesus himself. What can we offer that no one else can? The one true God.

We have the good news of forgiveness of sins and all the entailments of eternal life precisely because we have Jesus. The church must be good, but it is not by being good that the church principally demonstrates its uniqueness and benefit to the world; the church shows its benefit to the world by its belief in and proclamation of Jesus Christ. What a waste it would be to serve up good works but no Lord who saves apart from them!

The reality settles in and sobers us up. It's possible to do "Jesusy" stuff without knowing Jesus. It's possible to do good as part of some religious self-salvation project and not out of the joy of being saved. And that is another way the parable of the foolish builder is connected to the parable of the foolish steward—meticulously and carefully building a foundation upon our good works is a foolishly ignorant preparation.

The rock to build on, then, is not the doing of Jesus's words but the work of Jesus already done, namely his sacrificial death and glorious resurrection. The rock to build on is Jesus himself. When we really hear and do, we are showing that he is our foundation. Our righteousness, when it is not his righteousness imputed to us, is just so much sand.

Jesus tells us in John 14:6 that he is the way, he is the truth, and he is the life. He presents himself as the be-all and end-all. He is the embodiment of wisdom, the only wise God (Rom. 16:27). Who can know best the way things really are but the one who is the great I AM? Let the wise take heed.

4

# Three Times Found

> Now the tax collectors and sinners were all drawing near to hear him. And the Pharisees and the scribes grumbled, saying, "This man receives sinners and eats with them." (Luke 15:1–2)

The horror, the horror! Didn't Jesus's mama teach him any better? What possible good could come from consorting with these undesirables?

Certainly no good to the self-righteous religious establishment. But plenty of good to the undesirables. The Messiah is only making good on the ancient promises of God:

> I will have mercy on No Mercy,
> and I will say to Not My People, "You are my people";
> and he shall say, "You are my God." (Hos. 2:23)

When Jesus went around extending the right hand of fellowship to tax collectors, prostitutes, adulteresses, lepers, demoniacs, and half-breeds, the Pharisees and scribes could sense that their monopoly on "God's favor" was in serious jeopardy. Jesus clearly taught with authority and clearly commanded serious power, and now he was tapping into a virtually untouched demographic. It was in fact his primary demographic. Jesus was enjoying popularity among a great number of the common folk; now he was enlarging his constituency by treating outsiders like—gasp!—normal people. Which is to say, he treated all people like they needed forgiveness for sins and approval from God and like they could get both directly from him.

It is difficult to convince a man to believe something that his very livelihood is dependent upon his not believing. So most of the religious experts rejected Jesus. If he was the Way, their way was obsolete. By personally restoring the ceremonially unclean and by establishing the ubiquity of sinfulness in every human heart, he was systematically dismantling the Rube Goldberg justification machine the religious leaders had made out of the law. You'd be grumbling too if you suddenly discovered that Jesus was redrawing the inner circle, making it rather wide indeed, but that you found yourself, by virtue of your virtue, outside its perimeter.

That was kind of the point. Jesus Christ went around healing, feeding, comforting, and forgiving, and specifically among the "least of these." If you were full of yourself, you would feel no need for Jesus. He received tax collectors and sinners and ate with them to show that the gospel of the kingdom is good news for sinners—and sinners only.

Let's remember that, by Jesus's own explanation, the parables are designed to obfuscate as much as to enlighten (Matt. 13:13). With this in mind, it is rather interesting that he responds in Luke 15 to this grumbling about the gospel with three of these Spirit-powered stories. He is answering the grumblers in a way that is rather plain to those with receptive hearts and yet is guaranteed to compound the consternation of the unreceptive.

On a purely artistic basis, the ensuing triptych is simply beautiful. The parables of the lost sheep, the lost coin, and the lost son are symmetrical in concern, but each is distinct in perspective. Each makes the same point, and each makes its own point. As a development of thought, they build into each other, giving us three different angles on the same basic purpose of the kingdom—to bring the lost to God. As a narrative presentation, the two short tales set the stage for the longer one, like serials airing before the main feature.

There is also a striking difference between the first two stories and the third, something very obvious that many people miss, for many years myself included. We will get to that shortly, but first let's look at each piece of this masterful composition.

## The Lost Sheep

Jesus begins the first parable with a direct question. Breaking the cardinal rule of exegesis, he starts with the application. He's being very pointed about who's on which side while at the same time appealing to the grumblers' sense of logic:

> So he told them this parable: "What man of you, having a hundred sheep, if he has lost one of them, does not leave the ninety-nine in the open country, and go after the one that is lost, until he finds it? (Luke 15:3–4)

Jesus has simply appealed to their logic and shown them to be hypocrites. "Make the connection," he says. "If you lose a sheep, you go after it, don't you?" That's all Jesus is doing. When they lose a sheep, they don't simply cut their losses, and neither does he. He is determined to lose none of those whom the Father has given him (John 6:39). The sheep belongs in the fold; that's why it's called "lost." "If this had happened to your sheep, you'd do the same thing" is the point Jesus is making, and again, what he's done is appeal to their logic and familiarity while at the same revealing how arrogant it is to complain about what the Lord does with his own stuff.

But the story continues:

> And when he has found it, he lays it on his shoulders, rejoicing. And when he comes home, he calls together his friends and his neighbors, saying to them, "Rejoice with me, for I have found my sheep that was lost." Just so, I tell you, there will be more joy in heaven over one sinner who repents than over ninety-nine righteous persons who need no repentance. (Luke 15:5–7)

What Jesus means by "righteous persons who need no repentance" is difficult to ascertain. Is he speaking hypothetically, about so-called righteous people who don't think they need to repent? Or is he speaking of actually righteous people who are already "found" and therefore no longer need that initial repentance in saving faith? David Wenham suggests the former:

> There is . . . no need to infer that Jesus' reference to "ninety-nine righteous persons who need no repentance" means that he saw the Pharisees and their ilk as really righteous. It is obvious from other things he said, for example from the parable of the Pharisee and the tax-collector . . . that he did not. But Jesus' words are both an explanation of his ministry to those who saw themselves as the ninety-nine—which was logical on their own premises—and also an explanation of God's priorities as they truly are, since he really does rejoice more over the bringing back of the lost than over anything else.[1]

It would appear that Jesus is placing the grumblers in the category of the ninety-nine, as he has used their own categorization of tax collectors and sinners as outsiders in service of his prioritization of the lost. If this is the case, he must be speaking hypothetically, as Wenham explains, because obviously the grumblers needed to repent. In addition, unless we qualify the "righteous persons who need no repentance" as referring to saved persons who no longer need the initial repentance of saving faith, the category doesn't really work, because all people require repentance every day. What I mean is, Luther's first thesis was right: "When our Lord and Master, Jesus Christ, said 'Repent,' he called for the entire life of believers to be one of repentance." Is it possible that Jesus is making a relatively minute point about initial saving repentance in this broadside parable? Craig Blomberg appears to say yes, arguing the counterpoint:

> [I]f Jesus had the Pharisees and scribes in mind as those who were not rejoicing at the salvation of sinners, how could he

[1] David Wenham, *The Parables of Jesus* (Downer's Grove, IL: InterVarsity Press, 1989), 101.

> refer to them so positively? Many assume that Jesus' reference to those who do not need to repent reflects irony or sarcasm; by the "righteous" he really meant the "self-righteous." Yet this interpretation flies in the face of the consistently positive meaning of . . . "righteous" elsewhere found in the Gospels (cf., e.g., Mt 5:45, 10:41; Mk 6:20) and renders the conclusion that God rejoices more over the convert than over the hypocrite so self-evident as to be trite. There is certainly nothing in the depiction of the ninety-nine sheep or nine coins to suggest they were in any way blemished or counterfeit.
>
> In Luke's Gospel, moreover, the "righteous" consistently refers to those who are already right with God, the pious in Israel expectantly awaiting their salvation (cf., e.g., Lk 1:6, 2:25, 23:50). The word does not refer to people who are sinless but to those who place their hope in God.[2]

The best interpretation is likely the middle way, a blend of these two perspectives. Sheep and coins are not "characters" anyway, simply objects in the object lesson. But as they correspond with the self-righteous judgmentalism of the older brother in the third scene in the triptych, it is quite possible Jesus means for the ninety-nine persons who need no repentance to both positively refer to saved sinners already in the sheepfold (as the father assures the older brother that all he has is his) and negatively refer to the smug self-satisfaction of the grumbling Pharisees and scribes who believed they needed no repentance. This is another example of the way Jesus's parables confound and subvert those without the ears to hear.

The more direct picture is this: the kingdom is for sinners from both sides of the tracks. It is for the Jew first, but also for the Gentile. "I have other sheep that are not of this fold," Jesus says. "I must bring them also, and they will listen to my voice. So there will be one flock, one shepherd" (John 10:16). Paul elaborates:

[2]Craig L. Blomberg, *Interpreting the Parables* (Downer's Grove, IL: InterVarsity Press, 1990), 182.

> But now in Christ Jesus you who once were far off have been brought near by the blood of Christ. For he himself is our peace, who has made us both one and has broken down in his flesh the dividing wall of hostility by abolishing the law of commandments expressed in ordinances, that he might create in himself one new man in place of the two, so making peace, and might reconcile us both to God in one body through the cross, thereby killing the hostility. And he came and preached peace to you who were far off and peace to those who were near. For through him we both have access in one Spirit to the Father. So then you are no longer strangers and aliens, but you are fellow citizens with the saints and members of the household of God. (Eph. 2:13–19)

The promise of the gospel is for those near and for those far away. And ironically enough, in the economy of the kingdom, those farthest away turn out to be those "Hebrews of Hebrews" (see Phil. 3:5) huddled around the Torah.

The reaction of the shepherd to finding the lost sheep may have struck Jesus's first-century audience as a bit odd. "Make it walk back, for goodness' sake; that'll teach it to wander off," they might have said. But no. The shepherd puts the sheep on his shoulders and rejoices. He's not put out. He doesn't take out his anger on the stray. The response seems way out of proportion to the occasion.

"What man of you, having a hundred sheep, if he has lost one of them, does not leave the ninety-nine in the open country, and go after the one that is lost, until he finds it?"

Well, all of us. All of us would do that.

"And what man of you, when you find it, would lay it on your shoulders, rejoicing?"

Um. None of us, more than likely. That seems weird.

Perhaps a lamb could stir some kind of affection in the shepherd—because sheep are cute—but Jesus isn't talking about finding your beloved labradoodle Fifi. The first-century agrarian didn't think of sheep the way your kids probably do. Jesus is talking about livestock. I don't know if throwing a party to celebrate finding a lost sheep would strike any of his interlocutors as appropriate. It gets weirder in the next parable, when the woman throws a party after finding one lost coin.

The dissonance reveals there is something deeper at work, a key insight into the nature of the kingdom of God and the beating heart of our Shepherd-King. Good tidings of great joy. More on that shortly.

Through the prophets, God charges Israel's established shepherds as derelicts. "You have scattered my flock and have driven them away, and you have not attended to them" (Jer. 23:2). "My people have been lost sheep. Their shepherds have led them astray, turning them away on the mountains. From mountain to hill they have gone. They have forgotten their fold" (Jer. 50:6). Jesus recalls this sad state of affairs with his indictment of "hired hands" in John 10, the same space where he declares himself as the good shepherd. The condemnation from the prophets is accompanied by a rather startling commitment:

> He will tend his flock like a shepherd;
> he will gather the lambs in his arms;
> he will carry them in his bosom,
> and gently lead those that are with young. (Isa. 40:11)

> And he shall stand and shepherd his flock in the strength of the LORD,
> in the majesty of the name of the LORD his God.
> And they shall dwell secure, for now he shall be great
> to the ends of the earth. (Mic. 5:4)

If you are full of your own righteousness, lavishing a celebration on the recovery of the lost sheep will seem stupid. "Rejoice with me," Jesus nevertheless commands.

And those who see with the eyes of heaven will.

## The Lost Coin

What is implied in the parable of the lost sheep is explicit in the parable of the lost coin: namely, the nature of the search. We do not know all that the shepherd has undergone to find the lost sheep, only that he searches until he finds it. We can assume it was a great exercise. I picture the shepherd wandering over hill and over dale, all along the dusty trail. In the tale of the lost coin, the woman is sweeping up a dusty trail herself, "seeking diligently." Here's what Jesus says:

> Or what woman, having ten silver coins, if she loses one coin, does not light a lamp and sweep the house and seek diligently until she finds it? And when she has found it, she calls together her friends and neighbors, saying, "Rejoice with me, for I have found the coin that I had lost." Just so, I tell you, there is joy before the angels of God over one sinner who repents. (Luke 15:8–10)

In the first parable we see the need for the search, and in the second we see the nature of it. The whole house is lit up, and every inch is swept. The woman seeks diligently until she finds it. She is thorough. Like the shepherd, she doesn't stop until she finds the object of her search. It's always in the last place you look, anyway.

If the aim of God is that the knowledge of his glory will cover the earth like the waters cover the sea, inspecting between the cracks in the floor makes total sense. Our God is the God of the universe. And he is the God of square inches.

Like the shepherd, the woman rejoices when she finds the object of her search. She invites the neighbors over. Jesus says this is what happens when tax collectors and sinners repent and enter the kingdom. All heaven rejoices. And if the Pharisees and scribes are grumbling? Well, I guess he just put them in their place again.

## The Lost Son

Now comes the final vignette in the triptych, the climactic masterpiece. You are likely quite familiar with the story, but let's read it again. It is glorious:

> And he said, "There was a man who had two sons. And the younger of them said to his father, 'Father, give me the share of property that is coming to me.' And he divided his property between them. Not many days later, the younger son gathered all he had and took a journey into a far country, and there he squandered his property in reckless living. And when he had spent everything, a severe famine arose in that country, and he began to be in need. So he went and hired himself out to one of the citizens of that country, who sent him into his fields to feed pigs. And he was longing to be fed with the pods that the pigs ate, and no one gave him anything.
>
> "But when he came to himself, he said, 'How many of my father's hired servants have more than enough bread, but I perish here with hunger! I will arise and go to my father, and I will say to him, "Father, I have sinned against heaven and before you. I am no longer worthy to be called your son. Treat me as one of your hired servants."' And he arose and came to his father. But while he was still a long way off, his father saw him and felt compassion, and ran and embraced him and kissed him. And the son said to him, 'Father, I have sinned against heaven and before you. I am no longer worthy to be called your son.' But the father said to his servants, 'Bring quickly the best robe, and put it on him, and put a ring on his hand, and shoes on his feet. And bring the fattened calf and kill it, and let us eat and celebrate. For this my son was dead, and is alive again; he was lost, and is found.' And they began to celebrate.
>
> "Now his older son was in the field, and as he came and drew near to the house, he heard music and dancing. And he called one of the servants and asked what these things meant. And he said to him, 'Your brother has come, and your father

> has killed the fattened calf, because he has received him back safe and sound.' But he was angry and refused to go in. His father came out and entreated him, but he answered his father, 'Look, these many years I have served you, and I never disobeyed your command, yet you never gave me a young goat, that I might celebrate with my friends. But when this son of yours came, who has devoured your property with prostitutes, you killed the fattened calf for him!' And he said to him, 'Son, you are always with me, and all that is mine is yours. It was fitting to celebrate and be glad, for this your brother was dead, and is alive; he was lost, and is found.'" (Luke 15:11–32)

A few quick notes. First, when the son asks for his inheritance, he is essentially saying to his father, "I wish you were dead"—so serious is the offense in asking early for what would be due only upon the father's death. He severs ties with his family from the very beginning, in a sense, cutting himself off. Secondly, his time with the pigs is yet another sign of his utter separation. Swine were unclean to Jews by law, and here he finds himself dependent upon them, practically one of them! He has hit the bottomest bottom. He is now utterly alien to his people. Jesus is setting up the lost son as emblematic of all the untouchables and undesirables to whom he is bringing the kingdom. Thirdly, we see in the lost son's "coming to himself" the evidence of ignorant humility; he is not going to go claim his place as son, but in repentance is interested in working for his father, prevailing upon his father's mercy in becoming just another hired hand. How many Christians make this mistake! Seeing our great debt to our great God, we automatically assume, even after learning that salvation is available, that we must begin paying it off. We are so grateful for God's welcome, we assume the Lord has recruited us as a hired hand rather than receiving us as a beloved child whose debt has been paid by the blood of Jesus.

But perhaps the most important thing we ought to say about the parable of the lost son is that it is much more about the older brother than the younger. Jesus's subversive teaching is, in effect, who exactly is lost now? Who is it that is really far from the kingdom? All along he has been hinting at this spiritual poverty among the grumblers, and here it becomes clear as day—to those with sight, that is. The older brother is grumbling. Jesus's parables here are an answer to the complaints, and in the story of the lost son, the extended point is more about the older brother's legalism than the younger brother's hedonism. We are spared the details of the lost son's rebellion, but not of his brother's resentment.

In a brilliant way, Jesus is suggesting a fulfillment to a familial dysfunction at work throughout the biblical generations. If you're at all familiar with the narrative of the Scriptures, you are probably familiar with the younger brother/older brother dynamic that recurs throughout. According to Jewish custom, the oldest son is the honor-bearer of the family. His legacy has primacy. We see this, for example, in the law of levirate marriage, which says that if a man dies and leaves a childless widow, the next younger brother is obliged to marry the woman and thereby continue the lineage of his older brother. In fact, their firstborn would be considered the dead brother's firstborn. (This may be one reason why what's-his-name hands the kinsman redeemer dibs over to Boaz in the book of Ruth.) The older brother is the one owed the birthright.

But if you're familiar with the family stories in the Old Testament, you also know that the honored older brothers throughout the Scriptures tend to be blithering idiots. Family after family shows us the younger brothers outwitting, outlasting, and outshining the older brothers. The failure of the older brother to live up to his honorable position begins with Cain, proceeds through Esau to Joseph's brothers and to David's brothers, and culminates in the older brother in the parable of the prodigal son. It is not that the younger siblings are all that great themselves, of course, but one way God reinforces his penchant for shaming the wise with the foolish and the strong with the weak (1 Cor. 1:27) is by making the older serve the younger (Gen. 25:23; Rom. 9:12).

What we see is a gospel template gleaming beneath the

religious/custom template in each story. God routinely chooses the b-stringers, the scrubs, the alternates, the lowly, the foolish, the weak, and the unassuming to keep the all-stars humble. Older brother after older brother, then, exhibits failure after failure.

Then we get to the lost son story, and the older brother is put in place not just to show us again the shameful self-righteousness of those whose own honor seeks the dishonor of others, but to show us the desperate need for—finally, for once in history—*a good older brother*. There is that big difference between the third story and the first two: In the accompanying parables of lost coin and lost sheep, someone goes looking for the item lost. In the lost son parable, no one goes, certainly not the older brother, who is busy in his room writing that hit song, "Alone in My Principles." So who will go? Who will seek out the lost and rescue him?

The good older brother. The only good older brother. Jesus. He will wander out into the wilderness, wherever he must go to search out the lost sheep. "Those who are well have no need of a physician," Jesus reasons, "but those who are sick" (Matt. 9:12). "For the Son of Man came to seek and to save the lost" (Luke 19:10). That's why he came. That's his business. He will light up the house, put the chairs up on the tables, and sweep every floorboard and into every corner to find that one lost coin. He will go searching in every gambler's den, whorehouse, and pigsty until he finds every sinner God is calling home. And over and over again we see in the Gospels, as Jesus extends the welcome of the kingdom to the lowest of the low, he scandalizes the older brothers. They gasp and clutch their pearls while Jesus is handing the pearls out.

Finally, an older brother worthy of the honor! Finally, an older brother who serves the younger willingly, joyfully, and redemptively, for the glory of God in the reconciliation of all God's children to himself. And we are his family, if we will submissively acknowledge his birthright. Jesus is the older brother who does his job. Everyone else is the other guy.

Once again Jesus is turning the world of the religious self-justifiers on its head. He does this with the absence of a searcher in the lost son story, indicting the legalists' missional disobedience, and he does this with the identity of the searchers in the first two parables. Although the shepherd was a cherished image of God's care for his people throughout the Scriptures, by the first century the average Jew thought of shepherds as somewhat shady characters. They were sketchy types, the stereotypical longshoremen or "cursing sailors" of their day. And in his opening inquisition, Jesus asks the Pharisees to identify themselves with the shepherds. Then, he suggests they put themselves in the place of a woman. How rude.

But really, by making a shepherd and a woman the heroes of the parables, Jesus is identifying *himself* with these people, which is the big problem the Pharisees and scribes have with him at this moment. He is not standing above the untouchables, lording the kingdom over them. He is debasing himself, holding their hands, to say that the kingdom is specifically for them. Jesus is providing an even fuller picture of the lengths to which he will go to reach the despised and marginalized. He is willing to be put in their place, in *our* place. He is willing to be numbered among the transgressors (Isa. 53:12; Luke 22:37), not just to take the curse but to become the curse (Gal. 3:13). He was willing to become like us, that we might become like him.

## God, the Big Spender

Some have said that the most significant character in the parable of the lost son is the father. He corresponds to our heavenly Father, who overflows with lovingkindness to all generations, whose love is steadfast and equally abundant in riches to younger brother and older, Gentile and Jew, hedonists and legalists, the rebellious and the religious. The father in the story, like our heavenly Father, operates on the kingdom economy, not the world's. He is a giver of grace! When the lost son returns, the father imprudently runs to greet him. And then he throws a party. For the kid who wished he was dead, who shook his fist at him with every licentious spending spree during his exile. Like the joy for the found sheep and the found coin, the joy for the found son seems disproportionate to the occasion. And it *is* if your heart, like the older brother's heart, is set to law, not gospel.

And here is something peculiar about the parable of the lost son, which is very often called the parable of the "prodigal son." The word *prodigal* is an adjective referring to profuse expenditures, reckless abundance, a sense of "wastefulness." This applies of course to the lost son as he "squandered his property in reckless living" (Luke 15:13). But as Tim Keller has helpfully shown us, it is the father in the story who is the most prominent prodigal.[3] He is "wasting" his affection on his disgraced son, lavishing his goodness upon the one deserving of his condemnation. So Keller says the image of the gospel we receive in the parable of the prodigal son is actually of the prodigal God who loves us with reckless abundance, who, zealous for his own joy, is jealous for us, and who, with his Son, generously gives us all things (Rom. 8:32).

Were those older-brother Pharisees getting all this? You can almost hear these other words of Jesus echoing in the subtext: "Pay attention to what you hear: with the measure you use, it will be measured to you, and still more will be added to you" (Mark 4:24). If you persist in being resentful and judgmental like the older brother, that is how you will be measured yourself, since it is clear that you pride yourself in your self-righteousness. (That's what "Judge not, that you be not judged" [Matt. 7:1] really means.) But if you truck in grace, grace will keep on truckin' (John 1:16).

The lost son came to the point of seeking first his father's kingdom, and everything else was added to him. He used up his father's love, but still more was added.

The prosperity-gospelists pervert this promise, turning it into the lamest of proverbs, into legalistic voodoo, as if God can be manipulated like the gods of the pagans and as if his kingdom is some kind of vending machine you just need the passwords for. The

[3]Timothy Keller, *The Prodigal God* (New York: Dutton, 2008).

prosperity-gospelists misread the "more added to you" like the kid who is happy you've brought more dirt for his mud pies.

But the "more" we get is more of Christ and his multitudinous riches. Our God is no miser. He graciously gives us the best gifts, the ones that last. God is not stingy! Through Christ comes a universe of blessings so that our hearts might be filled to overflowing! Take note:

> "He has granted to us his precious and very great promises [*plural*]." (2 Pet. 1:4)
>
> "From his fullness we have all received, grace upon grace." (John 1:16)
>
> We have been "abundantly" pardoned. (Isa. 55:7)
>
> We are transformed from one degree of glory to another. (2 Cor. 3:18)
>
> "I came that they may have life and have it *abundantly*." (John 10:10, emphasis added)
>
> He has lavished the riches of his grace upon us. (Eph. 1:7–8)

On this theme of God's wild generosity, William Hendriksen writes,

> God's gifts are always most generous. He is forever adding gift to gift, favor to favor, blessing to blessing. He gives not only "of" his riches—as a billionaire might do when he gives a dollar to charity—, but "according to" his riches, the riches of his grace (Eph. 1:7). He imparts "grace upon grace" (John 1:16) . . . He delights in lovingkindness (Mic. 7:18). . . . When he loves, he loves the world; and when he gives, he gives his only begotten Son (John 3:16). That Son, moreover, not only intercedes for his people but "ever lives to make intercession for them" (Heb. 7:25). Truly, "He giveth and giveth and giveth again."

> "More besides shall be given to you." When Abraham's servant asks Rebekah for a drink, she not only quenches *his* thirst but *in addition* also that of the camels. . . .
>
> This is only a faint reflection of what God in Christ is doing constantly:
>
> He not only grants Solomon's wish for wisdom, but *in addition* promises him riches and lengths of days (1 Kings 3:9–15).
>
> He not only accedes to the centurion's request to heal the latter's servant, but *in addition* pronounces a blessing upon the centurion (Matt. 8:5–13).
>
> He not only answers the plea of Jairus, restoring to life his daughter, but *in addition* sees to it that the child gets something to eat (Mark 5:21–24, 43).
>
> He, the resurrected Christ, not only fulfils his promise to meet the disciples in Galilee (Matt. 26:32; 28:7, 16–20), but *in addition* meets and blesses them even earlier, in Jerusalem (Luke 24:33–48).
>
> He not only pardons the sinner—as a governor might grant pardon—but, *in addition*, adopts him and grants him peace, holiness, joy, assurance, freedom of access, super-invincibility.[4]

I can't help but picture the scene of the lost son returning, demoralized and broken. Is his father standing on the porch, arms crossed, tapping his foot? No, he runs to him. Does he hand his son work clothes and make him start at the bottom rung? No, he covers him in fine dress. Does he show him where the refrigerator is? No, he throws him a feast. All the boy wanted was a chance to pay back his debt, to earn his father's respect again and perhaps a place in the business. His dad gave him back everything and more.

And here we come with our battered, feeble, tattered faith. It isn't much to look at. But the Father receives it warmly and in exchange gives us the fullness of the riches of the eternal Christ.

[4] William Hendriksen, *The Gospel of Mark*, New Testament Commentary (Grand Rapids, MI: Baker, 1990), 164–165.

We are no more secure in Christ with a strong faith than with a small faith, so long as that small faith is true faith. Into our empty hand is placed the infinite blessings of our sovereign Savior.

When you have Christ and his kingdom, you have everything. You have him and therefore *all*: the eternal riches of his glory. So we receive not just that hell insurance and ticket to heaven, but also union with Christ, by which we are "seated with him in the heavenly places" (Eph. 2:6) and hidden with him in God forever. We receive the adoption as sons and daughters. We receive the indwelling Spirit. We are totally justified. We are cleansed, declared holy, set apart, and we receive in addition the promise of the fruit of the Spirit and more holiness to come. We receive the promise of the blessed hope, the glorification we will share with Christ, and the resurrection of the body to everlasting bliss in the new heavens and new earth.

To be forgiven by Jesus is to be forgiven seventy times seven, to be justified and rewarded seventy times seven. Completely, perfectly, irrevocably. The fullness of God works in the concert of his triune perfection to save us (1 Pet. 1:2). There is an echo of this truth in the triptych of Luke 15: we aren't just found, we are *perfectly* found, three times found!

So let's pay attention to what we hear in the gospel. If we lend God our ears, he will fill our eyes with the transforming vision of his glorious Son. When he fills our eyes with that vision, he fills our hearts. When he fills our hearts, he fills our souls, till we are overflowing in praise and love and moving out on mission to shine the light of Christ far and wide, that the knowledge of his glory might cover the earth like the waters cover the sea.

# 5

# Justice and Good Sinners

Jesus's revolutionary campaign of sabotage continues in perhaps the most simultaneously understood and misunderstood of all his parables. It usually goes by the title "the good Samaritan." The phrase "Good Samaritan" has become part of modern language. Even the biblically illiterate are familiar with the designation. The Good Samaritan helps those in need out of the goodness of his heart. And so, as so often happens, the world has taken what is inherently scandalous and tamed it for sentimental sensibilities.

President Obama often invokes the parable of the good Samaritan in his speeches on national health care, socialized medicine, and social justice in general,[1] which doesn't exactly miss the point but sort of clumsily grasps at the most obvious one. When it comes to the Bible, our president is like almost every other Westerner: a cherry picker. But there's sour grapes in the story of the so-called Good Samaritan, and they begin with the fellow who prompted the parable in the first place:

> And behold, a lawyer stood up to put him to the test, saying, "Teacher, what shall I do to inherit eternal life?" He said to

[1] Here is just one example: Barack Obama, "Remarks by the President to the Clinton Global Initiative," United Nations General Assembly (September 25, 2012), http://www.whitehouse.gov/photos-and-video/video/2012/09/25/president-obama-speaks-united-nations-general-assembly#transcript.

> him, "What is written in the Law? How do you read it?" And he answered, "You shall love the Lord your God with all your heart and with all your soul and with all your strength and with all your mind, and your neighbor as yourself." And he said to him, "You have answered correctly; do this, and you will live."
>
> But he, desiring to justify himself, said to Jesus, "And who is my neighbor?" Jesus replied, "A man was going down from Jerusalem to Jericho, and he fell among robbers, who stripped him and beat him and departed, leaving him half dead. Now by chance a priest was going down that road, and when he saw him he passed by on the other side. So likewise a Levite, when he came to the place and saw him, passed by on the other side. But a Samaritan, as he journeyed, came to where he was, and when he saw him, he had compassion. He went to him and bound up his wounds, pouring on oil and wine. Then he set him on his own animal and brought him to an inn and took care of him. And the next day he took out two denarii and gave them to the innkeeper, saying, 'Take care of him, and whatever more you spend, I will repay you when I come back.' Which of these three, do you think, proved to be a neighbor to the man who fell among the robbers?" He said, "The one who showed him mercy." And Jesus said to him, "You go, and do likewise." (Luke 10:25–37)

The story of the good Samaritan is a parable about justice and anthropology. It relocates a person's "center of the universe" by jostling his dearly held assumptions about the people in it.

The first thing we can say about the parable is that it does indeed speak to what is often called "social justice." We are told that Jesus's inquisitor was a lawyer (to be understood as an expert in the religious law, a professional theologian, if you will), that he wanted to know what to do to inherit eternal life, and that he was seeking to justify himself. This is a man clearly interested in righteousness/justice. Like the young rich ruler, he wants to know which i's need to be dotted and which t's crossed so that the right thing is done.

He is not really thinking in terms of the kingdom bringing heaven to earth, but of the kingdom bringing him to heaven. His sense of justice is self-centric. Simon Kistemaker explains the normality of this vision in the day:

> The Jew lived in a circular world: he placed himself at the center, surrounded by his immediate relatives, then his kinsmen, and finally the circle of all those who claimed Jewish descent and who were converts to Judaism. The word *neighbor* has a reciprocal meaning: he is a brother to me and I to him. Thus the circle is one of self-interest and ethno-centrism. The lines were carefully drawn to ensure the well-being of those who were inside and to deny help to those who were outside.[2]

Jesus then comes along, coloring, in the kingdom way, outside the lines. It is extremely difficult these days to understand the import of this scandal. In various places at various times, we see opportunities for modern applications. The story could take place between oppressed blacks and empowered whites in the tumultuous days of the fight for civil rights, or between Jews and Palestinians today. Referring to another parable—the tax collector and the Pharisee in the temple (Luke 18:9–14)—Craig Blomberg attempts to apply the ancient Jewish appraisal of tax collectors to modern religious sensibilities by calling it "The Parable of the Recovering Homosexual."[3] Indeed, if we wanted to get a sense of how the "good Samaritan" would have sounded to first-century Jewish ears, we might today call the story "the good homosexual." But we are getting ahead of ourselves.

The parable of the good Samaritan is most definitely about social justice (or what we might more simply call "active love for our neighbors"). It is definitely about more than that, but it is certainly not about less. The parable still stands today as one of Jesus's most direct rebukes to the idea that the gospel of the kingdom has nothing

---

[2] Simon J. Kistemaker, *The Parables: Understanding the Stories Jesus Told* (Grand Rapids, MI: Baker, 2002), 141.
[3] Craig L. Blomberg, *Preaching the Parables: From Responsible Interpretation to Powerful Proclamation* (Grand Rapids, MI: Baker, 2004), 156–168.

to do with taking care of the poor, sick, naked, or hungry. And you do not have to embrace the false "social gospel" to affirm that.

## The Kingdom and Social Justice

We are pendulum people, constantly overcorrecting from one error into an error on the other side. So when some come along preaching a gospel of social justice, others will rashly deny the necessity of the thing in the first place. The consequence is a small gospel, scaled only to the individual. We've veered away from the cliff and right into a ditch on the other side, and there we lie with the half-dead man from Jerusalem.

Jesus is combating the lawyer's narrowing of the kingdom to the fine point of his own justification, and the very inclusion of the couldn't-care-less passersby in the parable reinforces the assault. The priest and the Levite walk on by. Why? Perhaps for lots of practical and theological reasons, but primarily one overarching reason: self-interest. And self-interest would be the defeat of a church called to rescue the perishing among every tongue, tribe, race, and nation, among every social and economic class, and among every subculture and spirituality. But the gospel we believe and proclaim swallows up self-interest. It is scaled to eternity, made to fit the full extent of sin's systemic fallout. So if we love God, we love our neighbor. You cannot have the former without the latter, precisely because the gospel's full scope is shalom (peace on earth). Good works, then, give witness to the righteousness of God brought to bear in the gospel. Therefore, proclamation of the gospel of the kingdom inevitably entails the corroborating evidence of what we will call "social justice." And there are still more reasons why social justice is not expendable:

1. God doesn't merely *suggest* we care for widows and orphans; he *commands* we do so. And not just a few times.

2. In Jesus's miracles we see signs of God's in-breaking kingdom, which is to say not just that they signify God's power in Christ's lordship but that they signify that God's kingdom is restor-

ing righteous order to the world. Acts of social justice, in much the same way, are also signs of the kingdom. They are foretastes of the day when God will set all to rights.

3. In his letter to the Galatians, when Paul was confirming that "his" gospel was on the same page as the gospel of Peter, James, and John, he recalls how those pillars of the faith reminded him to care for the poor, which Paul says is the thing he was eager to do (Gal. 2:10). So even within the contextualized mission of taking the gospel to different cultures/tribes, care for the poor is a constant.

4. Christian social justice gives witness to the right-side-upness of God's kingdom.

5. When we are saved, we are changed from self-worshipers to God-worshipers, and as God equates love of our neighbor with demonstrated love of him, acts of social justice are proof of our redemption.

6. When you read through the Old Testament law, you find an astounding number of strictures not just on right relations with the community but also about meals, about work, about forgiveness of debt, about rest days, even about how to treat livestock. This tells us that there is a righteous order God expects his righteous people to live within. The work of social justice testifies to this order.

7. Caring for "the least of these" is caring for Christ (Matt. 25:40).

And for those who would say we should absolutely care for the poor, but for the *Christian* poor, not necessarily the poor of the world, I offer the objection of grace itself: The mission of Jesus Christ was to love you and me while we were most decidedly *not* Christians. We were poor in spirit, enemies of Christ and his kingdom, and he offered his body for us anyway. Is it even Christian, then, to say we will care only for those who are like us? For some reason it doesn't occur to us to question foreign missionaries who give of themselves, even to the point of death, for the lost and the pagan overseas. But Stateside we will give the unbeliever only scraps from the table. But the law actually commands us to love our neighbor as ourselves.

What shall we do, also, with the parable of the good Samaritan, in which the "bad guy," the outsider, is made the hero of the story? This parable is given in response to the question "Who is my neighbor?" Doesn't this story, even if it were all we had as a clue regarding to whom we should care for, say something radical about our scope of concern?

Yes, the riches of Christ is all the wealth a sinner truly needs, and we must never obscure or dilute that good news, even with works that are good. If silver and gold have we none, "such as we have" is nonetheless eternally precious. But if we have the silver and gold, shouldn't we give that too? Some may think that to be so free is to obscure the real pearl of great price. But in a delicious biblical irony, loving generosity doesn't show that we think money is important, but rather that we find money cheap in comparison to the treasure of Christ.

There is something the good Samaritan understands about justice that the religious experts can't see, that they refuse to see:

> Is not this the fast that I choose:
>     to loose the bonds of wickedness,
>     to undo the straps of the yoke,
> to let the oppressed go free,
>     and to break every yoke?
> Is it not to share your bread with the hungry
>     and bring the homeless poor into your house;
> when you see the naked, to cover him,
>     and not to hide yourself from your own flesh?
>         (Isa. 58:6–7)

And yet we find it necessary to be as clear as possible about what the gospel for the half-dead man in the ditch actually *is*.

## What Is Good News for the Poor?

If Christ and his kingdom are all that matters, we find money and material possessions put in their proper place. They are not rejected as evil, of course, but they find their orbit around Christ as the true treasure. This kingdom framework helps us in understanding the challenging things Jesus says about wealth and also about caring for the poor.

In Luke's version of the Beatitudes, we learn that Jesus had alternate versions to the clause on poverty. "Blessed are you who are poor, for yours is the kingdom of God" (Luke 6:20). Matthew's Gospel, written primarily for a Jewish audience, focuses on poverty of a different kind ("poor in spirit"; Matt. 5:3), but Luke, writing primarily for Gentiles, wants us to know that the kingdom's coming has real implications for the materially poor too. And yet, the gospel for the poor is still not money. As we've seen, there is plenty in the Scriptures to commend the need for social justice initiatives as implications of the gospel, but almost nothing to commend them as the gospel itself. The gospel for the materially poor is not financial justice, although that is a valid implication of the kingdom's coming to bear in the world; it is, instead, the same as the gospel for the poor in spirit: eternal life in Christ Jesus. Why must we hold this distinction between gospel content and gospel entailments as it relates to poverty? Here are nine reasons:

1. The gospel is the news of the work of Christ—sinless life, sacrificial death, bodily resurrection—which is to say, the gospel is not the news of anything we've done or can do. The gospel is also "the kingdom" that was coming in and through Christ's ministry, inaugurated in his life, death, and resurrection. But whether we use the gospel definition of 1 Corinthians 15 or the kingdom gospel framework of the synoptic Gospels, the gospel is still news of something that Christ has done or is doing. Therefore, anything that happens now and is done by us—including, but not limited to, what we might call social justice—is not the gospel message itself, but is the Christian's living as if that gospel message is true. I maintain that the gospel's content ends and the gospel's implications begin when we start "doing stuff."

2. If the gospel's content includes economic justice for the poor, it means that the gospel includes work that Christians do, and if

the gospel includes work that Christians do, we end up "preaching ourselves" and stealing the glory of the gospel that is due God alone. Paul writes in 2 Corinthians 4:5, "For what we proclaim is not ourselves, but Jesus Christ as Lord, with ourselves as your servants for Jesus' sake." We are the servants of others—including in the work of caring for the poor—but we preach as the gospel Christ only, and this distinction is held for Jesus's glory.

3. Economic justice is a sign of the good news, but not the news itself, in the same way that Jesus's miracles of the healing of the blind or raising of the lame were not the good news, but signs pointing to the gospel of the redemption of creation. We see this delineation perhaps most starkly in John 6 when the crowds were eager to eat the signs (bread) but demurred on eating the signified (Christ's flesh).

4. Economic justice is temporal justice. This is perhaps the most crucial point to be made. The gospel's justice is eternal. None of us gets to take money with us into eternity. Loving our neighbor by providing for the poor demonstrates that our treasure is not monetary. But to argue that social justice is gospel content, not gospel implication, is to muddle the eternal treasure of Christ with treasure that rusts and decays. The miracles were not permanent. Those who were healed still died. Those who were raised from the dead died again. Those given food and money were hungry and in need again. Even marriage, one of the most glorious and direct representations of the gospel, gives way at the consummation of the kingdom into the wedding feast of the Lamb. We won't need marriage or sex to have happy lives when heaven takes over earth, and we certainly won't need money or possessions or medicine for that reason either. Given all that Jesus says related to earthly treasures rusting and decaying, we do the gospel of eternal life no favors by making money and material possessions part of its announcement.

5. Related to that, interpreting "good news for the poor" as economic justice is to misdirect focus off Christ as the super-fulfillment of the Old Testament prophecies; it is to make the same mistake as most of Jesus's Jewish audience, whose messianic expectation

pictured him literally overthrowing the Roman occupation and establishing political kingship in Jerusalem. Now, of course, Jesus *did* do that. He was proclaiming his lordship—and in effect denying Caesar's—but as we have said, the way he was doing that was not immediately literal. That Jesus is Lord has profound effects on how Christians live, including economically, but those are *effects* of Christ's lordship, not the *content* of his lordship. Or, to put it another way, a poor person can have eternal life while remaining poor. Some would suggest this view merely "spiritualizes" the promises of God, and while there is a way some do that in disharmony with the Scriptures, we should at least reiterate that what the Bible calls "spiritual" is not un-real.

Further, I would not go so far as to say that Jesus merely spiritualized the kingdom; he was really there, he was really Lord, he really offered his tangible self to follow and trust and to die, and this incarnational reality and sacrifice and resurrection is not unreal at all. Indeed, there is nothing un-real about the promise of a risen Lord securing new bodies for us in a new heavens and new earth to come.

But if we reduce the gospel to its implications, we will have to make sense of how the gospel proclaiming "liberty to the captives" would have encouraged John the Baptist while he languished in prison, awaiting execution. And we must ask how it could encourage any believer struggling financially or materially. To force the issue gives way to the perniciousness of the prosperity gospel.

6. The "good news for the poor" that Jesus preaches is not economic justice, or else his own ministry was fairly a failure, as we don't see too many examples of the disciples providing money for the poor. In fact, they were occasionally lacking for things like food and money themselves. It would also make Peter and John's gospel encounter with the lame man in Acts 3 a consolation prize. They had no silver and gold, but they had something far better.

7. "Good news for the poor" necessarily meaning "economic justice for the poor" is an eisegetic reading. Take a look at Luke 7:22, for instance:

> And he answered them, "Go and tell John what you have seen and heard: the blind receive their sight, the lame walk, lepers are cleansed, and the deaf hear, the dead are raised up, the poor have good news preached to them."

Notice that Jesus doesn't say "the poor receive finances." The blind get sight back. The lame get mobility. The lepers get restored flesh. The dead get life. But the poor don't get un-poor. They have the good news preached to them. This good news is not money, but the treasure of Christ, the satisfaction of Christ. Indeed, Jesus said elsewhere that we will always have the poor with us (Matt. 26:11).

8. True justice for the poor consists in realizing that poverty is no hindrance to gaining the treasure of all-surpassing worth. This is not out of step with the larger paradigm of "the gospel of the kingdom." It makes perfect sense of the Beatitudes, for instance, which promise, "Blessed are you who are poor, for yours is the kingdom of God" (Luke 6:20). How does it promise the kingdom to the poor? Not in giving money, but in turning the tables on how the haves and have-nots are regarded. No, the promise to the poor is not that they will be rich monetarily but that they will receive the far greater blessing of eternal life in Christ, the approval of God, the status of coheir with Jesus. In the world's fallen economy, the poor are at the bottom of the barrel because they don't have the power of money. But in God's economy, money is *not* power, and therefore the rich, the powerful, the lords of the earth are humbled, and the humble are exalted.

If the gospel for the poor is economic parity, aren't we preaching the gospel of middle class–ness? Or a wealth gospel? The reason the gospel of the kingdom is good news for the poor is not because the Son of Man comes handing out cash and prizes, but because it upturns the economic values of the world. In God's kingdom, the rich man has his reward now and he will perish later, but the poor are elevated, saved, made "rich toward God" (Luke 12:21).

9. If the gospel's content includes economic justice, it makes little sense to say we believe in this gospel with the gift of faith.

I don't need faith to believe I will receive money, merely an open hand. The requirement of the spiritual open hand of faith for grasping of the gospel demands that the gospel promises something (as of yet) immaterial.

With all that said, we must reiterate that care for the needy (whether poor or hungry or naked or ill) is a command of God binding on his people and to be obeyed as joyful gospel witness. Like all good works, seeking justice for the poor or otherwise underprivileged is a worshipful response to the gospel of Christ's finished work, but our good works are not the gospel itself. This is a supremely important point, because the danger persists that those who insist that social justice is the gospel are "seeking to justify themselves." As we see again, Jesus really is bringing good news to the poor, but he is at the same time subverting our concept of good news. He brings the richness of himself and holds nothing of himself back, and in doing so he redefines wealth for us.

That is the point easily missed in the commonest readings of the good Samaritan. The "go, and do likewise" (Luke 10:37) is crucial. But so is the casting. The parable is a scandal to the self-centered in its widening of the boundaries of "neighbor," but it is scandalous in its underlying doctrinal assertion, not merely in its straightforward practical application.

## The Doctrinal Scandal of the Good Samaritan

What is the real point of this story? The primary point is in answering the law-expert's question: "Who is my neighbor?" So when Jesus gets to the end, the moral imperative "Go, and do likewise" is a direct command not to be ignored by the inquisitor, or by us.

We see what everyone from the president of the United States to the president of the nearest hospital sees in the parable: A God-loving Christianity, which is the only real kind of Christianity, is neighbor-loving Christianity, and the category of "neighbor" is not limited to those who look, think, and live like us. Our neighbors, in fact, include our enemies. So we see the strains of kingdom-proclaiming social justice in the narrative.

But if Jesus just wanted us to know that we're supposed to care for people who are not like us, he could have just as easily had the man from Jerusalem be the hero and the Samaritan be the victim. That, in fact, would be a more direct parallel to the flat moral imperative for Jewish lawyers to show mercy to Samaritans, or for Christians to show mercy to non-Christians. Instead, he makes the Samaritan the hero. Why?

There is a doctrinal point in the parable, an indicative accompanying the imperative. It's why we see in the context that the inquisitor is "desiring to justify himself." It's why, I think, we get the details of the priest and the Levite passing by. These plot points are a poke in the eye of the religious establishment, of course, but casting the Samaritan as "the good guy" is a five-finger exploding-heart death punch. Jesus knew the Samaritan was a heretic, but he's not saying heresy is okay! Jesus is not calling sin good, not then and not ever. But by consorting with tax collectors and Samaritans, he is showing how sinners can be called good.

The movie *Fred Claus* (2007) is a mediocre Christmas movie at best, but there is one short scene in the film that is gleaming with gospel brilliance. It gets me every time. Fred, the brother of Santa Claus, in a fit of empathetic mercy to all the rough-around-the-edges kids in the world, starts going through the "naughty list" and stamping every entry with the label NICE. It's a scandalous act of unjust justice. An efficiency expert assigned to the struggling North Pole operation is mortified. And there you have it.

Jesus has the audacity (and the authority) to sovereignly make naughty kids nice, and the religious efficiency experts have been up in arms about it ever since.

Making the half-breed heretic the hero of the story is a piercing pinprick to the gaseous bladder of Christless piety. The parable of the good Samaritan makes it abundantly clear that justification cannot come from ethnicity or religion or any other earthly badge of honor. By making the bad guy "good," Jesus shows us how any sinner is ripe for righteousness because the ground is level at the foot of the cross. It is a similar point to Jesus's forgiving of the woman caught in adultery (John 8:1–11). He isn't saying the woman didn't deserve death for her sin; he's saying that everyone else in the crowd did, too. Spiritually speaking, they were all adulteresses. And spiritually speaking, the self-righteous Jews were all Samaritans.

"For all have sinned and fall short of the glory of God" (Rom. 3:23).

Who indeed has loved his neighbor, who has shown mercy, more than Jesus? Who brings righteousness by sabotaging self-righteousness? Jesus.

It is Jesus—the good and faithful Jew—who puts himself in the place of the sinner, so that the justice of God may be satisfied, so that his will may be done on earth as it is in heaven.

The lawyer seeks to justify himself by being a good person. "Who is my neighbor?" "How much is enough?" That's what he really wants to know. The anthropological point of Jesus's parable is the premise of Paul's claim that "neither circumcision nor uncircumcision counts for anything" (Gal. 5:6).

Most people assume there are really two categories: good people and bad people. There are people who are trying and people who aren't. Most religions, including some identifying as Christian, operate according to these two categories. There are religious people and irreligious people.

There's a local cult group here in Vermont called the Twelve Tribes that teaches that, in the afterlife, bad people go to hell, people in the Twelve Tribes go to heaven with Jesus, and good people who don't know Jesus occupy a renewed earth. (It's somewhat like the Jehovah's Witnesses that way.) They want to accommodate the two categories in their creation of three categories, because they know "good people" and "bad people" are the categories that "work."

But Jesus and his Bible put a red *X* on this categorization. All people are born condemned. We all know apathetic licentiousness won't rectify that. But the Scriptures tell us being good won't solve the problem either. There is only one category for us.

We don't need a "good people" category. We need a whole new category. Christ supersedes our plausibility. The gospel is the other category, because only Christ counts for anything.

6

# The Dreadfulness of Death after Death

Your wickedness makes you as it were heavy as lead, and to tend downwards with great weight and pressure towards Hell; and if God should let you go, you would immediately sink and swiftly descend & plunge into the bottomless gulf, and your healthy constitution, and your own care and prudence, and best contrivance, and all your righteousness, would have no more influence to uphold you and keep you out of hell, than a spider's web would have to stop a falling rock. Were it not that so is the sovereign pleasure of God, the earth would not bear you one moment; for you are a burden to it; the creation groans with you; the creature is made subject to the bondage of your corruption, not willingly; the sun don't willingly shine upon you to give you light to serve sin and Satan; the earth don't willingly yield her increase to satisfy your lusts; nor is it willingly a stage for your wickedness to be acted upon; the air don't willingly serve you for breath to maintain the flame of life in your vitals, while you spend your life in the service of God's enemies. . . .

And the world would spew you out, were it not for the sovereign hand of him who hath subjected it in hope. There are the black clouds of God's wrath now hanging directly over your heads, full of the dreadful storm, and big with thun-

> der; and were it not for the restraining hand of God it would immediately burst forth upon you. The sovereign pleasure of God for the present, stays his rough wind; otherwise it would come with fury, and your destruction would come like a whirlwind, and you would be like the chaff of the summer threshing floor.
>
> The wrath of God is like great waters that are dammed for the present; they increase more and more, & rise higher and higher, till an outlet is given, and the longer the stream is stop'd, the more rapid and mighty is its course, when once it is let loose. 'Tis true, that judgment against your evil works has not been executed hitherto; the floods of God's vengeance have been withheld; but your guilt in the mean time is constantly increasing, and you are every day treasuring up more wrath.[1]

No one really preaches like that anymore. And some say, "Good!" I say it's because we've really lowered the stakes. In the age of *Love Wins*, we've relocated hell solely to earth and convinced ourselves there's nothing worse than losing one's body (Matt. 10:28).

Hell just doesn't sound like a good God. Especially when we've redefined goodness.

But some avoid preaching hell not because they don't believe in it but because they find it impolite and untoward. It is the disagreeable part about God, the part to obscure. And in obscuring the bad news, it is no wonder so many churches in the West have forgotten the good. It makes less sense. Man's chief problem, they assume, is lack of success, scarcity of happiness; therefore, our message ought to be 7 Steps to a Victorious Whatever. And thus we offer shiny new laws that only increase the trespass (Rom. 5:20).

Jesus was not skittish about preaching hell because he knew the stakes were that high. "Sin no more, that nothing worse may happen to you," he tells the healed paralytic (John 5:14). Because

[1] Jonathan Edwards, "Sinners in the Hands of an Angry God," in *"Sinners in the Hands of an Angry God" and Other Puritan Sermons*, ed. David Dutkanicz (Mineola, NY: Dover, 2005), 177.

he knows there are worse things than being paralyzed. He knows there are worse things than dying.

## The Sheep and the Goats

As we prepare to examine the parable about the rich man and Lazarus, let's look at one of Jesus's direct references to the afterlife (in Matt. 25:31–46). Following the barrage of high-stakes parables concluding the Olivet Discourse (Matthew 24), this word about the eternal destinies of the righteous and the unrighteous contains elements of a parable (separating people like sheep and goats; Matt. 25:32–33) but it is largely a circling back around to answer the disciples' question about the end of the age (Matt. 24:3). Why be alert and diligent, so as to be found faithful? Because the stakes couldn't be higher:

> Then he [the Son of Man] will say to those on his left, "Depart from me, you cursed, into the eternal fire prepared for the devil and his angels. For I was hungry and you gave me no food, I was thirsty and you gave me no drink, I was a stranger and you did not welcome me, naked and you did not clothe me, sick and in prison and you did not visit me." Then they also will answer, saying, "Lord, when did we see you hungry or thirsty or a stranger or naked or sick or in prison, and did not minister to you?" Then he will answer them, saying, "Truly, I say to you, as you did not do it to one of the least of these, you did not do it to me." And these will go away into eternal punishment, but the righteous into eternal life. (Matt. 25:41–46)

This passage does not, as some suppose, teach a works righteousness. We need only hold it up with the similar teaching in which Jesus sent the doers of good works (in his name!) to the same eternal punishment as these non-doers of works (Matt. 7:21–23). J. C. Ryle explains:

> The last judgment will be a judgment *according to evidence.* The works of men are the witnesses which will be brought

> forward, and above all their works of charity. The question to be ascertained will not merely be what we said, but what we did—not merely what we professed, but what we practiced. Our works unquestionably will not justify us. We are justified by faith without the deeds of the law. But the truth of our faith will be tested by our lives. Faith which has not works is dead, being alone. (James 2:20)[2]

What the "sheep" are receiving at the end of their faithful lives is the inheritance prepared for them at the foundation of the world (Matt. 25:34), before they had done anything either good or bad. Their lives of goodness, of tending to Christ, as it were, are the evidences of their having tended to Christ's church—"the least of these my brothers" (v. 40). This is not to say, of course, that the mission of the church does not include such care for those outside the church; as I argued in the previous chapter, it does. It is only to say that the sheep receiving the inheritance are those who have been "blessed by my Father" (v. 34), have been promised the blessing before time (v. 34), and have made the care of Christ through the care of his people a chief concern of their lives (v. 40).

Like the parable of Lazarus and the rich man, this teaching then shows us the dreadfulness of the death after death. "Then he will say to those on his left, 'Depart from me, you cursed, into the eternal fire prepared for the devil and his angels'" (Matt. 25:41).

Jesus is not talking about a fiery garbage dump outside Jerusalem. It has been common to think that, since Jesus surely could not mean to send people into a fiery hell for eternity, the "historical context" shows us instead that he is just speaking metaphorically of the eternal annihilation of unbelievers with yet another allusion to Gehenna (explicit in Matthew 5:22, 29–30; 10:28; 18:9; 23:15; Mark 9:43), the Valley of Hinnom outside the city where trash was continually burning. But this claim is, if you'll forgive the term, rubbish. There is virtually no evidence from the time in question to support such a claim about the Valley of Hinnom, and

[2] J. C. Ryle, *The Gospel of Matthew* (1856), http://www.gracegems.org/Ryle/Matthew.htm.

what has become a sort of biblical urban legend today—similar to the old chestnut, since debunked, about the "eye of the needle" being a gate into the city through which camels must walk on their knees—actually originates well into the thirteenth century. George R. Beasley-Murray is one of many scholars addressing the claim:

> The notion, still referred to by some commentators, that the city's rubbish was burned in this valley, has no further basis than a statement by the Jewish scholar Kimchi made about A.D. 1200; it is not attested in any ancient source.[3]

Further, we should find it suspect that those who deny hell along these lines do not similarly metaphorize Jesus's words about heaven. The place of punishment? An exaggeration; doesn't exist. Heaven? Realer than can be. Eternal punishment is a myth, while eternal life is a reality. An obvious case of double-mindedness.

No, when Jesus speaks of eternal punishment he means just that. He means that hell is real. Of course, our perceptions of it may be inaccurate, but our belief in it is well grounded in the Scriptures. It is a place prepared for the Devil and his angels, so it cannot simply refer to the graves of the mortal. Likewise, since Jesus is highlighting two destinations in this passage, not one, we know he cannot be referring to the grave of death, nor is he teaching universalism.

The language Jesus uses to describe hell may be symbolic, of course, but the thing about symbols is that they have referents. They correspond to real things, and biblical symbols often pale in comparison to the realities to which they point. In other words, when Jesus says there will be weeping and gnashing of teeth in the place of eternal punishment, it is not likely that he means it will be not so bad as all that; more likely he means it will be much worse.

Similarly, to even use the phrase "eternal" in relation to this punishment, to this place of fiery condemnation, is to tell us that it is exactly that: eternal. Hell is forever. The destruction is eternal

[3] G. R. Beasley-Murray, *Jesus and the Kingdom of God* (Grand Rapids, MI: Eerdmans, 1986), 376–377.

(2 Thess. 1:9). The fire is eternal (Jude 7). The "gloom of utter darkness" is "reserved forever" (Jude 13). Jesus refers to the fires of hell as being "unquenchable" (Matt. 3:12; Mark 9:43). And in case we are led to believe that the eternal destruction refers to an irreversible annihilation, Revelation 14:11 tells us that "the smoke of their torment goes up forever and ever."

Simply (and bluntly) put, hell is real and eternal because God's holiness is real and eternal. The unrepentant workers of iniquity will serve to showcase God's justice for all eternity. This *should* make us uncomfortable. It should make us uncomfortable enough to make our calling and election sure.

Because the frightening thing is that, to enter hell, all one has to do is nothing.

"Truly, I say to you, as you did not do it to one of the least of these, you did not do it to me" (Matt. 25:45). All you have to do to go to hell is not rock the boat. Accept the status quo. Hell is quite easy to enter. Because outside of Christ we stand condemned already (John 3:18), we need simply do nothing. As Edwards says, there is nothing between the reprobate and hell but air. The only thing preventing the breathing unbeliever's entrance into hell at this very moment is the patience of God.

"The gate is wide and the way is easy that leads to destruction, and those who enter by it are many" (Matt. 7:13).

You few, you happy few, enter by the narrow gate.

## Lazarus and the Rich Man

Now we turn to Jesus's parable about this place called hell. It is one of his more detailed stories, enhanced by the inclusion of proper names (Lazarus, Abraham), the only time Jesus does this in a recorded parable. Some have surmised this is because it is not a parable at all, but a real incident. It is more likely that the inclusion of proper names is to heighten the reality of what is being described—to emphasize that real people with real lives go to heaven or to hell—although perhaps there is some significance to the fact that Jesus names the rewarded while the condemned man goes nameless:

> There was a rich man who was clothed in purple and fine linen and who feasted sumptuously every day. And at his gate was laid a poor man named Lazarus, covered with sores, who desired to be fed with what fell from the rich man's table. Moreover, even the dogs came and licked his sores. The poor man died and was carried by the angels to Abraham's side. The rich man also died and was buried, and in Hades, being in torment, he lifted up his eyes and saw Abraham far off and Lazarus at his side. And he called out, "Father Abraham, have mercy on me, and send Lazarus to dip the end of his finger in water and cool my tongue, for I am in anguish in this flame." But Abraham said, "Child, remember that you in your lifetime received your good things, and Lazarus in like manner bad things; but now he is comforted here, and you are in anguish. And besides all this, between us and you a great chasm has been fixed, in order that those who would pass from here to you may not be able, and none may cross from there to us." And he said, "Then I beg you, father, to send him to my father's house—for I have five brothers—so that he may warn them, lest they also come into this place of torment." But Abraham said, "They have Moses and the Prophets; let them hear them." And he said, "No, father Abraham, but if someone goes to them from the dead, they will repent." He said to him, "If they do not hear Moses and the Prophets, neither will they be convinced if someone should rise from the dead." (Luke 16:19–31)

In connection with the rest of the Bible's teaching about eternal condemnation, including the teaching on the sheep and the goats, we see again here that (1) hell is real, (2) hell is eternal, and (3) hell is very easy to get to.

Some will say, "Oh, it's just a parable." Okay, but a parable about what? Like symbols, parables have referents. They correspond to things—things that are bigger and more real than their examples. What Jesus refers to as "torment" and "anguish" cannot mean an unconscious void. Nor, more obviously, can it mean "everyone goes to heaven." Nor can it refer to "hell on earth," since the rich man is clearly in a postmortem place, unreachable from heaven.

Similarly, Jesus draws on the traditional Jewish designations for the afterlife: Abraham's bosom and Hades (or the grave of the wicked). He is not essentially making a practical point about being nice to each other but a theological point that confirms and clarifies earlier divine revelation.

The chasm between heaven and hell is fixed. It is irrevocable. The anguish will be forever, and from it there will be no relief. Whatever may be gathered from the narrative as speculative, this point certainly is not hazy. Jesus is teaching through the figure of Abraham, receiver of the everlasting covenant, that God's promise of condemnation is everlasting.

We see here again how frighteningly easy it is to go to hell. Like the rich man, simply mind your own business. The very short description of his life reveals the depths of his excess. He "feasted sumptuously every day." This rich man loved himself a lot. This is very, very easy for anyone to do, and it is very, very easy to be self-involved all the way into self-destruction.

It is quite easy to go to hell. You don't even have to believe what you see! Abraham tells the man that witnessing a miracle—someone going to the living from the dead, presumably Lazarus—will achieve nothing for those who do not believe in the Law and the Prophets. Basically, seeing with the eyes of the body will not result in belief until seeing with the eyes of the soul does. Abraham is saying about the rich man's relatives, "If they won't believe the word of God about the Messiah, miracles won't do them any good."

Do you remember Jesus's response to skeptical Thomas?

> Now Thomas, one of the Twelve, called the Twin, was not with them when Jesus came. So the other disciples told him, "We have seen the Lord." But he said to them, "Unless I see

> in his hands the mark of the nails, and place my finger into the mark of the nails, and place my hand into his side, I will never believe."
>
> Eight days later, his disciples were inside again, and Thomas was with them. Although the doors were locked, Jesus came and stood among them and said, "Peace be with you." Then he said to Thomas, "Put your finger here, and see my hands; and put out your hand, and place it in my side. Do not disbelieve, but believe." Thomas answered him, "My Lord and my God!" Jesus said to him, "Have you believed because you have seen me? Blessed are those who have not seen and yet have believed." (John 20:24–29)

Jesus condescended in mercy to let Thomas see, but he is emphatic: "Blessed are those who have not seen and yet have believed."

In this sense, the parable of Lazarus and the rich man affirms what Jesus has said about the parables as a whole: Spiritual regeneration precedes the exercise of faith.

## Preaching Hell Is a Great Kindness

Perhaps like me, the first time you read Jonathan Edwards's classic sermon "Sinners in the Hands of an Angry God" was in a high school English class. The sermon was presented as a snapshot of Puritan theology. My high school English and history teachers got the Puritans mostly wrong, positing them as dour and dull pathologically religious killjoys. Certainly "Sinners" is one of Edwards's most somber sermons—I maintain it is not his best—but the presumption that Edwards wrote it because he relished psychologically torturing his congregation is unfair and uncritical. It is also historically tone-deaf to Edwards's context and spiritually tone-deaf to the Bible.

Today, the preaching of hell is often characterized as nothing less than spiritual abuse. When John Piper preached his last sermon as senior pastor of Bethlehem Baptist Church in Minneapolis, the local paper introduced a feature story on his retirement with this line: "John Piper will not be in the pulpit, promising God's judgment against sinners, for much longer."[4] Does John Piper preach God's judgment against sinners? Well, sure, given some qualifications. John Piper preaches the gospel. He is a very serious preacher; influenced heavily by Edwards himself, he may in fact be the Edwards of our day. And as with Edwards, many confuse Piper's heavy sober-mindedness about the wrath of God as judgmentalism, as a case of being wound up way too tight. But to characterize the primary theme of Piper's ministry (or Edwards's) as "judgment against sinners" is to mischaracterize it. These men preach the salvation of sinners through Jesus Christ alone, who took that horrible judgment upon himself. Let those with the ears to hear *hear*.

Today, however, every evangelical is considered a fundamentalist (in the pejorative sense), and to preach grace comes with the expectation of playing nice with all people in all circumstances. One fellow in our little town once characterized the theme of my message using that very word. "Every preacher has their thing," he told me, as we both shivered one winter afternoon in his woodshop. "Your thing is grace." I was heartened at the time that he had so easily seen this. But one Sunday, as I issued a warning that we all should watch our doctrine closely, I criticized prosperity-gospelists from the pulpit, and I was instantly on the outs with this man. Even after numerous conversations on the issue, he has never returned to our church. Why? Because in his mind to call out heresy is not Christian. The biblical writers had no such compunctions. They knew the stakes are too high.

My ex-supporter mistakenly believed that preaching grace precluded preaching judgment. Certainly some Christians have made quite a tradition out of preaching hell without preaching the gospel, which is just as stupid as not preaching hell at all. Some preach hell as if it were more horrible than heaven is wonderful, as if it were more fascinating than Christ is beautiful. Some can preach hell out of morbid fascination, legalistic fearmongering, and spiritual

[4] Rose French, "Fiery Preacher Leaving Pulpit, but This Won't Be His Last Word," *Minneapolis Star Tribune* (December 29, 2012), http://www.startribune.com/lifestyle/185174322.html?refer=y.

manipulation. But the proper response to foolishness is never more foolishness.

*If* hell exists—and I know that's a big "if" in the estimation of some—it is entirely reasonable to speak and act as if it were the gravest danger facing anyone. It would certainly be more dangerous than bodily death, if Jesus's logic is to have any influence.

You don't even have to be a Christian to understand this. Perhaps you've seen Penn Jillette's YouTube video rant on Christian proselytization, which went viral a couple of years ago. Jillette, one-half of the celebrated illusionist duo Penn and Teller, is an atheist. He does not believe hell exists. But he says pointedly to Christians in his rant that if *you* believe hell exists, it would not be hateful at all to warn him about it. It would in fact be hateful *not* to. This is what we should all call *being logical*. Jillette uses the illustration of a speeding bus. If he's standing in its way and doesn't see it coming, the loving thing to do is to push him out of its way. He then asks, "How much do you have to hate someone *not* to proselytize?"

Again, we should absolutely talk about hell in gracious ways, which is to say, we should not be "bad news" people but "good news" people. We should not preach hell the way some of our fundamentalist forebears did, as if hell were the *only* reality. We ought to say it is real and it is a danger to those apart from Christ, and then we ought to hold out Christ as the glorious, wonderful, hell-proof hope.

Preaching hell in the context of the gospel is not hate. And getting angry about the denial of hell or the preaching of heresy that sends people there is not blood thirst: it is what logical people do when someone says that the giant waterfall your canoe is heading for isn't really there. It is an anger born not of hate, but love.

Here is that snarling killjoy Edwards on the subject:

> If there be really a hell of such dreadful and never-ending torments, as is generally supposed, of which multitudes are in great danger—and into which the greater part of men in Christian countries do actually from generation to generation

> fall, for want of a sense of its terribleness, and so their danger of it, and so for want of taking due care to avoid it—then why is it not proper for those who have the care of souls to take great pains to make men sensible of it? Why should they not be told as much of the truth as can be? If I am in danger of going to hell, I should be glad to know as much as possibly I can of the dreadfulness of it. If I am very prone to neglect due care to avoid it, he does me the best kindness who does most to represent to me the truth of the case, that sets forth my misery and danger in the liveliest manner.[5]

The stakes couldn't be higher. If you're reading this yet unsure of your eternal destiny, I urge you, flee to Christ. There is glad escape from eternal condemnation in the safety of the Savior who has taken the condemnation for sins upon himself and conquered death and hell—yes, for even you, if you want him.

## Hell Is Conquered in Christ

"And these will go away into eternal punishment, but the righteous into eternal life" (Matt. 25:46).

What should the rich man and his relatives have heard and believed from Moses and the Prophets? The saving grace of Messiah, according to Jesus, who showed the disciples on the road to Emmaus all the things about himself from Moses and the Prophets (Luke 24:27). And according to Philip (John 1:45), and according to Paul (Acts 26:22–23; 28:23), and according to the author of Hebrews (chapters 7–8).

How does one become righteous? By being born again. By dying with Christ and therefore being raised to new life in Christ. By being *in Christ*. This is the only way to avoid hell:

> He said to them, "But who do you say that I am?" Simon Peter replied, "You are the Christ, the Son of the living God." And

[5] Jonathan Edwards, "The Distinguishing Marks of a Work of the True Spirit," in *Jonathan Edwards on Revival* (Carlisle, PA: Banner of Truth, 1994), 106.

> Jesus answered him, "Blessed are you, Simon Bar-Jonah! For flesh and blood has not revealed this to you, but my Father who is in heaven. And I tell you, you are Peter, and on this rock I will build my church, and the gates of hell shall not prevail against it." (Matt. 16:15–18)

Once again, we see that saving faith comes as a result of divine revelation to the heart. Peter didn't confess Christ as Savior and God because he'd crunched the spiritual numbers but because the Father granted it to him to believe. Satan's saboteurs work in code, but Peter has been given the key. It is the first benefit of regeneration.

And now the benefits stream in. From Christ's fullness there is grace upon grace (John 1:16). On the confession of faith, Christ will build his church. And the church is called the body of Christ precisely because its true confessors are united to Christ. And because the true confessors are united to Christ, they are as secure as Christ is, which means, among a multitude of things, that they have his Spirit and are secured against hell, its Devil, and his schemes.

You and I, although we are sinners, may conquer hell if we are in Christ, because Christ has conquered hell. Here is something provocative, dissolving of the pernicious dualism masquerading sometimes as Christian faith: hell does not belong to Satan. As the place of condemnation, it is a realm under our sovereign God's jurisdiction. Satan himself will suffer there, just like the rest of the condemned.

And so it is more precise to say in the long run that in the last day, God wins. He wins even now. He has never failed. Oh, we could say that in the end love wins too, so long as we are acknowledging along with the Bible that those who love themselves, and thereby hate God, will suffer eternal defeat in hell. Hate loses. Those, then, who love the Lord their God with all their heart, soul, mind, and strength—and their neighbors as themselves—win. Infinitely. Irrevocably. Invincibly:

> There is therefore now no condemnation for those who are in Christ Jesus. For the law of the Spirit of life has set you free in Christ Jesus from the law of sin and death. For God has done what the law, weakened by the flesh, could not do. By sending his own Son in the likeness of sinful flesh and for sin, he condemned sin in the flesh . . . (Rom. 8:1–3)

The fall brought sin, and sin brought justifiable condemnation, but Christ the conqueror defeats death and hell. The parables Jesus tells are themselves glimpses into the warfare. They are dispatches from the spiritual battlefield, postcards from the revolution. They show us what is happening as God's kingdom breaks into the world, as heaven invades earth, as the Father's will is done here as it is done there. Call them propaganda posters, if you like, but they are portraits of inevitable and inaugural reality. The new king is the ancient of days, and he's finally setting the world to rights, bringing the great shalom that creation has been groaning for, in and through Jesus the Christ, who is the Prince of Peace who has come to break the bonds of injustice, to bind the strongman, to kill sin, and to conquer the grave. To be rescued into Abraham's bosom, then, is even then merely the foretaste of the infinite joys of the new heaven and new earth to come after.

Get yourself then to Christ and *into* Christ. He is storing up wrath even now for the unrepentant, and will not fail to dispense it at the day of judgment. But there is escape from the Judge *in* the Judge.

This Christ is our refuge! This Christ is our security! This Christ is our salvation!

The righteous will enter into eternal life on that coming day. Perhaps it is for you only a breath away. Nothing separates you from judgment but air. If Christ is your righteousness, you may have the confidence to die as one assured of the inheritance prepared for you before the foundation of the world.

I have found great joy in this bit of verse from the Scottish minister Robert Murray M'Cheyne. It is all about the claiming of the glorious Christ as the Lord Our Righteousness (*Jehovah-Tsidkenu* in the Hebrew), leading to that eternal life *after* life after death:

(The watchword of the Reformers)

I once was a stranger to grace and to God,
I knew not my danger, and felt not my load;
Though friends spoke in rapture of Christ on the tree,
Jehovah Tsidkenu was nothing to me.

I oft read with pleasure, to soothe or engage,
Isaiah's wild measure and John's simple page;
But e'en when they pictured the blood-sprinkled tree
Jehovah Tsidkenu seemed nothing to me.

Like tears from the daughters of Zion that roll,
I wept when the waters went over His soul;
Yet thought not that my sins had nailed to the tree
Jehovah Tsidkenu—'twas nothing to me.

When free grace awoke me, by light from on high,
Then legal fears shook me, I trembled to die;
No refuge, no safety in self could I see—
Jehovah Tsidkenu my Savior must be.

My terrors all vanished before the sweet name;
My guilty fears banished, with boldness I came
To drink at the fountain, life-giving and free—
Jehovah Tsidkenu is all things to me.

Jehovah Tsidkenu! my treasure and boast,
Jehovah Tsidkenu! I ne'er can be lost;
In thee I shall conquer by flood and by field—
My cable, my anchor, my breastplate and shield!

Even treading the valley, the shadow of death,
This "watchword" shall rally my faltering breath;

For while from life's fever my God sets me free,
Jehovah Tsidkenu my death-song shall be.[6]

I beg of you, friend, trust this Christ and his righteousness as your Christ and your righteousness. Flee hell by trusting the loving grace of God in the sin-killing, death-conquering, hell-proof Jesus. "Escape for your life. Do not look back or stop. . . . Escape to the hills, lest you be swept away" (Gen. 19:17).

---

[6] Robert Murray M'Cheyne and Andrew A. Bonar, *Memoir and Remains of the Rev. Robert Murray M'Cheyne* (Edinburgh, London: Oliphant Anderson & Ferrier, 1894), 574.

7

# Jesus Is for Losers

Jesus is for losers.

That's how I read the Gospels, anyway. The kind of people attracted to Jesus in the pages of Scripture are not those with everything going for them. Those who felt like they had the world on a string did not tend to care much for the man who held the world in his hands. Instead, it was the broken, burdened, and beaten-down who seem most attracted to Jesus. There are exceptions, of course, but when the outwardly successful find Christ, it is always because they recognize their inward failure.

Jesus's teaching in fact tended to draw a sharp distinction between the humble poor in spirit and the prideful rich in self-righteousness. He is constantly polarizing. The magnetic tension created by Jesus's ministry produces a stark separation between those who love him and those who oppose him. This is not just the by-product of Jesus's teaching but often its purpose. Consider these provocative statements by Jesus:

> No servant can serve two masters, for either he will hate the one and love the other, or he will be devoted to the one and despise the other. You cannot serve God and money. (Luke 16:13)

> Whoever is not with me is against me, and whoever does not gather with me scatters. (Matt. 12:30)

> Do not think that I have come to bring peace to the earth. I have not come to bring peace, but a sword. For I have come to set a man against his father, and a daughter against her mother, and a daughter-in-law against her mother-in-law. And a person's enemies will be those of his own household. Whoever loves father or mother more than me is not worthy of me, and whoever loves son or daughter more than me is not worthy of me. (Matt. 10:34–37)

Jesus is not forming a fan club. He is demanding allegiance.

## The Great Banquet

The parable of the great banquet (or great feast) is prefaced in Luke 14 by a real-life Sabbath encounter between Jesus and some Pharisees in which our Savior, who is dining with these experts, asks them whether it is lawful to heal on the Sabbath. They do not reply. Filling in his own blanks, Jesus heals a man with dropsy right there on the spot. Then he says something so refreshingly obvious: "Which of you, having a son or an ox that has fallen into a well on a Sabbath day, will not immediately pull him out?" (Luke 14:5). No one is more logical than Jesus. With one statement he demonstrates he has authority from the Father, a sense of loving care from the Father, and a ruthless rationality from the Father. If a son—or even an ox!—falls into a pit, you don't tell him you'll come back later. That would be ridiculous. And God is not ridiculous. If your son falls into a pit on Saturday, you pull him out the same as if it were Tuesday.

In both fulfilling and explaining the law, Jesus helps us see that the law has not been given out of some sense of spiritual sadism. Man has not been made for the Sabbath, but the Sabbath for man (Mark 2:27). It is entirely lawful to do good on the day of rest, because we are not to take a rest from worship.

The connection between this incident and the ensuing parable is of particular interest. Jesus confounds the legalists, who specialize in elevating empty behavior over sincere belief and therefore looking good over doing good, by restoring a man who has endured painful swelling for who knows how long, and on the Sabbath. Jesus has satisfied the law, actually, by ushering the afflicted man into rest. This healing right before the blind eyes of the legalists is exactly what the parable illustrates: the giving of kingdom benefits to those with no social or religious currency with which to purchase them, and the denial of kingdom benefits to those who cannot see them as beneficial:

> He said also to the man who had invited him, "When you give a dinner or a banquet, do not invite your friends or your brothers or your relatives or rich neighbors, lest they also invite you in return and you be repaid. But when you give a feast, invite the poor, the crippled, the lame, the blind, and you will be blessed, because they cannot repay you. For you will be repaid at the resurrection of the just."
>
> When one of those who reclined at table with him heard these things, he said to him, "Blessed is everyone who will eat bread in the kingdom of God!" But he said to him, "A man once gave a great banquet and invited many. And at the time for the banquet he sent his servant to say to those who had been invited, 'Come, for everything is now ready.' But they all alike began to make excuses. The first said to him, 'I have bought a field, and I must go out and see it. Please have me excused.' And another said, 'I have bought five yoke of oxen, and I go to examine them. Please have me excused.' And another said, 'I have married a wife, and therefore I cannot come.' So the servant came and reported these things to his master. Then the master of the house became angry and said to his servant, 'Go out quickly to the streets and lanes of the city, and bring in the poor and crippled and blind and lame.' And the servant said, 'Sir, what you commanded has been done, and still there is room.' And the master said to the servant, 'Go out to the highways and hedges and compel people to come in, that my house may be filled. For I tell you, none of those men who were invited shall taste my banquet.'" (Luke 14:12–24)

The man giving the banquet is the Father. Through his proclaimed word the invitation is given to all. "Come, for everything is now ready" is akin to "Repent, for the kingdom of heaven is at hand." Then come the excuses. Many are called. But few are chosen.

There are two main features of this parable, surrounding the two types of invitees (no surprise, given Jesus's plan to separate everyone into the categories of sheep and goats). The first group makes excuses for not coming to the banquet. There is nothing particularly insightful about these excuses; they are placeholders for any old excuse one might make to reject Christ and his kingdom. Their commonality is common today: they are utterly mundane. Blomberg writes, "What all three share is an extraordinary lameness."[1]

Of course they never appear so to the one making them. Those obsessed with business and home and family justify themselves, mentally calculating that these are good, valuable things, and therefore understandable as trade-ins for the kingdom of God. Certainly Jesus's own family thought so:

> And his mother and his brothers came, and standing outside they sent to him and called him. And a crowd was sitting around him, and they said to him, "Your mother and your brothers are outside, seeking you." (Mark 3:31–32)

Jesus's family worried he'd gone crazy (v. 21). How blind do you have to be to be told by an angel that your son would be the Messiah and later worry he's gotten too big for his britches? How blind do you have to be to grow up with Jesus, pick up somehow that he has committed no sins, and yet still not believe in his claims? Somewhere along the way, the journey of Jesus's family had taken them from joy to fear. Giving Mary the benefit of the doubt, we can chalk up her concern to being protective. Perhaps she simply fears for Jesus's life, in which case she is being a good mom but a bad Christian.

---

[1] Craig L. Blomberg, *Interpreting the Parables* (Downer's Grove, IL: InterVarsity Press, 1990), 234.

Where Jesus goes and what Jesus calls us to do as we follow him is very daunting.

Many see the temptation to this very fear when one of their kids answers the call to foreign missions. It is admirable. We are glad some people do that. But we hope for something less risky for our own children. "Can't you serve Jesus somewhere else?"

So why have Mary and the siblings come to stop Jesus? Because the trajectory he is on is scary, disruptive, unsafe, for him and for others. But Jesus will not be deterred:

> It is interesting to note the quiet, firm perseverance of our Lord in the face of all discouragements. The slanderous suggestions of enemies and the well-meant remonstrances of ignorant friends were alike powerless to turn him from his course. He had set his face as a flint towards the cross and the crown. He knew the work he had come into the world to do. He had a baptism to undergo, and was distressed until it was completed (Luke 12:50).
>
> So let it be with all true servants of Christ. Let nothing turn them for a moment out of the narrow way, or make them stop and look back. Let them take no notice of the ill-natured remarks of enemies. Let them not give way to the well-intentioned but mistaken entreaties of unconverted relations and friends. Let them reply in the words of Nehemiah, "I am carrying on a great project and cannot go down" (Nehemiah 6:3). Let them say, "I have taken up the cross, and I will not throw it down."[2]

Jesus prized something more than even the good things of the world, including his family. He wanted the will of his heavenly Father to be done. And here's where we get into that tricky stuff Jesus says, like, "Whoever loves father or mother more than me is not worthy of me, and whoever loves son or daughter more than me is not worthy of me" (Matt. 10:37), and "Follow me, and leave the dead

[2] J. C. Ryle, *Mark*, Crossway Classic Commentaries, ed. Alister McGrath and J. I. Packer (Wheaton, IL: Crossway, 1993), 44–45.

to bury their own dead" (8:22). Jesus ever proclaims that the kingdom must be sought first, before fields and oxen and even wives.

Christ is to be our prized possession. Remember the parables of the treasure and the pearl! We are to consider all things as loss for the sake of knowing him (Phil. 3:8).

When his family has come to put a stop to his shenanigans, Jesus says, "Who are my mother and my brothers?" (Mark 3:33). It is a disruptive, defining question. Jesus reframes the entire conversation, bringing the kingdom of God into it.

There is something bigger happening here, he's saying, bigger than biological family. Certainly bigger than fields and oxen. The parables are homespun tales, but the home they refer to is of another world. All of these things? They are passing away. Including marriage (Matt. 22:30).

Now, Jesus doesn't hate his family. He just loves the Father more. And because he loves the Father more, he knows that the family that will endure for all eternity is the family of God. And so the parable of the banquet is not about neglecting family and the obligations of ordinary life. It's about crucifying idols, whether they come from your family or anywhere else, and about prizing Christ as all-satisfying. It's about surrendering the plausible arguments we make for finding the kingdom of God inconvenient.

And this is why it's not the man with dropsy making excuses. He has nothing left to offer. He is well aware of his need, while those of us able to medicate ourselves with accumulations and achievements keep our sense of need at bay. The man giving the banquet orders that all the poor and crippled and blind and lame be brought in to the feast. The kingdom is for such as these.

Why invite people to dinner who cannot repay you? Because it pictures the gospel in a way the mutual admiration society doesn't.

## The Gospel As Middle and Better Way

To treat anyone on the basis of what they may provide to you in return is relational legalism. It is an objectification of people, a using of them, a treating of them like vending machines. It doesn't have to be the poor or otherwise needy we treat this way. It can be our spouse or our church family. When we give and serve only for the anticipated gratitude, we engage in legalism.

But the gospel changes the way we think of others and the way we think of things. It refocuses for us the glory of God in Christ's loving and serving of us. When we focus on the satisfaction Christ brings to our worshiping souls, it changes the way we view the wares of the world.

Consider these polar opposites: legalism and license, Pharisaism and hedonism, religion and anarchy, self-righteousness and unrighteousness. The items in each of these pairs are more alike in essence than they appear—because they each reflect our innate need to worship and the self-interest that our passions, religious or irreligious, tend to spring from, but between these polarities lies the gospel of Jesus Christ. It is the middle and better way.

The gospel is the middle way because it provides the centering of God's powerful grace, freeing us from the condemnation of works righteousness on the one hand and the condemnation of disobedience on the other. It announces the "at hand"–ness of the kingdom, the manifest presence of God's sovereignty, which fulfills the old covenant and inaugurates the new covenant, thereby superseding the way that is passing away with the Way that is here to stay.

The gospel is the better way because it takes the excesses of the hedonistic polarity and applies them in Spiritual power to the aims of the religious polarity: Jesus posits that disciples may be required to go with someone for a mile. License would have us disobey the command altogether—running in the other direction. Legalism would have us obey what is required—going one mile. The grace in the gospel, however, trains us (Titus 2:11–12) to do the minimum *and more*: a second mile. They want your coat? Give 'em your shirt too.

Similarly, think of the marriage relationship. If we simply followed the law, we would treat our spouses fairly, kindly, well. But captured by Christ in his gracious gospel, husbands don't just avoid being mean to their wives; they cherish them, loving them sacrificially, selflessly. Wives don't just respect their husbands; they submit to them. The affectionate excess of licentiousness is channeled by grace to super-fulfillment of the law. God in Christ did not simply tolerate us; he lavished the riches of his grace upon us (Eph. 1:7–8).

The gospel is not a bare minimum thing. Apply it to the area of financial giving. Paul urges the middle and better way of the gospel in 2 Corinthians 9:7. The lawful thing to do would be to give. Ten percent sounds about right. The disobedient thing would be not to give at all. The gospel goes to the heart first, not the hands. How generous was God in Christ? As Tim Keller says, "Jesus didn't tithe his blood."[3] He gave what was needed, for the joy set before him, even though it killed him. So the gospel provides the grounds for sacrificial, joyful giving. Don't give under compulsion; don't give under reluctance. Give according to the measure of the gospel's dominion over your heart. The excessive passion of the "all out" of stinginess is applied to the requirement to give so that it becomes a zealous "all in" generosity.

In repentance I pursue holiness as zealously as I pursued sin in unrepentance, with much more affection for God than I afforded my idols, even in the panting passions of my lust. Only the gospel can empower this.

Over and over, Jesus shows us this middle and better way. "You have heard not to kill. I say not to hate." "You have heard not to commit adultery. I say not to lust." Not killing or committing adultery are certainly ways to obey the law. Not objectifying people made in God's image in the depths of our hearts is a way to go deeper, to go the second mile in response to the law's demand for the first. So Jesus says, "Love your enemies and bless those who persecute you." The law would only have us tolerate, avoid, and in some cases prosecute.

---

[3]Tim Keller, "The Gospel-shaped Life," message delivered to The Gospel Coalition New England Regional Conference (October 19, 2012), http://www.centerforgospelculture.org/resource/plenary-1-the-gospel-shaped-life/.

The gospel explodes niceness. "Outdo one another in showing honor," it says (Rom. 12:10).

The gospel would have us turn the impulse for revenge inside out until it's a gracious forgiveness. For that's what Jesus did for us. He has not just met the requirements of the law; he has signaled the end of it. He has not just justified us; he has sanctified and glorified us. He has not just pardoned us; he has united us to himself. He has given us not just life, but life abundant (John 10:10).

So now we look through the gospel at the law and see it differently. Not as a burden, but as a delight. We see others not as projects or impediments, but as image-bearing opportunities to make Jesus look very big.

And this is why the Father himself specializes in sinners. This is why Jesus is for losers. We have all the makings of being liabilities to his mission, not assets, and yet he has chosen us, like Israel, so that he may shame the strength and wisdom of the world with the weak and the foolish in the glorification of his amazing grace. So the Father brings the poor and the lame and the crippled to the feast to make his gospel look very, very big.

And he knows that the poor and the lame and the crippled will be more impressed with a feast anyway.

## The Wedding Feast

The primary points of the parable of the great banquet are present in the parable of the wedding feast, with one peculiar exception:

> And again Jesus spoke to them in parables, saying, "The kingdom of heaven may be compared to a king who gave a wedding feast for his son, and sent his servants to call those who were invited to the wedding feast, but they would not come. Again he sent other servants, saying, 'Tell those who are invited, "See, I have prepared my dinner, my oxen and my fat calves have been slaughtered, and everything is ready. Come to the wedding feast."' But they paid no attention and went off, one to his farm, another to his business, while the rest

> seized his servants, treated them shamefully, and killed them. The king was angry, and he sent his troops and destroyed those murderers and burned their city. Then he said to his servants, 'The wedding feast is ready, but those invited were not worthy. Go therefore to the main roads and invite to the wedding feast as many as you find.' And those servants went out into the roads and gathered all whom they found, both bad and good. So the wedding hall was filled with guests.
>
> "But when the king came in to look at the guests, he saw there a man who had no wedding garment. And he said to him, 'Friend, how did you get in here without a wedding garment?' And he was speechless. Then the king said to the attendants, 'Bind him hand and foot and cast him into the outer darkness. In that place there will be weeping and gnashing of teeth.' For many are called, but few are chosen." (Matt. 22:1–14)

The invitation is similar to that of the previous parable. The excuse-making is less explicit but still there. We have misbehaving servants in this case, much like the unfaithful servants in other parables. But in this story we encounter something strange: a guest at the party without the proper attire.

It is probably best not to overanalyze. The point of the parable, really, is that there will be no one in heaven who got there by mistake. You cannot sneak in. There is only one way, and it is to receive the invitation and obey its restrictions, which include clothing yourself in righteousness. And to be clothed in righteousness is to be clothed in Christ alone (Eph. 4:24; Gal. 3:27). Therefore, union with Christ through faith is the only way in.

The legalist expects to attend the wedding feast dressed in his personal best. He would be astounded to find his earthly lessers there, dressed much finer than he. As it turns out, the garb of the self-righteous is pretty ragged anyway (Isa. 64:6).

Those whom we categorize as "bad" as well as those we consider "good" will be in the kingdom of heaven, so long as they are dressed in the wedding garment of the gospel. And so we find, like the Pharisees in Jesus's view, we have as much goodness to repent of as badness. Like Paul, we must consider even our goodness as loss. Jesus is for losers.

The premise at the heart of the parables of the great banquet and the wedding feast is made very plain in the parable of the Pharisee and the tax collector:

> He also told this parable to some who trusted in themselves that they were righteous, and treated others with contempt: "Two men went up into the temple to pray, one a Pharisee and the other a tax collector. The Pharisee, standing by himself, prayed thus: 'God, I thank you that I am not like other men, extortioners, unjust, adulterers, or even like this tax collector. I fast twice a week; I give tithes of all that I get.' But the tax collector, standing far off, would not even lift up his eyes to heaven, but beat his breast, saying, 'God, be merciful to me, a sinner!' I tell you, this man went down to his house justified, rather than the other. For everyone who exalts himself will be humbled, but the one who humbles himself will be exalted." (Luke 18:9–14)

In religious terms, what did the Pharisee have that the tax collector didn't have? Lots.

What did the tax collector have that the Pharisee didn't have? Nothing except money, which he at this point considers nothing.

The Pharisee brought all his religious currency to the market and found that his money was no good there. Instead the tax collector walked away justified, because he "owned" his spiritual poverty (Matt. 5:3); he copped to the bottomlessness of his need. He brought nothing to the table and therefore was "rich toward God" (Luke 12:21).

The prophet calls: "Come, everyone who thirsts, come to the waters; and he who has no money, come, buy and eat! Come, buy wine and milk without money and without price" (Isa. 55:1).

The tax collector understood these economics. Those who enter the kingdom understand. We confess our spiritual poverty and lameness, our utter sinfulness. We bring it to Jesus, trusting in his gospel; having lost all, ready to give all. The cry of our bankrupt hearts becomes, "Lord, have mercy on me, a sinner!" We want nothing but salvation. We cry out like the hymnist:

> Nothing in my hand I bring,
> Simply to the cross I cling;
> Naked, come to Thee for dress;
> Helpless look to Thee for grace;
> Foul, I to the fountain fly;
> Wash me, Savior, or I die.[4]

Having lost all, we give all. And, we receive all!

And let us not miss two key features of the parables of the great banquet and the wedding feast: they are about banquets and feasts!

It is not as if God is offering some piddling meal in exchange for all. That would certainly be worth making excuses to avoid. The feast God offers in Christ is not the lentil stew, good for a temporary quelling of a hunger pang, but all the attendant honors of the birthright, good for an eternity of unassailable joy. When people reject the gospel it is precisely because they do not perceive the reality of the kingdom it proclaims. Sometimes this is due to the way we "pitch" the gospel, as if it were all cross and no resurrection. But the gospel's blessings are vast and unfathomable. Ray Ortlund writes,

> God doesn't merely remove our defect. He restores us to something better. He not only takes away our problem ("Forgive all our sins"), but he also does us good ("receive us graciously"). God's moral calculus is factored very much to our advantage.[5]

God offers life abundant through Jesus. And the alternative to Christ's abundant life is not a pretty good life nor merely a medio-

---

[4] Augustus Toplady, "Rock of Ages" (1776).

[5] Raymond C. Ortlund, Jr., *When God Comes to Church: A Biblical Model for Revival Today* (Grand Rapids, MI: Baker, 2000), 72.

cre life, but a condemned one, a deadly devastation. This is always where idolatry leads, even if the things we worship are generally good things. Anything we choose at the expense of allegiance to Christ becomes poison, the means of our death.

And yet Christ does not call us to deny good things, but only to put him above them (Matt. 6:33). Clothed in his righteousness alone, we find he has prepared a place for us, and a feast in that place, and a multitude of joys around the banquet table that make the treasures of this world pale. This is why it is called "the gospel of the kingdom."

The bread of life and the living water really satisfy, forever and ever. Those agreeable to losing all for Christ will in him find all.

# 8

# The Parables before the Parables

Identifying parables in the Old Testament is an intellectually arduous and frustrating task. The varied use of poetic forms, metaphors, symbols and types, the apocalyptic, dreams, and so on and so forth render the search as time-intensive as one would care to make it, depending on how "parable" is being defined.[1] Certainly much of old covenant prophecy could be labeled parable (Hos. 12:10). Recall that the Hebrew word for parable (*mashal*) in the Old Testament is used for proverbs, stories, riddles, and similes. In addition, throughout the Old Testament, in both the historical and the poetical texts, we find types and shadows of Christ and his new covenant.

For our purposes, however, we will look primarily at some key stories that connect to the unfolding gospel story in the New Testament, and we will focus on intentional fictions meant to convey God's prophetic truths. That is, we will not look at historical events—things that actually happened—that may also be interpreted as parables of the kingdom (things like Noah's ark or water flowing from desert rocks or ravens delivering bread to Elijah), but instead at narrative or poetic stories that in a parabolic way reveal truth to or conceal truth from their hearers.

---

[1] Defining "parable" rather generously, Herbert Lockyer compiles a fine and impressive survey in his book *All the Parables of the Bible* (Grand Rapids, MI: Zondervan, 1963).

## Jotham and the Cry for a King

The world of the book of Judges is a sordid, nasty, utterly broken place. Some of the most horrific accounts of sin detailed in the Bible are found in the book of Judges. We are told quite plainly, "In those days there was no king in Israel. Everyone did what was right in his own eyes" (Judg. 14:7; 17:6). In Judges 9, the people of Israel are beginning to reap what they've sown in discord and disobedience. After the death of Gideon (referred to as Jerubbaal in Judges 9), the nation has descended into apostasy, and God's judgment looms. But it is not, as so often, judgment in the guise of an invading army; it is more along the lines of what we see detailed in Romans 1:24, or Psalm 81:12: "So I gave them over to their stubborn hearts, to follow their own counsels."

Abimelech, a son of Gideon by one of his concubines, saw an opportunity to fill a void in power, and making an appeal to his family for support, he made a shrewd and self-interested case for the establishment of himself as a king. "Would you rather be ruled by seventy men?" he argued (Judg. 9:2), referring to the totality of Gideon's sons, "or by one?" What ensued was a succession of hits that makes *The Godfather* look like *Strawberry Shortcake*. Using money from a house of Baal-worship, Abimelech hired seventy assassins. "Worthless and reckless fellows," Judges 9:4 calls them. Together they murdered all of Abimelech's brothers "on one stone" (v. 5). All, that is, except one. The youngest, named Jotham, escaped.

The brazen act of murder, nearly sacrificial in its overtones, is certainly devil worship, whether explicitly or implicitly. The root of pride if left unchecked will grow into a murderous tree. Through this wicked use of force, Abimelech was made king.

We pick up the story here:

> When it was told to Jotham, he went and stood on top of Mount Gerizim and cried aloud and said to them, "Listen to me, you leaders of Shechem, that God may listen to you. The trees once went out to anoint a king over them, and they said to the olive tree, 'Reign over us.' But the olive tree said to

> them, 'Shall I leave my abundance, by which gods and men are honored, and go hold sway over the trees?' And the trees said to the fig tree, 'You come and reign over us.' But the fig tree said to them, 'Shall I leave my sweetness and my good fruit and go hold sway over the trees?' And the trees said to the vine, 'You come and reign over us.' But the vine said to them, 'Shall I leave my wine that cheers God and men and go hold sway over the trees?' Then all the trees said to the bramble, 'You come and reign over us.' And the bramble said to the trees, 'If in good faith you are anointing me king over you, then come and take refuge in my shade, but if not, let fire come out of the bramble and devour the cedars of Lebanon.'" (Judg. 9:7–15)

Jotham's story is a crypto-parable. His employment of trees and vines and fire are elemental to several of Jesus's more prominent parables. Jotham includes three symbols of national flourishing that lay at the—for lack of a better word—root of Jesus's own promises and warnings. They are the olive tree, the fig tree, and the grapevine. Each, personified by Jotham, is asked by the trees to come and reign over them. In general, Jotham is indicting the people's God-offending demands for a king. They should have no king over them but *YHWH*, yet still they stamp their feet. More specifically, however, there is a lesson to learn in each of the parable's would-be rulers.

The trees ask the olive tree, renowned for its "fatness," its abundance, to rule over them because idolatrous people will easily be ruled by extravagance and consumption. Wanting to be ruled by the olive tree is making an idol of materialism, of riches. It is parallel to the New Testament's "their god is their belly" (Phil. 3:19).

The trees next ask the fig tree to reign over them. The fig tree serves in the Jewish mythos as the national symbol of safety and security and of stability. We see this symbolically in the prophetic "shade" the fig tree offers (1 Kings 4:25; Mic. 4:4). Remember also that it was with fig leaves that Adam and Eve first sought to cover their shame. The cry of the trees for the reign of the fig tree is a seeking of ultimate hope in temporary safety and peace. It is the symbolic equivalent of the false prophets crying "Peace, peace" where there is no peace (Jer. 6:14; 8:11).

The trees next ask the vine to reign over them. The vineyard and its grapevines are symbols of national abundance and fruitfulness, of luxurious provision, and generally of God's favor. Here the trees asking for the vine's presence reveals the arrogant audacity of the people asking for God's favor despite their idolatry. It is a foreshadowing of Paul's words in Romans 6:1: "Are we to continue in sin that grace may abound?" The trees—and the idolatrous nation detailed in the book of Judges—would say, "Why not!"

But of course God's favor does not work in any of these ways. The cry for these kings goes unheeded. The olive tree, the fig tree, and the vine all decline the request made of them. Indeed, what we may gather is embedded in Jotham's parable is that a repentant nation focused on *YHWH* as their only hope and glory might actually have enjoyed the abundance of the olive tree, the security of the fig tree, and the libation of the vine. That, after all, was the original significance of these biblical symbols!

Jotham then drills down into the heart of the matter: "Then all the trees said to the bramble, 'You come and reign over us'" (Judg. 9:14). The bramble is Abimelech. And the people are going to get what they ask for.

For what is a bramble? A dry, thorny bush. An invasive and offensive weed, really. Suitable only for the machete and the bonfire.

"Come, get under my shade," the bramble calls. "I will take care of you."

The bramble promises destructive fire if the trees will not comply. But it's a trick. Like the Devil tempting the Lord with the provision of bread or the security of the angelic helpers or the abundance of the nations, the promise belies that the fire is not outside Abimelech's reign but inside. The threats of Abimelech draw the people in, where they are in the most danger.

Examined like this, we can see in Jotham's parable the gospel application for us today. Our hearts are desperate for a king. We will make an idol of nearly everything, and indeed, the abundance of possessions and the security of comfort and the assumption of God's favor for our self-righteousness are the most common of our idols. But God's gifts are good gifts and terrible gods. In the end, if we will not serve God as God, we will find our refuge no refuge at all but a house of brambles—dry and thorny and reserved for the fires of hell. Several of Jesus's parables make the same point, and it is not for no reason that he curses the fig tree and tells stories about dead trees ready for the fire. His warning is Jotham's, and vice versa.

We cry out for a king, and Jesus answers the call. For all who will trust him, he is eternal provision, everlasting security, and infinite favor. He is the vine (John 15:5); all else is bramble.

## Nathan and Taking Sin Personally

Jotham's parable declares the condemnation of the Shechemite idolaters. But with the Spirit's assistance, it perhaps could have convicted some hearers of their sin. Jesus's parables often revealed the hardness of heart of the Pharisees and the Sadducees, although they did not often understand that—precisely because their hearts were too hard. On the other hand, the parable of Nathan in 2 Samuel 12 sets up its subject nicely for the victory blow of conviction.

Remember that David has taken Uriah's wife, Bathsheba. Surrendering to his lusts and abusing his power in this brazen act of adultery (and in his subsequent calculations in the murder of Uriah), David brings shame to Israel and to Israel's God. The prophet, however, understands the delicacy in rebuking the king for his sin. In an interesting turn of events, the subtle use of parable actually has a more powerful effect than an outright rebuke might have accomplished:

> And the LORD sent Nathan to David. He came to him and said to him, "There were two men in a certain city, the one rich and the other poor. The rich man had very many flocks and

> herds, but the poor man had nothing but one little ewe lamb, which he had bought. And he brought it up, and it grew up with him and with his children. It used to eat of his morsel and drink from his cup and lie in his arms, and it was like a daughter to him. Now there came a traveler to the rich man, and he was unwilling to take one of his own flock or herd to prepare for the guest who had come to him, but he took the poor man's lamb and prepared it for the man who had come to him." (2 Sam. 12:1–4)

The sense is straightforward. The rich thief of the poor man's lamb is King David. The king does not at first see himself in the parable, but he sees the injustice straightaway. And he mistakes the story for reality:

> Then David's anger was greatly kindled against the man, and he said to Nathan, "As the LORD lives, the man who has done this deserves to die, and he shall restore the lamb fourfold, because he did this thing, and because he had no pity." (2 Sam. 12:5–6)

Nathan, in so many words, says, "Hey, man: that's you!"

David has seen the sin but not the sinner. Nathan helps him find his place in the story. The result, by God's grace, is David's repentance. The consequences of the king's sin continue throughout the book, and indeed throughout David's life. Yet God continues to use him, to identify with him (1 Sam. 13:14; Acts 13:22), and to promise the Messiah through his offspring. David repents, "and the rest of the book relates how David triumphed through suffering brought on by his sin."[2] We see throughout the Bible's chronicle of David how faithful God is to sinners—even sinners who need a lot of help in repenting of their sin. We do not often see ourselves the way we ought; these planks in our eyes are so close we don't notice them.

---

[2] James M. Hamilton, Jr., *God's Glory in Salvation through Judgment: A Biblical Theology* (Wheaton, IL: Crossway, 2010), 421.

By beautiful contrast, in considering the story of mankind's brazen theft of God's glory—a story which does not indict him *in the least*—Jesus, unlike David, immediately and totally identifies himself with the sinner anyway. The sinless Son of Man takes the sin personally. He owns what is not his so that we might own what is not ours (2 Cor. 5:21). This gospel is foreshadowed in 2 Samuel itself:

> David said to Nathan, "I have sinned against the Lord." And Nathan said to David, "The Lord also has put away your sin; you shall not die." (2 Sam. 12:13)

When we will own our sin in repentance, when we will take it personally in godly sorrow, the God of justice applies the punishment to his Son. The wrath is stilled; propitiation is made. When Jesus comes preaching the gospel of the kingdom in sermon and parable, he means for us to take the whole thing personally. We cannot be bystanders to the in-breaking of the kingdom, because it necessarily involves us. Will its proclamation find purchase in our hearts? Or are we shallow-soiled, short-rooted?

We are condemned according to our sin; to be aficionados of Jesus or admirers of Jesus or simply an audience for Jesus will not keep us from the wrath to come. We cannot be apathetic about this eternal life-and-death situation. "The kingdom of heaven has suffered violence, and the violent take it by force" (Matt. 11:12).

Therefore, time and time again, we are commanded to do things like "lay it to heart" (Deut. 4:39; Mal. 2:2) or "take hold" (1 Tim. 6:12, 19). We have to make the faith our own by making our sin our own. Only in that way will Jesus take it as his. Nathan's parable reminds us to work on the planks in our eyes, to take up the planks of our cross daily in identification with the sinless Savior who identified with us.

## Isaiah and the Song of the Broken Garden

Nearly all of the Old Testament parables lay out the world as it is after the fall and before the new creation: broken. God's pre-Christian stories compile reminder upon stark reminder that all creation is groaning for redemption. They leave the gate open for the triumphal entry of the Messiah, who will set all things right by exposing how hopeless and cursed the situation is without him. Like Jotham's parable and Nathan's parable, Isaiah's lyrical parable of the destruction of *YHWH's* vineyard reveals the sad state of creation's affairs:

> Let me sing for my beloved
> my love song concerning his vineyard:
> My beloved had a vineyard
>     on a very fertile hill.
> He dug it and cleared it of stones,
>     and planted it with choice vines;
> he built a watchtower in the midst of it,
>     and hewed out a wine vat in it;
> and he looked for it to yield grapes,
>     but it yielded wild grapes.
> And now, O inhabitants of Jerusalem
>     and men of Judah,
> judge between me and my vineyard.
> What more was there to do for my vineyard,
>     that I have not done in it?
> When I looked for it to yield grapes,
>     why did it yield wild grapes?
> And now I will tell you
>     what I will do to my vineyard.
> I will remove its hedge,
>     and it shall be devoured;
> I will break down its wall,
>     and it shall be trampled down.
> I will make it a waste;
>     it shall not be pruned or hoed,
>     and briers and thorns shall grow up;
> I will also command the clouds
>     that they rain no rain upon it. (Isa. 5:1–6)

The parable, like many prophecies, operates on various levels. First, it recalls the fall of creation through Adam's disobedience. God made the world and all in it, and he made it all "good." When man fell, the original design for the garden was stunted. Adam and Eve went their own way; they went rogue, "wild," seeking fruit forbidden them rather than the fruit desired for them by God. The result, of course, was a spiritual wasteland. God exiled them from the garden and handed them over to the encroaching wilderness.

On the more immediate level of meaning, Isaiah is referring to the state of Israel's contemporary affairs. The nation is once again in turmoil, having turned from *YHWH* to its own duplicitous ways. Where God commands justice, the people deal in bloodshed, and where God speaks righteousness, the people complain (5:7).

When Isaiah experiences the glory of the Lord in the temple in Isaiah 6, he is commissioned to bring the word of God to a hard-hearted people. There lies the prototype for Jesus's audience: their ears are heavy and their eyes are blind (6:10). In the parable of Isaiah 5, the prophet reveals the source of the kingdom's shoddy state. Without the walls of God's protection and the rain of God's favor (5:5–6), the devastation will be staggering (6:13). It is no less foreboding with Jesus's warnings in the Gospels.

That is the third level on which Isaiah's parable operates. Since Jesus has co-opted the language of Isaiah 6 to explain how his parables work (Matt. 13:13), we know that Jesus is proclaiming the gospel of the kingdom to a generation as wicked and adulterous as Isaiah's. When Jesus speaks of blind guides and ravenous wolves and sneaky thieves and hired hands who don't care about the sheep, he is referring to the same kind of environment as exposed in Isaiah 5.

And yet the promise of Christ's justice in the gospel winds its prophetic way through Isaiah as well. In Isaiah 27, the vineyard that is in shambles in Isaiah 5 is said to flourish because *YHWH* keeps it himself directly. And the devastated remnant, the stump of Isaiah 6:13, puts forth a shoot, a righteous branch that finally bears fruit (11:1).

Like Jotham's parable, Isaiah 5—for those who have the ears to hear—stokes the repentant heart's longing for the true vine, in whom there is life and life abundant. Who will build up the walls again? Who will rebuild the ancient devastations? Who will bring the spring rain of God's righteousness? Christ the Lord.

## The Prophet Ezekiel's Parables and the Prophet Ezekiel As Parable

We conclude our survey of Old Testament parables with a cursory look at the prophet Ezekiel. His book is so rich with *mashal* that we cannot do it anywhere near justice. Nearly every chapter of this complex revelation contains a parable of some kind. Ezekiel himself sighs, "Ah, Lord God! They are saying of me, 'Is he not a maker of parables?'" (Ezek. 20:49). Yes, we answer back; yes, you are!

This is not a commentary, of course, so I cannot examine each parable in Ezekiel. But there is plenty to consider about the gospel of Jesus in the following texts:

Jerusalem's siege (Ezek. 4:1–3)
Jerusalem's iniquity (4:4–6)
Jerusalem's confinement (4:7–8)
Jerusalem's starvation (4:9–12)
Jerusalem's sinfulness (5:1–4)
The two eagles and the vine (17:1–10)
The lion's whelps (19:2–9)
The two harlots (23:2–21)
The boiling pot (24:3–5)
The cedar in Lebanon (31:3–18)
The sea monster (32:1–16)
The shepherds and the flock (34:1–24)
The valley of dry bones (37:1–14)
The living waters (47:1–12)

As you can see, what was said of Jesus—"he said nothing to them without a parable" (Matt. 13:34)—could easily be said of

Ezekiel as well. You can see in the general descriptions some symbols familiar to Jesus's stories: vine, lion, shepherds, living water. Again, each is revelatory in its own way, but I will focus here on two of these parables in particular: the two eagles and the vine (Ezek. 17:1–10) and the valley of dry bones (37:1–14).

In the parable of the eagles and the vine, Ezekiel prophesies the riddle of Judah's troubles until the inauguration of the messianic kingdom:

> The word of the Lord came to me: "Son of man, propound a riddle, and speak a parable to the house of Israel; say, Thus says the Lord God: A great eagle with great wings and long pinions, rich in plumage of many colors, came to Lebanon and took the top of the cedar. He broke off the topmost of its young twigs and carried it to a land of trade and set it in a city of merchants. Then he took of the seed of the land and planted it in fertile soil. He placed it beside abundant waters. He set it like a willow twig, and it sprouted and became a low spreading vine, and its branches turned toward him, and its roots remained where it stood. So it became a vine and produced branches and put out boughs.
>
> "And there was another great eagle with great wings and much plumage, and behold, this vine bent its roots toward him and shot forth its branches toward him from the bed where it was planted, that he might water it. It had been planted on good soil by abundant waters, that it might produce branches and bear fruit and become a noble vine.
>
> "Say, Thus says the Lord God: Will it thrive? Will he not pull up its roots and cut off its fruit, so that it withers, so that all its fresh sprouting leaves wither? It will not take a strong arm or many people to pull it from its roots. Behold, it is planted; will it thrive? Will it not utterly wither when the east wind strikes it—wither away on the bed where it sprouted?" (Ezek. 17:1–10)

Verses 11–21 help us interpret the parable thus: The cedar from Lebanon is representative of Israel herself. The first great eagle is

Nebuchadnezzar, who, in taking the top of the tree, has taken Judah's nobles and brought them captive to Babylon. Though in captive exile, Judah is expected to demonstrate its submission to God's chastening through the Babylonians by remaining humble and loyal to Nebuchadnezzar. What God has set up, in his inscrutable sovereignty, is Judah's flourishing in the land of its enemies (Ezek. 17:5–6; see also the complementary Jer. 29:4–7). The top of the tree clipped off, indeed, becomes a seed planted in the soil of Babylon which becomes a flourishing vine.

Enter the second eagle. This is Pharaoh Hophra of Egypt. The vine turns its branches toward this eagle instead of the first, representing the treachery of Judah's king (Zedekiah), who has plotted with the Pharaoh to overthrow Nebuchadnezzar. God promises to judge Zedekiah for his distrust, saying he will die in exile in Babylon. And he does.

Similar is the outcome for all who will distrust the Lord's sovereign plans for his exiled children and instead turn to trust in "chariots and . . . horses" (Ps. 20:7). The danger was similar in Jesus's day, as the Jewish people lived under Roman occupation and oppression. Rather than seek to live faithfully to *YHWH* while in this exile, some sought to bring the kingdom themselves, through physical violence. The zealots, for instance, routinely sought to overthrow the pagan authorities in one way or another. And they often ended up nailed to crosses, examples to warn off any other would-be revolutionaries floating about.

The tension is not as high but eerily similar in our day, particularly in the West. As we experience a persistent cultural downgrade, the Christian's sense of exile increases. Rather than seeking to trust God's call to be salt and light, to be "in the world but not of it," many Christians seek to push the cause of Christendom through the abuse of power and the delegation of the kingdom to government legislation. We lash our hearts to the elections of certain politicians rather than to our own election by God from the foundation of the world. We forget that the kingdom does not come through political plotting but through the proclamation of the gospel. We stretch our branches to the wrong king.

But God is faithful even if we are not. Ezekiel 17 ends with the promise of the dawn of the coming kingdom. As Lamar Cooper sums it up,

> The concluding statement of the chapter affirms the certainty of the Lord's promised restoration. Although some have understood it to have been fulfilled in the restoration of Judah under Zerubbabel, Ezra, and Nehemiah, the language goes beyond such limited scope (cf. Ezra 9:8–9) to a time yet future when Israel will have its perfect King, the Messiah, reigning on the earth in righteousness.[3]

This will happen because God promises to do the work of restoration *himself*! He will take a sprig off the top of the cedar and will plant it on the top of a high mountain (Ezek. 17:22),

> and all the trees of the field shall know that I am the LORD; I bring low the high tree, and make high the low tree, dry up the green tree, and make the dry tree flourish. I am the LORD; I have spoken, and I will do it. (v. 24)

God will rescue his people himself; he will plant them himself; he will care for them himself. He himself will be their king. We are seeing the glints of Christ's glory breaking through Ezekiel's allegorical shades.

In parables before this and after, Ezekiel remains himself a character as perplexing as his prophecies. Indeed, we know almost nothing about him historically. He is not quoted very widely in the New Testament; most of the more obvious connections are concentrated in Revelation.

God required quite a bit from Ezekiel. He was called not just to prophesy but to live the prophecies. Every prophet, of course,

---

[3] Lamar Eugene Cooper, Sr., *Ezekiel*, New American Commentary, ed. E. Ray Clendenen, vol. 17 (Nashville: Broadman & Holman, 1994), 184.

had some skin in the game, but Ezekiel found himself just as often experiencing the parable as much as telling it. For instance, God forbade him to mourn the death of his wife (Ezek. 24:15–16). At the beginning of the book, Ezekiel is made to eat the book (3:1–3). He is both prophet and priest (1:3). When he sees visions, he is actually transported in the Spirit to the realm in which to see them (37:1). The resulting composite portrait is not simply of Ezekiel as parable-teller but of Ezekiel *as a parable* himself. In this way, he is a type of Christ, the living parable (see chapter 9), who is his truer and better. For the mourning due the groom for his dead bride is granted to Christ, who in his sorrow raises his bride to redeem her, in order to rejoice over her. In the gospel, the mourning becomes dancing. In the gospel, Christ has subsisted not on bread alone but on every one of the Father's words; but he has not just consumed the scroll: he speaks it through the revelation of the kingdom and the Lamb's book of life. Jesus is prophet and priest, as well, but also king. And the true and better Ezekiel in the Gospels is not transported to the valley of dry bones simply in the Spirit, but in the flesh as well, having incarnated himself as the central miracle in the work of substitutionary atonement.

We turn now to the wonderful promise contained in that most famous parable of Ezekiel.

## Dry Bones and Revival, Then and Now

In Ezekiel 37 we read a rather fascinating parable of . . . well, what exactly? We are not sure. The obvious overtone is that of the resurrection of the dead at the consummation of history, the consummation of the firstfruits of Christ's own resurrection. But scholars do not entirely agree that what is envisioned is the future bodily resurrection.[4] In the subsequent interpretation (37:11–14), the immediate sense—not ruling out, of course, application to the future resurrection of the dead in Christ—is more along the lines of the restoration of the fortunes of exiled Israel. The people are in

[4] Ibid., 319–322.

despair; they suffer from rejection and hopelessness, and from their own rebellion. There is a dark cloud looming over the land. What the parable first indicates is what we might call *revival*.

What Ezekiel is prophesying in the parable is the day when God's Spirit reinvigorates his people for the sake of his own glory:

> The hand of the LORD was upon me, and he brought me out in the Spirit of the LORD and set me down in the middle of the valley; it was full of bones. And he led me around among them, and behold, there were very many on the surface of the valley, and behold, they were very dry. (37:1–2)

The immediate referent corresponding to the valley full of bones is the remnant of people slain in the conquest of Israel. These are the victims and the martyred heroes of the long-gone days of glory. The bones are "very dry," which means their lives are but a distant memory. More than that, it means that the halcyon days of Israel's fortunes are so far gone that the current situation appears utterly hopeless.

As a pastor in New England, I know many Christians in our region who feel the same way. Many more in the larger West are beginning to feel this way. We are now living in a post-Christian era. For Christians in Europe or in America's northeast, there is often a profound sense of dryness, of even hopelessness. What once was the hotbed of vibrant evangelical Protestantism is now a vast wasteland, liberal and Christless and pagan. I sometimes see the historic white-steepled churches dotting rural New England highways and byways as our images of the dry bones. Too many are empty now, or getting there. Too many pulpits where the gospel was once preached now proclaim universalism, moralistic deism, pluralistic utopian feel-goodism. Some aren't houses of religion at all but have become antique stores, cafes, community centers, or vacant relics of town history.

I walk around my town and the surrounding towns and see a spiritual dark cloud hovering over the place like the covering and veil mentioned in Isaiah 25:7. I hear the Lord asking me what he asked Ezekiel:

> And he said to me, "Son of man, can these bones live?" And I answered, "O Lord God, you know." (Ezek. 37:3)

God's provocative question cuts to the quick of our soul, sorting its affirmations from its denials. Given not just what we know of the darkness of a place but also what we know of the light of the world, what is our perspective on our places of ministry? Can there be revival here, of all places?

Notice Ezekiel's humility: "O Lord God, you know." He does not trust in a church program, ministry technique, or missional strategy. He trusts in the living God. Would God bring revival to Israel? Will God bring revival to New England? Will the Spirit once again refresh with mighty power your nation, your town, your church? Only God knows, because only God gives. Contrary to popular religious sentiment, you don't bring revival by hanging up a sign announcing one. The Spirit is not beholden to our calendars.

But our God is a reviving God. He will do it in his own timing, not ours, and by his own power, not ours—but when he says he will do it, he will do it:

> Then he said to me, "Prophesy over these bones, and say to them, O dry bones, hear the word of the Lord. Thus says the Lord God to these bones: Behold, I will cause breath to enter you, and you shall live. And I will lay sinews upon you, and will cause flesh to come upon you, and cover you with skin, and put breath in you, and you shall live, and you shall know that I am the Lord." (37:4–6)

What is the thing needed first? "O dry bones, hear the word of the Lord!" God commissions Ezekiel to proclaim his word. Now, as then, it is not our wisdom or eloquence but the powerful word of God that "makes things happen." Jesus, remember, did not shout seven helpful tips for successful living into Lazarus's tomb. He commanded him to "Come forth!" And as Jesus speaks in parables, he is not giving advice or making suggestions. He is proclaiming the realities of God's manifest sovereignty, and those with the ears to hear *hear*.

Because the gospel of Jesus Christ is Spiritually powerful, we should never write off a person or place as too far gone or too much dead. Bringing dead things to life is kind of Jesus's whole deal. The very dry bones are no match for the living water. Since the reality of revival presupposes deadness, a dead place should be considered ripe for revival!

As the gospel is preached faithfully, the Spirit revives those whom the Father has chosen. "I will cause breath to enter you," he promises. The breath here is a symbol of God's Spirit. We recall the moment of man's creation, as God made man out of the very dry dust of the ground and breathed life into him. That is the picture of creation; here in Ezekiel is a picture of renewal, of restoration.

Notice that as Ezekiel is proclaiming the word of God over the bones, it is the Lord who is *breathing*, who is causing things to happen. We preach, but we don't bring the wind! Charles Finney, by contrast, thought revival could be achieved somewhat mathematically:

> It is not a miracle, or dependent on a miracle, in any sense. It is a purely philosophical result of the right use of the constituted means—as much so as any other effect produced by the application of means. There may be a miracle among its antecedent causes, or there may not. The apostles employed miracles, simply as a means by which they arrested attention to their message, and established its Divine authority. But the miracle was not the revival. The miracle was one thing; the revival that followed it was quite another thing. The revivals in the apostles' days were connected with miracles, but they were not miracles.

> I said that a revival is the result of the *right* use of the appropriate means.[5]

I say that Finney is dead wrong. Dangerously wrong.

But Finney's words here serve as the philosophical precursor to countless church growth strategies today and the prevailing church growth framework in general. As a sort of churched version of "If you build it, they will come," this approach to the expectation of revival renders the supernatural natural and the providential pragmatic. Finney and his many modern spin-offs conflate the work of the preacher with the work of the word. They confuse the minister's required work with the Lord's free prerogative. It is God who says, "I will cause breath to enter you" (Ezek. 37:5), and that, when he does, "You shall know that I am the LORD" (v. 6). When the result is worship of God, the credit does not go to the prophet but to God. The entire prophetic enterprise, the entire purpose of revival, is the knowing of God and the enjoying of his sovereign lordship.

By way of contrast to Finney, enter the wisdom of Martyn Lloyd-Jones:

> A revival is a miracle. It is a miraculous, exceptional phenomenon. It is the hand of the Lord, and it is mighty. A revival, in other words, is something that can only be explained as the direct action and intervention of God. It was God alone who could divide the Red Sea. It was God alone who could divide the waters of the river of Jordan. These were miracles. Hence the reminder of God's unique action of the mighty acts of God. And revivals belong to that category. . . . These events belong to the order of things that men cannot produce. Men can produce evangelistic campaigns, but they cannot and never have produced a revival.[6]

This knowledge ought both to humble us and to embolden us. Ezekiel obeys:

[5] Charles G. Finney, *Lectures on Revivals of Religion*, 2nd ed. (New York: Leavitt, Lord, 1835), 12.
[6] D. Martyn Lloyd-Jones, *Revival* (repr., Wheaton, IL: Crossway, 1987), 111–112.

> So I prophesied as I was commanded. And as I prophesied, there was a sound, and behold, a rattling, and the bones came together, bone to its bone. And I looked, and behold, there were sinews on them, and flesh had come upon them, and skin had covered them. But there was no breath in them. (37:7–8)

Now he's got a crowd gathered. Sometimes preaching the gospel will do that. Jesus certainly gathered a crowd now and again. But crowds can be deceiving. And thus a warning: It is possible to look successful, to look alive, and yet not be filled with the Holy Spirit of God. It is possible to assemble a great lumbering mechanism of people, gathered under religious pretenses even, but there be no breath of life in them, just the appearance of life.

A common story passed around among preachers is the one about the Korean pastor who once visited the States, and upon his reaching the last day of his visit, he was asked what he thought about American churches. "It is remarkable," he is reported to have said, "how much the American church gets done without the Holy Spirit."

The rattling of the bones, the assembling of the sinews, all into a mass of lifeless structure is a reminder that God wants us to be alive with him, not just busy. It is a reminder that revival is not the sudden eruption of religious busywork. Paul writes, "For we know, brothers loved by God, that he has chosen you, because our gospel came to you not only in word, but also in power and in the Holy Spirit and with full conviction" (1 Thess. 1:4–5).

I once watched a video of a motocross bike jumping over a pastor on stage. It was of course only the umpteenth demonstration of spiritualized showmanship I've seen—that we've all seen—coming out of evangelical churches. And I'm not saying these churches or their pastors don't have the Holy Spirit. But I *am* saying that setting up a dirt bike track in your sanctuary is profoundly stupid.

What is profoundly stupid is the sheer amount of innovation, creativity, energy, ambition, and astounding levels of human wherewithal that go into crafting the most amazing worship experiences

Americans have ever seen inside churches where the gospel isn't preached. There's only one thing we hold that the New Testament calls "power," and that's the gospel.

In Ezekiel 37:8 we have something that looks alive but isn't.

Is this what we've crafted with many of our ecclesiastic enterprises? Have we only set loose an army of shiny, platitude-dispensing golems?

Is this also true even of churches with "sound doctrine," where human ingenuity and personality and tradition reign?

What, then, is the prescription for this active lifelessness?

> Then he said to me, "Prophesy to the breath; prophesy, son of man, and say to the breath, Thus says the Lord God: Come from the four winds, O breath, and breathe on these slain, that they may live." So I prophesied as he commanded me, and the breath came into them, and they lived and stood on their feet, an exceedingly great army. (37:9–10)

The prescription is the life-giving proclamation that pleads for the Holy Spirit and his reviving wind. There is a preached word and a prayerful openness to the power of the Spirit. And the result is a church *alive*, fired with gospel militancy and mobilized for kingdom mission.

Church, let's not settle!

Let's not settle for big churches.

Let's not settle for busy churches.

Let's not settle for the favor of men.

Let's not settle for what passes these days for success.

Let's not settle for ministerial markers that could be shared by religious organizations that don't preach Christ crucified.

Let's instead preach the gospel stubbornly and long for the Spirit's power expectantly. Let's press in, bang on heaven's door, and plead for revival. Let's ask for God's glory. Let's acknowledge that only he brings revival, and let's beg him for it.

What would it look like if the church in New England were

stirred up in revival by God's Holy Spirit? Oh, I don't rightly know, but I am asking the Lord to show me. Many believers native to this region have been tugging on Christ's royal robe for years on end to see such a thing. We pray the prayer of Habakkuk 3:2:

> O LORD, I have heard the report of you,
> and your work, O LORD, do I fear.
> In the midst of the years revive it;
> in the midst of the years make it known;
> in wrath remember mercy.

Through the church's stubborn fixation on the prophetic word of the gospel and a hopeful expectancy for the Spirit's reviving work, the Lord just might hijack the agenda of our neighborhood. He just might change the subject in our churches and towns:

> Then he said to me, "Son of man, these bones are the whole house of Israel. Behold, they say, 'Our bones are dried up, and our hope is lost; we are indeed cut off.'" (Ezek. 37:11)

I see in the cry of Israel here a reminder of the unrevived church's posture in too many cities. A despair, a hopelessness, a sense of abandonment can pervade and settle in. It can become the default setting for far too many. In some regions, churches have become so wearied by cultural downgrade and their own disobedience to God's mission, they have instead circled their wagons and occupy themselves with religious self-interest.

Many of us lack a sense of brokenness over our burnt-over districts. I think of Nehemiah weeping over the destroyed walls of Jerusalem, a hundred years after the fact! When was the last time any of us were so undone by the spiritual state of our cities that we wept? Too often, we are too busy being self-righteously angry to realize that but for the grace of God, so go we.

There is a reminder implicit in the desperation of Israel that we today may see hope break our cities open when our churches manifest a brokenness for them.

This is certainly the position of Jesus, who looked out upon the teeming crowds of sinners and felt compassion for them, seeing them as sheep without a shepherd.

The Lord repeats the vision message:

> Therefore prophesy, and say to them, Thus says the Lord God: Behold, I will open your graves and raise you from your graves, O my people. And I will bring you into the land of Israel. And you shall know that I am the Lord, when I open your graves, and raise you from your graves, O my people. And I will put my Spirit within you, and you shall live, and I will place you in your own land. Then you shall know that I am the Lord; I have spoken, and I will do it, declares the Lord. (Ezek. 37:12–14)

Ezekiel's prophetic vision here has a fulfillment more immediate than the days of Jesus's ministry, but we can see the tones of the Messiah's revolution all over the prophecy. When Jesus began his public work, the people of Israel were once again desperate and distracted. They too felt cut off. They too longed for God to redeem them from their affliction. They too longed to be restored to their land, or more accurately, to have their land restored to them.

And Jesus was of course doing all of this, in and through himself. But he did not do it in the ways most Jews expected. Those with the eyes to see could see.

They could see Jesus.

Those with the ears to hear the shepherd's voice, knowing they belong to him, could hear in his parables and sermons that he was restoring Israel by creating a people for himself. New life was afoot in his words and deeds. They could see that to have this life meant having first and foremost Jesus himself. Any who were willing to trade in all other aspirations could have the king and his kingdom.

The takeaway today, as then, is that a longing for revival is really a longing for Jesus. It is not a longing for an experience or a refresh or a reboot. It is a longing for the Redeemer.

One of the important things to remember about Ezekiel 37 is that while Ezekiel experiences the vision, he does not get to experience what is envisioned. The things God promises to do, the things he has just shown the prophet, will take place after Ezekiel has died and become dry bones himself. The revival shown is simply the coming attractions of days to come.

This may be true for us as well. God has given many of his faithful servants today a vision for revival in their churches and regions. We ought not let that go. We ought to stoke the fires of this vision as often as we can. And given the reality that God brings revival in his own time, understanding that he may not bring it in ours, and he may not bring it until the day of our grandchildren's grandchildren, we ought to press on in prayer and expectation anyway.

Many things the Lord foretold in the days of his public ministry have yet to come to pass. One repeated reminder found in his parables is this: Be ready. Stay watchful, stay alert. Let us do so in prayer. Let us do so in prayer for revival. Let us be sober-minded about the insidious idolatry of our awesomeness-driven churches. Let us turn in repentance to the centrality of the gospel of Jesus, and nag God daily to send fresh wind from heaven. Maurice Roberts offers wise rebuke and stirring encouragement:

> It is to our shame that we have imbibed too much of this world's materialism and unbelief. What do we need more than to meditate on the precious covenant promises of Holy Scripture until our souls have drunk deeply into the spirit of a biblical supernaturalism? What could be more profitable than to eat and drink of heaven's biblical nourishment till our souls become vibrant with the age-old prayer for revival, and till we find grace to plead our suit acceptably at the throne of grace?
>
> The Lord has encouraged us to hope in Him still. O that He would teach us to give Him no rest day or night till He rain righteousness upon us![7]

[7] Maurice Roberts, "The Prayer for Revival (Psalm 89)," Life Action Ministries blog (October 1, 2000), https://www.lifeaction.org/revival-resources/heart-cry-journal/issue-14/prayer-revival-psalm-89/.

In the days of the Old Testament parables, the longing of the heart was for the salvation only Jesus brings. Jesus has brought it. As the sheep did who could hear Jesus's voice in the days of the New Testament parables, let us behold the Lamb of God who takes away the sin of the world.

# 9

# Jesus, the Living Parable

Strictly speaking, the "I am" statements found in the Gospel of John are not parables. But as we've seen, it is difficult to speak strictly about what fits into this genre in the first place. The scope of *mashal* seems quite malleable in the Old Testament. A less flexible but not inflexible scope persists into the New Testament. Some scholars and preachers will include the similitudes of Matthew 5:13–14 (salt and light) in the genre of parable. The metaphors Jesus uses there complement the symbolic mechanism of many parables. And while I have not made space in this book to include the detailing of every clearly identified parable of Jesus, much less every significant instance of metaphor and symbol found in the Gospels, the seven peculiar statements from the Johannine narrative demand inclusion because of the way they resemble the parables' subjects and object. That is to say, the "I am" statements are like the parables because they are complex comparisons that reveal the glory of God in Christ to those who have the ears to hear. They reveal truth to the hearts of some and confound the minds of others.

Jesus employs the phrase "I am" multiple times in John's Gospel, and we will cover all the more prominent instances, but the central focus of this chapter will be on the following seven:

- I am the bread of life.
- I am the light of the world.
- I am the door.
- I am the good shepherd.
- I am the resurrection and the life.
- I am the way, and the truth, and the life.
- I am the vine.

As we saw in the last chapter, the prophetic deployment of parables in speaking for God was not an innovation of Jesus but originated in the Old Testament. And as with the Old Testament parables, these seven parabolic statements highlight *YHWH's* special relationship with Israel, as her God, as her Father, as her life, as her everything. The Old Testament parables we explored revealed the expectation of messianic deliverance and vindication. God himself would be Israel's king. In the New Testament, as in the Old, we learn that Israel's king is both a supreme and a subversive king, ruling in multifaceted and often unexpected ways. He rules over all, and he will judge all, but his sovereign rule is typified by sharing, by feeding, by serving, by sacrificing. And so on.

The seven "I am" statements give us glimpses into God's faithfulness to his people. And like the parables, these seven statements serve as more than illustrations. One does not simply hear or not hear prophecy; one receives it or rejects it. One is softened by it or hardened by it. The parables, as we've seen, serve as both announcements of the kingdom and the prophetic means of the kingdom. As N. T. Wright says, "The parables are not just 'about' the return of Israel's god into her history, to judge, redeem and restore her; they are also agents of that all-important event."[1] Accordingly, these seven special declarations of Jesus are both "about" the kingdom and the agents of the kingdom. They reveal both the subject of the kingdom and the object, the means of our entry, who happens to be the King himself. Like all the other parables, only in

[1] N. T. Wright, *Jesus and the Victory of God* (Minneapolis: Fortress, 1996), 181. For explanation as to Wright's use of the lowercase "god," see his *The New Testament and the People of God* (Minneapolis: Fortress, 1992).

these forms more directly, the "I am" statements reveal and center on Jesus Christ himself. It is for this reason I say that the "I am" statements reveal that Jesus is himself a parable.

The "I am" statements also reside as points upon the Gospel's narrative trajectory, serving John's evangelistic purpose (John 20:31). Each builds upon the other, increasing the intensity of the revealing of the light who is life. See each one as another level of illumination as in the rising of the sun. The development of these seven statements in John's Gospel gives us the shape of the gospel—God himself inhabiting man to bring life to man.

## I Am the Bread of Life

"I am the bread of life; whoever comes to me shall not hunger, and whoever believes in me shall never thirst" (John 6:35).

John 6 details a fascinating episode in the ministry of Jesus. It is a long chapter and a complex one, beginning with the miraculous feeding of the five thousand. As with all miracles, we are meant to see them as pointers to the signified, Christ himself and his kingdom. Like the parables, the miracles are windows into the life of the in-breaking kingdom of God. But many wanted Jesus to be their performing magician, like a trained miracle monkey or some such blasphemy. The Pharisees often sought signs from him in this way, as later did Herod (Luke 23:8). The average Joes of Jesus's day were rather a mixed bag. It is difficult to know if even all the people he physically healed were born again. Certainly many were given faith and therefore had the eyes to see and the ears to hear Jesus as the Lamb of God who takes away the sins of the world. They received both the sign and the one signified. Others, however, seemed content to seek Jesus only for his benefits and not for himself. We see this very clearly in John 6, as Jesus moves from demonstrating to preaching:

> "Truly, truly, I say to you, whoever believes has eternal life. I am the bread of life. Your fathers ate the manna in the wilderness, and they died. This is the bread that comes down from

> heaven, so that one may eat of it and not die. I am the living bread that came down from heaven. If anyone eats of this bread, he will live forever. And the bread that I will give for the life of the world is my flesh."
>
> The Jews then disputed among themselves, saying, "How can this man give us his flesh to eat?" So Jesus said to them, "Truly, truly, I say to you, unless you eat the flesh of the Son of Man and drink his blood, you have no life in you. Whoever feeds on my flesh and drinks my blood has eternal life, and I will raise him up on the last day." (John 6:47–54)

Even the disciples grumbled after Jesus said all that.

There are several things Jesus is doing in this miracle and the discourse following. In the miracle, he is first demonstrating his presence as the provision of daily bread from the Father. He is also making the connection between the manna received by the children of Israel in the desert and this provision. But he goes further to say that he doesn't just provide the manna; rather, he *is* the manna. In this way he is also raising the specter of antinomianism with many, because faithful Jews weren't supposed to consume blood.

The way Jesus constantly redirects his culture's understanding of the old covenant Scriptures is an implicit assertion of his authority over not just the culture but their Scriptures! Indeed, when the crowd marvels that Jesus taught as one with authority (Matt. 7:28–29), they aren't just seeing the kind of authority that results from years of study and theological training but the kind of authority that results from being the very author of what is being taught.

Jesus's audience was likely familiar with the words of Deuteronomy: "man does not live by bread alone, but man lives by every word that comes from the mouth of the Lord" (Deut. 8:3). We have read that Jesus is the Word of God (John 1:1). Putting one and one together, we get the dual meaning of God's provision in his word and God's provision of himself as the incarnate Word of God revealed in the written word of God. It is not bread alone that gives life but the bread of life.

And what fascinating bread! "I am the bread of life; whoever comes to me shall not hunger, and whoever believes in me shall never thirst" (John 6:35). Never thirst? How is it that bread might satisfy thirst? The bread of life is clearly all-satisfying.

Jesus has elsewhere referenced his supply of living water (John 4:10), an explicit connection of himself with the promises of Jeremiah 17:13 and Zechariah 14:8. But there is no such explicit connection here. Perhaps it is implied. Or else, Jesus is stating just how sufficient the nourishment of his flesh actually is. In context, he widens his command to include both eating his flesh and drinking his blood. There are certainly foreshadowings of the Eucharist here, but at this point Jesus has yet to institute the Lord's Supper, and, furthermore, it seems better to say the Eucharist corresponds to John 6 rather than that John 6 corresponds to the Eucharist. Calvin appeals to the Hebrew custom of using the word "bread," as in daily bread, as a figure of speech to mean more generally "dinner" or "supper."[2] If this is the case, the kind of bread Jesus says he is has a multiplicity of effects. To come to him in hunger is to be satisfied not just in hunger but also in thirst. The supreme and preeminent Lord of All is in fact the bread that is an everlasting meal, an eternal feast for the soul.

And while Genesis 3:19 prescribes bread procured through the sweat of the brow, the gospel promises bread given freely through the bloody brow of the Son.

## I Am the Light of the World

"I am the light of the world. Whoever follows me will not walk in darkness, but will have the light of life" (John 8:12).

While the parabolic bread of life has an ancient connection to the Old Testament stories of manna and Passover and miracle cakes (1 Kings 17:8–16), the light of the world has a primordial connection:

---

[2] John Calvin, *John*, Crossway Classic Commentaries, ed. Alister McGrath and J. I. Packer (Wheaton, IL: Crossway, 1994), 160.

> In the beginning, God created the heavens and the earth. The earth was without form and void, and darkness was over the face of the deep. And the Spirit of God was hovering over the face of the waters.
>
> And God said, "Let there be light," and there was light. (Gen. 1:1–3)

John's echoes of the opening pages of God's word are rather easy to see:

> In the beginning was the Word, and the Word was with God, and the Word was God. He was in the beginning with God. All things were made through him, and without him was not any thing made that was made. In him was life, and the life was the light of men. The light shines in the darkness, and the darkness has not overcome it. (John 1:1–5)

We must not see what John isn't showing, however. He is not saying that the Word of God who is the light of the world was created like the first light of creation. Rather, he is saying that the Son was present at the creation of the world, that he was integral to the emanation of the first light. It makes sense. Light begets light. And as God sends forth light in the dawn of creation, making something out of nothing, separating land from water and shaping order from nothingness, he comes at the dawn of new creation as light into darkness, bringing forth new life, sifting order from the disorder of sin and the injustice it has wrought.

Jesus's kind of light is rather specific. It is not the kind of light you merely see, but the kind of light *you follow*. Like the light at the end of a tunnel. Or, more biblically speaking, like a pillar of fire in the wilderness (Ex. 13:21). The old covenant connection reminds us that Jesus's very existence demands a response. There is no such thing as apathy to Jesus. If you are not with him, you are against him (Matt. 12:30). Thus, as the bread of life requires that Christians eat, the light of the world requires that Christians follow. Jesus has not announced himself thus to simply be appreciated; rather, he asserts himself at the center of the universe of need, requiring the orbit of worshipful obedience around him. Herman Ridderbos elaborates:

> In these sayings the "I" receives so much emphasis that it no longer functions as the subject of the sentence (with, say, "light" as predicate) but, conversely, is itself the predicate with "light" as subject: "The light of the world am *I*." Therefore the point is not primarily to analyze what "light" means here—understanding of that concept is assumed—but that the light that the world needs and by which alone a person can escape the darkness is *Jesus*, and therefore that whoever follows *him* will not walk in darkness. In this focus of the revelational utterance everything is concentrated on the person of Jesus, which explains why, in the Pharisees' reaction (vs. 13), the issue is not light but Jesus' claim to be the light.[3]

By declaring "The light of the world am I," Jesus has equated everything good in the world with himself. All that is good is said to be light. And therefore as Jesus is the embodiment of goodness, he is the embodiment of light.

This goodness—real goodness, real righteousness, I mean—is sourced in God. That is why the light of the world existed before anything else existed. And it is why in the end, when darkness is climactically condemned to darkness, the Light will endure from everlasting to everlasting. In the end, "the city has no need of sun or moon to shine on it, for the glory of God gives it light, and its lamp is the Lamb" (Rev. 21:23). In the end, the light of life will prevail for days unending, because he who is "the radiance of the glory of God" (Heb. 1:3) will cover the earth "as the waters cover the sea" (Hab. 2:14).

## I Am the Door

"I am the door. If anyone enters by me, he will be saved and will go in and out and find pasture" (John 10:9).

[3] Herman Ridderbos, *The Gospel of John: A Theological Commentary* (Grand Rapids, MI: Eerdmans, 1997), 292–293.

A preface to Christ's claiming to be "the way" (John 14:6), John 10:9's reference to the door (or "gate," as in the entrance to the sheepfold), is contextually inextricable from the next "I am" statement in John 10:11, about his being the shepherd. There is a larger soteriological point we may learn here. Jesus is the door and therefore the entryway to salvation, and Jesus is the shepherd and therefore the sustainer of our salvation (see also Heb. 10:23; 12:2).

The door metaphor is similar to the light metaphor. Just as "the light of the world" is a Christ-centric statement, so also "the door" is one of Christ's Christ-centric statements. "You must follow me to find life," he is saying. "And you must go through me to get life." Jesus again makes himself the center of the universe. Notice he does not say "I am *a* door," but as John reflects in the Greek definite article ἡ (*hē*), "I am *the* door." He is not allowing for the existence of other doors through which or other names under which people may be saved. He makes no bones about it: if you would have salvation, you must have Jesus. "And there is salvation in no one else," Peter preached, "for there is no other name under heaven given among men by which we must be saved" (Acts 4:12).

## I Am the Good Shepherd

"I am the good shepherd. The good shepherd lays down his life for the sheep" (John 10:11).

Jesus has just said he is the door. In the very next breath he says he is the shepherd.

And what a bizarre shepherd! What kind of shepherd would lay his life down for sheep? To say that such a shepherd is good is the very least we could say. He would be unfathomably good. He would be perplexingly good. He would be seen as crazy, actually. Or, to the spiritually blind, not good but evil (John 10:20).

Jesus is on one level indicting the generations of hypocritical shepherds, self-interested shepherds, and evil shepherds. The guardians of the faith had for too long sold out the sheep, failed to protect them and to feed them (John 10:12–13). He now is finally the shepherd who does his job. Thinking this way, the shepherd who lays his life down rather than putting his own life first makes good sense.

On another level, Jesus is indeed pushing the limits of rationality. This shepherd is not good simply because of what he *does*—sacrificing himself—but because of who he *is*—God himself. "I myself will be the shepherd of my sheep, and I myself will make them lie down, declares the Lord GOD" (Ezek. 34:15). The shepherd does good, and the shepherd is good, because the one who says "I am the good shepherd" is the great I AM.

The great I AM incarnate is the gate to the sheep pen and a shepherd and a sheep (John 1:29). He will be all that he will be to save the lost sheep. At every point of our need, there stands Jesus as the meeting of that need and our vicarious doer of perfection. From A to Z, he has us more than covered. This is why he may say that he is not just life but *eternal* life, resurrection life.

## I Am the Resurrection and the Life

"I am the resurrection and the life. Whoever believes in me, though he die, yet shall he live, and everyone who lives and believes in me shall never die. Do you believe this?" (John 11:25–26).

At this point in the Johannine narrative, Jesus's "I am" statements become less material. Or do they?

It would seem that "the resurrection and the life" evokes a spiritual idea, an apparently less concrete metaphorizing than "door" or "shepherd." But in biblical theology, resurrection and life are not spiritual in the "less than real" sense but in the "more than real" sense. Jesus, like all orthodox Jews, believes in the future bodily resurrection. Jesus believes and teaches that eternal life means not disembodied bliss in an immaterial locale in outer space but tangible (new) life on a tangible (new) earth. When Jesus says, "I am the resurrection and the life," he is saying that if you want to have life in the eternal flesh, you must believe in him. When Jesus says, "though you die, yet will you live" (see John 11:25), he is not referring to the initial presence of the departed soul with him where God is but to the everlasting presence of the resurrected body in the new heavens and the new earth. Even if you die, you will live. Really live. Not in someone's heart or dreams or memories. On God's gloriously green earth. This is the ultimate eschatological hope of the Scriptures from Old Testament to New. It is Job the sufferer's hope (Job 19:25–27), and Paul's (1 Cor. 15:42–49).

How can the Nazarene carpenter's son make such amazing claims? The answer lies in the common thread to the "I am" statements, of course—the "I am." Orthodox Christians affirm that Jesus is the Son of God, the second divine person of the Trinity incarnate, but not many know that even these statements are more evidence for the doctrine of Christ's divine self-consciousness. The "I am" statements are parables in this way too: each of the seven statements has a certain metaphorical sense for readers with common sense, but they have a certain doctrinal sense for readers with an awakened Spiritual sense.

Jesus is self-assigning the divine name—*YHWH*, or I AM. Similarly "hidden" is Jesus's declaration as he comes walking on the roaring waves: "It is I" (Matt. 14:27; Mark 6:50; John 6:20). Who can command the waters with such authority? I AM:

> Christ is revealing the transcendent dimension of his nature. "It is I" (Greek, *ego eimi*) in Mark 6:50 echoes the identical words of Exodus 3:14, with its divine name, "I AM." So, too, the verb "pass by" (v. 48) is the same as used in the LXX of Exodus 33:19 and 34:6 for God "passing by" (i.e., revealing himself to) Moses. Job 9:8 and Psalm 77:19 provide further Old Testament background for Yahweh as the one who treads upon the sea. Christ is here disclosing his divine nature.[4]

The "I am" statements in substance *and in form* are Jesus's divine self-disclosures. Human rationality must obey the divine sensibility. Certainly only God could be the resurrection and the life!

[4] Craig L. Blomberg, *Jesus and the Gospels* (Nashville: Broadman & Holman, 1997), 273.

Assembling all that Jesus says along these lines, Don Carson finds the inevitable conclusion warranted by the evidence:

> The majority of the "I am" statements in John have some sort of completion: "I am the bread of life" (6:35), "I am the good shepherd" (10:11), "I am the true vine" (15:1) or the like. These are plainly metaphorical, and although they are reasonably transparent to later readers, they were confusing and difficult for the first hearers (e.g. 6:60; 10:19; 16:30–32): religious leaders did not customarily say that sort of thing. . . . And if the most dramatic of the sayings in John, "Before Abraham was born, I am" (8:58) is without explicit parallel, it is hard to see how it makes a claim radically superior to the Synoptic portrayal of a Jesus who can not only adjudicate Jewish interpretations of the law but radically abrogate parts of it (Mk. 7:15–19) while claiming that all of it is fulfilled by him (Mt. 5:17ff.); who forgives sin (Mt. 9:1ff.) and insists that an individual's eternal destiny turns on obedience to him (Mt. 7:21–23); who demands loyalty that outstrips the sanctity of family ties (Mt. 10:37–39; Mk. 10:29–30) and insists that no-one knows the Father except those to whom the Son discloses him (Lk. 10:22); who offers rest for the weary (Mt. 11:28–30) and salvation for the lost (Lk. 15); who muzzles nature (Mk. 4:39) and raises the dead (Mt. 9:18–26). Individual deeds from such a list may in some cases find parallels in the prophets or in the apostles; the combination finds its only adequate parallel in God alone.[5]

As Carson is showing here, as Lewis so cleverly stated,[6] there is simply no precedent among the religious teachers of Jesus's day for this self-application. No sane person would say this about himself. No "good teacher" would say these things about himself. And unless we want to say Jesus was a liar, we must see Spiritually that the accumulation of all that Jesus says about himself, reflected in

[5] D. A. Carson, *The Gospel according to John* (Grand Rapids, MI: Eerdmans, 1991), 58.
[6] In his now-famous "trilemma." See C. S. Lewis, *Mere Christianity* (New York: Macmillan, 1952), 45.

the apex of self-revelation here—"I am the resurrection and the life"—highlights Jesus's place as a living, breathing parable of God, as the living parable who reveals God and in fact *is* God.

He then goes on to expand upon his claim that he is life.

## I Am the Way, and the Truth, and the Life

"I am the way, and the truth, and the life. No one comes to the Father except through me'" (John 14:6).

The Lord is being awfully exclusive here, isn't he? He is not leaving much wiggle room for those who would like to find God in some other way. This is not a commonly cited saying of Jesus by those who prefer to think him seeker-friendly.

Do all roads lead to the same place? Yes: the judgment seat of Christ, where there lies a great fork. Two ways diverge at Jesus. One leads to the Father, the other to everlasting judgment.

Are all religions true? Not if they disagree with Jesus about himself or anything else, because he is the truth.

Is life all about finding your bliss, following your heart, doing your thing, dancing while no one's watching, achieving the American dream, getting all the toys, remembering the moments that take your breath away, just being a good person, staying young at heart, making the world a better place, being a better you, or discovering your miracle? No, life is ultimately and principally Jesus.

One thing this particular "I am" statement helps us to remember is that all the other "I am" statements are illuminations not of the virtues or the symbols but of the I AM. Jesus is reminding us that he is the divine personification of virtue. Of all the virtues. He is in fact life, so that to not have I AM is to not have life. To not have I AM is to not have the way and therefore to be lost. To not have I AM is to not have the truth and therefore to live a lie. As the one true God revealed in the flesh, Christ is the supreme good. We cannot have virtues without Christ, because Christ is the confluence and embodiment of all that is good. All that is good, in fact, emanates from him as a reflection of his perfect goodness. There is no such thing as *grace*, even—at least, not as a "thing"—but only Christ who is the grace of God for us. As Sinclair Ferguson so powerfully puts it,

> [R]emember that there isn't a thing, a substance, or a "quasi-substance" called "grace." All there is is the person of the Lord Jesus—"Christ clothed in the gospel," as Calvin loved to put it. Grace is the grace of Jesus. If I can highlight the thought here: there is no "thing" that Jesus takes from Himself and then, as it were, hands over to me. There is only Jesus Himself.[7]

And so we must be constantly following these parabolic symbols—way, truth, life—backwards to their revelatory source. The way is Jesus. The truth is Jesus. The life is Jesus. The danger so often in our journey of faith is that we cave to sentimentality and vague "spirituality" and thus forget that the symbols have a personal referent. We talk of these "things" as if they were impersonal life forces floating around the atmosphere. Some churches promote themselves as celebrants and distributors of "glory," "hope," "peace," "spirit," "victory," and, yes, even "grace," without the enfleshment the Bible demands of these things. They become cheerleaders of feelings rather than worshipers of God. One church I attended on an Easter Sunday once upon a time made almost no reference to the bodily resurrection of Jesus in the sermon but instead spoke of Easter as representing "new doors" for people to walk through, new opportunities, fresh starts. But Jesus is the door (John 10:9), so in the New Testament's peculiar metaphorical economy, disembodied doors lead only to hell.

So let us not toss around willy-nilly words like "spirit," "grace," "peace," and "hope." The Bible will not let us have these ideas merely as ideas, as things. They are personal. Thus: "He himself is our peace" (Mic. 5:5; Eph. 2:14) and "God is love" (1 John 4:8).

---

[7] Sinclair Ferguson, in Deborah Finnamore, "An Interview with Sinclair Ferguson," Ligonier Ministries blog (April 28, 2010), http://www.ligonier.org/blog/grace-alone-interview-sinclair-ferguson/.

Let's not ply in ethereal virtues, no matter how Christianly gauzed. Leave ethereal virtues to vague saviors. Our way, truth, and life can be known, and will be known face-to-face. Our Savior is incarnate!

## I Am the Vine

"I am the vine; you are the branches. Whoever abides in me and I in him, he it is that bears much fruit, for apart from me you can do nothing" (John 15:5).

Once again the Lord is declaring a new thing by fulfilling an image of old. Bread and light, sheep gates and shepherds. "The vine" is likewise in the Hebrew mythos. So let us remember that Jesus is not making all new things but is making all things new! (Rev. 21:5). Gerald Bilkes writes,

> [W]e find that vines are a common picture throughout the Old and New Testaments (see Psalm 80; Isaiah 5; Jeremiah 2; Ezekiel 17). Notably, every time the Lord compares His people to a vine or a vineyard in the Old Testament, it is to accuse them of fruitlessness, of failing to be what He expected them to be. Yet now, Christ makes clear how His people can and will bring forth fruit—through communion with Him, the true vine.[8]

Jesus tells us what will happen to the vegetation that does not produce fruit. In Matthew 7:15–20 he conflates the imagery on both sides, saying that the wolves in sheep's clothing are bad trees primed for casting into the fire. But the good shepherd is the good vine. (Jesus can mix his metaphors all he wants, because he is Jesus!)

The Lord is abundantly clear on the consequences of lack of abundance (see also Matt. 3:12). But no tree will bear good fruit if it has weak roots (Matt. 13:6), poor soil (Mark 4:5), lack of water (Job 8:11; Jer. 2:13), and no light (Eph. 4:18). Jesus, then, brings all these ingredients himself, and goes above and beyond in actually grafting us into himself. We aren't the tree, or the vine. He is.

---

[8] Gerald M. Bilkes, *Glory Veiled and Unveiled: A Heart-searching Look at Christ's Parables* (Grand Rapids, MI: Reformation Heritage, 2012), 214.

Therefore, the seven "I am" statements culminate to establish the overarching salvation theme of the New Testament: union with Christ. We are to be in him, and he in us. We are to be through him, and he through us. We will live ("abide") in each other, because through faith we will be mystically united to him, inseparably and irrevocably. This is true life and eternal life, because Jesus lives forever. If we are united to him, hidden with him in God (Col. 3:3) and seated with him in the heavenly places (Eph. 2:6), we are as secure as he is.

Should we seek this life in another way, we will be doomed to fail. Should we even seek to put Christ's teachings in the framework of some other guru or some other religion, we will only compound our brokenness. New wine needs new wineskins (Mark 2:22), or the whole thing will burst open. The situation is as dire as falling headlong into the rocks and having our guts spilling out. We cannot have the new way of Christ in the old way of doubt or works. We cannot have Christ in the way of privatized religion or dead institutionalism or any other way that would seek to dilute what it ought to magnify. What Christ brings in the declaration of himself in all parables and miracles and sermons and atonement is nothing short of newness upon newness, a ransacking of hell and a redeeming of earth in the rescue of sinners and the reverse of the curse. The "I am" statements are "I am" mandates. In the assertion of the seven positives, Jesus announces that he is the antidote to the Adamic poison:

- Where Adam's eating of the forbidden fruit was death, the eating of the bread of Christ's flesh is life.
- Where Adam's sin brought darkness into our hearts and therefore into the world, Jesus brings the light.
- Where Adam's disobedience earned the curse of exile from the garden, its way blocked forever to reentry, Jesus is the door to the eternal garden of new creation.
- Where Adam's disobedience brought into the world exploitation and murder, the un-keeping of our brothers, Jesus is the good shepherd who lays his life down for the sheep.

- Where Adam's disobedience brought corruption and death into the world, Jesus is the resurrection and the life.
- While Adam's disobedience means lostness, lies, and hell, the perfectly obedient Jesus is the way, and the truth, and the life.
- And where Adam's fall brought a curse to the earth, Jesus is the flourishing vine.

All of the "I am" statements reveal where life is found. We cannot have life without Jesus. Bread. Light. Door (through which we are saved). The good shepherd who lays his life down. The resurrection and the life; the way, and the truth, and the life. Now, the true vine.

Oh, Lord, give us this life! Give us the eyes to see and the ears to hear that we would get inside the life of Christ!

## The Living Parable

Jesus is himself a parable. Just as the parables' words may be heard but not heard, seen yet not seen, Jesus is the incarnate Word of God who is either received or rejected. Blessed are those who hear him and believe. Condemned are those who are offended by him and disbelieve.

He is a living parable because he is the inscrutable, eternal, ineffable God become a man, dwelling among men, tempted like men, sacrificed for men. As the parables contain the Spiritual power of awakening or deadening within stories of the human experience, Christ is the Spirit-conceived power of God undergoing the human experience.

Like the other parables, this parable is deceptively complex. The parable of the gospel of Christ is simple enough that a child may believe and deep enough to sustain the life of a countless multitude of saints for all eternity. Here is a mystery: he became one of us that we might become like him.

10

# The Unstoppable and Unfathomable Kingdom

From the outset, in terms of outward appearances, Jesus's ministry was probably not much to look at. The departed carpenter's son had a sketchy pedigree. He selected a ragtag band of young misfits to be his disciples. He preached a revolution not physically carried out. He was dedicated to the bottom rung of society. And yet, the way Mark's Gospel in particular describes his mission, Jesus and these misfits hit the ground running. They evinced a force that could not be contained. Confounding the critics, astonishing the skeptics, and winning the lost, Jesus's ministry is pictured as a juggernaut of Spiritual majesty and victory:

> And he said, "The kingdom of God is as if a man should scatter seed on the ground. He sleeps and rises night and day, and the seed sprouts and grows; he knows not how. The earth produces by itself, first the blade, then the ear, then the full grain in the ear. But when the grain is ripe, at once he puts in the sickle, because the harvest has come."
>
> And he said, "With what can we compare the kingdom of God, or what parable shall we use for it? It is like a grain of mustard seed, which, when sown on the ground, is the smallest of all the seeds on earth, yet when it is sown it grows up and becomes larger than all the garden plants and puts out

> large branches, so that the birds of the air can make nests in its shade."
>
> With many such parables he spoke the word to them, as they were able to hear it. He did not speak to them without a parable, but privately to his own disciples he explained everything. (Mark 4:26–34)

The first of these two complementary parables is unique to Mark's Gospel, and it encapsulates what Mark's Gospel is all about: big power from small beginnings. The idea is expanded in the second parable, which we find also in Matthew's and Luke's Gospels. The smallest seed becomes the largest plant.

Herein are vibrant images of the kingdom and its growth. In the womb of a virgin the God of the universe is conceived by the Spirit. The fullness of deity dwelled embryonically. Into the tiny backwater town of Bethlehem the Lord was delivered. In the village outskirts the Rabbi Jesus began his public ministry. Into a diverse group of young fishermen, tax collectors, and zealots Jesus poured his wisdom. In a hostile and broken world did Jesus's Jewish friends turn everything upside down, even the world itself (Acts 17:6). Why? Because at the cross, Jesus is victor, and from the grave, he is conqueror.

Jesus breaks all the normal rules. He can do this, because he makes the rules. And as he's writing the new chapter in human history with his blood, those accustomed to managing the rules—those "powers that be," those hired hands—are freaking out. Even the citizens of the kingdom are left scratching their heads!

No one could have anticipated this turnaround! We should have. It is forecasted throughout the Old Testament Scriptures. The kingdom of God was the worst-kept secret in history, but it still manages to surprise.

## The Kingdom Is Unfathomable because It Runs Counter to Our Wisdom

The scatterer of the seed "sleeps and rises night and day, and the seed sprouts and grows; he knows not how" (Mark 4:27). This is certainly one way life in the kingdom keeps a Christian humble.

Time and time again we think we know how this thing works, but time and time again we are wrong. Jesus's disciples thought they knew how revolution would come; you bring it by sword. But this is not how the revolution came, and Jesus rebuked those who tried to bring it with physical violence.

Time and time again the church thinks we know how people change. We just tell people to get their act together, of course. And then we are surprised when this doesn't seem to work. Why can't we nag someone into spiritual maturity?

But the more we lead with law, the more we stifle real growth. The more programs we throw at our church, the more inward it becomes. The more strategies we bring to the table, the less Spiritual wisdom holds sway. As that Korean pastor said, "It's amazing what you can accomplish without the Holy Spirit."

We stay busy, brooding, building, asking God to bless our efforts, and then pat ourselves on the back when the Spirit works in spite of our ignorant attempts to quench him.

Time and time again we think we have the killer program, the system, the strategy, the secret for achieving Christian maturity and church growth, but the Bible tells us the Spirit blows where he wills, like the wind (John 3:8). We cannot generate a move of God; otherwise it would be called a move of *us*.

The emphasis today mirrors the emphasis of yesterday. Reach the cream of the crop, plant churches in the power centers, send missionaries to the cultural influencers, convert the CEOs and celebrities, and then you will see "trickle-down" kingdom expansion. Seminary professors warn ministers-in-training away from rural areas and some inner cities. It would be a waste of their talents.[1] It is the same "winner's circle" evangelism strategy I remember from my youth. If you want to see the gospel take over your school, we were encouraged, you must reach the quarterback, the head cheerleader, and the student body president.

Of course, all of these power centers and power people need

---

[1] David Van Biema, "Rural Churches Grapple with a Pastor Exodus," *Time* (January 29, 2009), http://www.time.com/time/magazine/article/0,9171,1874843-1,00.html.

the gospel! We should not *not* take the message of salvation through repentant faith to them. But as a principle it seems to miss the tone of Jesus's ministry, which was largely on the outskirts, among the people on the fringes. Jesus is looking specifically for the forsaken. He is intentionally selecting the weak and foolish. And he builds his church not through entrepreneurial ideas or clever strategies but through his gospel.

This so disturbs us. We want to make things happen!

How do we get people to grow in Christ?

Scatter the seed, we are told.

How does it take root and grow in people's lives?

(shrug)

## The Kingdom Is Unstoppable and Unfathomable because It Grows in Spite of Us

"The earth produces by itself, first the blade, then the ear, then the full grain in the ear" (Mark 4:28).

The seed is scattered, but it grows—apart from pep talks and coaxing. The right conditions for growth are important (Mark 4:1–9), but no seed grows because the sower wills it to do so. "The earth produces by itself." This is a picture of the gospel, which is a power unto itself. It is like a seed that grows. It is purely a work of the Spirit.

The gospel is power:

> For I am not ashamed of the gospel, for it is the power of God for salvation to everyone who believes, to the Jew first and also to the Greek. (Rom. 1:16)

> Of this gospel I was made a minister according to the gift of God's grace, which was given me by the working of his power. (Eph. 3:7)

> [O]ur gospel came to you not only in word, but also in power. (1 Thess. 1:5)

> [T]he gospel . . . has come to you, as indeed in the whole world it is bearing fruit and increasing. (Col. 1:5–6)

You and I can't stop this thing or control it.

Reflecting on the growth of the church in Corinth, Paul writes, "I planted, Apollos watered, but God gave the growth" (1 Cor. 3:6).

Reflecting on the sweeping changes of the Reformation, Martin Luther wrote, "All I have done is to put forth, preach and write the word of God, and apart from this I have done nothing. While I have been sleeping, or drinking Wittenberg beer with my friend Philip and with Amsdorf, it is the word that has done great things. . . . I have done nothing; the word has done and achieved everything."[2]

Or as my friend Ray Ortlund has been known to say, "In Acts, they preached and awe came down. You can't put that in your worship order. 10 a.m.: awe comes down."

"But when the grain is ripe, at once he puts in the sickle, because the harvest has come" (Mark 4:29).

I have the great privilege of pastoring a great church in rural Vermont. One thing an outsider learns about New England rather quickly is that each New England state has its own personality and particular culture. Yet there is something all six New England states share: a general spiritual dryness. There are exceptional corners, of course, places experiencing extraordinary growth in the faith and perhaps even revival. But for the most part, Christians scattered throughout New England are trudging along while fighting off discouragement and praying for a fresh move of God in our region.

I don't know what the Spirit is doing in New England. I don't have a crystal ball. I don't know what he's doing in Rutland County, where my church is located. Sometimes I look around and groan inwardly. I go into the city of Rutland several times a week and the brokenness is palpable. As I mentioned in chapter 8, I see there a dark cloud hanging over the city, even on sunny days.

[2] Gerhard Ebeling, *Luther: An Introduction to His Thought* (Minneapolis: Fortress, 1970), 66–67.

Unemployment and poverty are increasing problems, and therefore so are drugs and other crimes. The young people in Rutland especially seem to share a helplessness, a stuck-ness. The temptation to throw in the towel and give over to hopelessness is huge.

All I know is, according to the parables of the kingdom, it's not my job or anyone else in the church's job to make stuff happen. It's our job to scatter the seed, to nurture the seed, to work hard at sowing the seed, and then to pray and love and laugh and rest while the Spirit does his job in the gospel.

The grain will grow ripe in God's timing.

"And let us not grow weary of doing good, for in due season we will reap, if we do not give up" (Gal. 6:9).

The grain isn't ripe yet, but it will be. The kingdom is unstoppable. No rocky soil of New England will be hard enough to stop it. No sheep of the good shepherd's will be too lost to be found by him. The kingdom of God runs counter to our wisdom and works in spite of us.

## The Kingdom Is Unstoppable and Unfathomable because It Confounds Our Logic

> And he said, "With what can we compare the kingdom of God, or what parable shall we use for it? It is like a grain of mustard seed, which, when sown on the ground, is the smallest of all the seeds on earth." (Mark 4:30–31)

The smallest of all the seeds? Well, not really, but remember the parables are not scientific treatises. They are stories, analogies, parallels employing figures of speech. The mustard seed is really small: that is the point.

Like you and me, the mustard seed is not much to look at. If you were designing a movement to take over the world and claim dominion over the universe, you would not come up with Christianity. Which is why every made-up religion has at its root self-help, self-determination, and self-righteousness. Only Christianity says, "You can't do it, friend. But God will do it for you."

This certainly doesn't appeal to the flesh. It would certainly not produce the grotesque self-worship of Joel Osteen on the "Oprah" show leading the audience in a chant of "I am strong. I am healthy. I am rich." I am being brainwashed.

Grace for sin? Who would have made this up?

The God who delights in making the "smallest seed" his primary means of miracle, that's who.

Israel says, "Gee, thanks for choosing us, God, but we are in the category of nations to sneeze at."

God says, "It was not because you were more in number than any other people that the LORD set his love on you and chose you, for you were the fewest of all peoples" (Deut. 7:7).

Proving the wonders of marvelous grace, God chooses the younger brothers, the spotty brides, the know-nothings and nobodies. He chooses the sinners. It is sinners the Father loves!

And the King?

> [H]e had no form or majesty that we should look at him,
> and no beauty that we should desire him.
> He was despised and rejected by men;
> a man of sorrows, and acquainted with grief;
> and as one from whom men hide their faces
> he was despised, and we esteemed him not. (Isa. 53:2–3)

When the disciples try to shuffle the children off to children's church, the King basically says, "No, let them come. The kingdom is for these nobodies" (Matt. 19:14).

Paul says he came "to preach the gospel, and not with words of eloquent wisdom, lest the cross of Christ be emptied of its power" (1 Cor. 1:17). In 1 Corinthians 2:1–5 he writes:

> And I, when I came to you, brothers, did not come proclaiming to you the testimony of God with lofty speech or wisdom. For I decided to know nothing among you except Jesus Christ and him crucified. And I was with you in weakness and in fear

> and much trembling, and my speech and my message were not in plausible words of wisdom, but in demonstration of the Spirit and of power, so that your faith might not rest in the wisdom of men but in the power of God.

Where ought our faith to rest? Certainly not in our missional logic.

We want to see the kingdom unstoppable and unfathomable, and so logically the emphasis in the evangelical church is on bigness. Big programs, big churches, big people.

Obsession with production, with coolness, with cultural credibility. We forget that Jesus is looking for losers. And what we end up revealing is our fundamental distrust of the gospel.

When you think of all we've thrown at the problem of evangelical decline, of the collegiate Christian dropout problem, of the pitiful level of charitable giving within the church, of the impotence of the church in contemporary society, you'd think we'd realize it's time to admit we are out of ideas and stop coming up with pathetic variations on the old ones. There is nothing new under the sun, brothers and sisters. There are only so many "God at the Movies" and television show tie-ins you can do before you have to stop calling yourself innovative and relevant. The world will always do entertainment better than we can. But it will never have what only we have. Where does our faith rest?

And the beauty of the gospel is that you don't have to be great to wield its power. As we have seen, it actually helps if you're *not* great. Because the gospel's greatness is enough.

Recall the well-worn anecdote about Charles Spurgeon's grandfather James introducing his grandson, saying, "Here comes my famous grandson, Charles. He can preach the gospel better than I can. But you can't preach a better gospel, can you, Charles?"

Commenting on the power and position of the preacher, Paul writes, "And from those who seemed to be influential (what they were makes no difference to me; God shows no partiality)—those, I say, who seemed influential added nothing to me" (Gal. 2:6).

Cheeky! "Sure, sure. Peter, James, and John, those pillars, they *seemed* like somebodies, I guess." I love it!

But is Paul being as disparaging as he appears? Not really, but sort of. Here's Luther on this verse:

> Paul disparages the authority and dignity of the true apostles. He says of them, "Which seemed to be somewhat." The authority of the apostles was indeed great in all the churches. Paul did not want to detract from their authority, but he had to speak disparagingly of their authority in order to conserve the truth of the Gospel. . . .
>
> He answered [the Judaizers]: "What they say has no bearing on the argument. If the apostles were angels from heaven, that would not impress me. We are not now discussing the excellency of the apostles. We are talking about the Word of God now, and the truth of the Gospel. That Gospel is more excellent than all apostles."[3]

"The gospel is more excellent than all apostles." Yes!

You know what? John Piper, Matt Chandler, Mark Dever, Tim Keller, David Platt—these guys and more are (probably) better preachers than you and I. But if your gospel is the Bible's gospel, their gospel isn't any better than yours. We have the same gospel. They can't improve on it any more than you can defuse it.

When we find our attractional lures failing to build, we think we need more aggressive leaders, cleverer visionaries, better talkers. When really what we need is a better word.

If you're a good preacher, you're probably a better speaker than Paul—because Paul himself acknowledged he wasn't an impressive speaker—but if your gospel is the Bible's gospel, it is not your speaking that wakens hearts but the same power that the "unimpressive" Paul set loose.

If you know and speak the gospel, you are a channel for God's destroying of strongholds and resurrecting of lives. Every

[3] Martin Luther, *Commentary on the Epistle to the Galatians*, section on Galatians 2:4–13.

Christian who can articulate the gospel has the launch code and access to the button.

If you preach the gospel, you wield the most powerful word in the universe. It's not the gnosis of the apostles. It's the resurrecting word entrusted to us all.

Through the news of the saving life, death, and resurrection of Jesus Christ, the same God who made us humans from dirt will make a mighty church out of dirty people.

"[W]hen it is sown it grows up and becomes larger than all the garden plants and puts out large branches, so that the birds of the air can make nests in its shade" (Mark 4:32).

Here is a picture of rest but also of the gathering of the resters. The tiny seed grows into a kingdom that will welcome people from every tongue, tribe, race, and nation.

And here is a truth that is humbling and empowering at the same time: God's will might be for our smallness, but it is not for his. So like the forerunner John the Baptist, we must agree to say, "He must increase, but I must decrease" (John 3:30).

The kingdom of God is unstoppable and unfathomable because it grows exponentially. Everywhere the gospel goes, the gospel is doing its work. As the sowers scatter the seed—preaching the gospel, testifying to its truth with their good works, making disciples, planting churches, sending out sowers to replicate the work in new places—the branches begin to grow out, spreading to embrace the sun of righteousness that gives them life. And the disciples make disciples who make disciples. And the churches plant churches that plant churches. And the gospel does not return void. The whole world will eventually be covered with the knowledge of the glory of God, every nook and cranny gleaming with the celestial beauty of our faithful Redeemer.

Isaiah says the holy seed may look like a stump (Isa. 6:13), what results from cutting a tree down; from that stump will come forth a shoot (Isa. 11:1), the righteous branch. Jeremiah says the righteous branch will reign as king (Jer. 23:5). Jesus says, "I am the vine"

(John 15:5). From humble and apparently dead beginnings comes the world-swallowing be-all and end-all.

## The Attitude and Latitude of Christ's Kingdom

> With many such parables he spoke the word to them, as they were able to hear it. He did not speak to them without a parable, but privately to his own disciples he explained everything. (Mark 4:33–34)

Here is a sweet glimpse into Jesus's pastoral heart. And it is a revelation of two senses of his ministry in relation to the disciples. "As they were able to hear it" shows us that they *were* able to hear it. It also shows us that Jesus spoke *when* they were able to hear it. The Word gave them the ears to hear the word.

Jesus is an unparalleled sower, and the kingdom is growing ultimately because Jesus is tending to its growth. Even now, through his Spirit, he is tending to the exponential growth of the kingdom. "When the Spirit of truth comes, he will guide you into all the truth" (John 16:13).

The Spirit of God is still building his people, still carrying them along, still equipping them for every good work, still ministering to them and helping them. Yes, he who began a good work in you will be faithful to complete it (Phil. 1:6). And the gates of hell will not prevail against it (Matt. 16:18).

In fact, the gospel is always scaled to eternity, even in our lean seasons and times of suffering. Eternal life means exactly that—eternal. Declared from the foundation of the world, promised in the covenant, secured by the incarnated and crucified and risen and glorified and ascended and reigning and returning Son, granted by the Holy Spirit, guaranteed in heaven where no moth or rust can destroy. Foreknown by the Father, merited by the Son, and sealed by the Spirit, there is eternity written in the Christian's heart, such that he *will* find it out. If you are in Christ now, you have that life *now*. You are now a citizen of heaven (Phil. 3:20).

With this reality in heart and mind, we can be tuned to the

deep joy of the in-breaking kingdom. This kind of happiness is at hand at all times. Even when the harvest seems pitiful, there is joy in heaven. Remember that found sheep, that found coin, that found son.

Brought by faithful sowers to the far places and the low, the gospel of Jesus conducts heavenly business, spreading heavenly happiness. Couched in heaven's invasion of earth and heaven's vindication of earth, how could it not? As Lesslie Newbigin writes, "Mission begins with a kind of explosion of joy."[4] The juggernauty growth of the gospel (Col. 1:6) requires newness all around. It is bursting through our lives and structures. It is utterly transformative. This is what we see in the breakneck pace with which Mark records the Gospel where we find these seed parables. He wants us to see (1) the absolute depths of joy and (2) the extraordinary wideness of transformation this joy has. The sheer authority of Jesus's teaching results in deliverance, healing, restoration, and resurrection. How come?

> Now John's disciples and the Pharisees were fasting. And people came and said to him, "Why do John's disciples and the disciples of the Pharisees fast, but your disciples do not fast?" And Jesus said to them, "Can the wedding guests fast while the bridegroom is with them? As long as they have the bridegroom with them, they cannot fast. The days will come when the bridegroom is taken away from them, and then they will fast in that day. No one sews a piece of unshrunk cloth on an old garment. If he does, the patch tears away from it, the new from the old, and a worse tear is made. And no one puts new wine into old wineskins. If he does, the wine will burst the skins—and the wine is destroyed, and so are the skins. But new wine is for fresh wineskins." (Mark 2:18–22)

How is this talk of cloths and wineskins connected to the question about fasts? I think it goes something like this:

---

[4] Lesslie Newbigin, *The Gospel in a Pluralist Society* (Grand Rapids, MI: Eerdmans, 1989), 116.

The Mosaic law really required only one regular fast. The others that occupied the Jewish calendar grew up around traditions—not bad things in and of themselves. It is possible that John's disciples were fasting because he had already been either imprisoned or executed. They likely fasted out of mourning. The disciples of the Pharisees likely fasted out of tradition, which became an idol for many of them (see Luke 18:12). One kind of fasting (grief, expectation) was legitimate, the other not. But Jesus's disciples weren't going with the flow of the traditions, mainly because they had nothing to grieve (yet) and no merit to glory in. They had Messiah, and having Messiah means having fullness of joy (John 15:11).

Jesus goes on to connect the man-made traditions and ceremonies to outdated structures not suitable for the new wine of the gospel. This joy is growing, going forth into the world and bearing fruit. It cannot be grafted onto brittle, inflexible institutions. The gospel is not just for Jews but for Greeks as well. It is for the unclean, the ungodly, and the outcasts. (It's for the losers!) All that came before is fulfilled now in Christ. The light by nature cannot be confined to the shadows. It must spill out, shine forth.

There is a time to fast (cf. Ecclesiastes 3), but those united to Christ are to be typified not by grief but by joy, even in hardship (Hab. 3:17–18; Rom. 12:12; Phil. 4:4; 1 Thess. 5:16; 1 Pet. 4:13). This means that joy must run *deep*. And if joy runs deep, it will overflow and run wide.

When we have this deep joy, we navigate seasons of suffering and brokenness with both the firmness of faith and the flexibility of it. We are able to confidently say, "This day"—with all its troubles—"is the day the LORD has made; let us rejoice and be glad in it" (Ps. 118:24). Because we know that the joy is so deep, it will buoy our souls for all eternity.

The ferment of the gospel needs the wineskin of the church, which shall be made up of all peoples. The Jewish ceremonial laws and temple system are no longer sufficient for the purposes of God's glory covering the whole earth as the waters cover the sea.

The ferment of the gospel needs the wineskin of missional

adaptability. Our traditions and structures must serve the joy of Christ and his kingdom, not the other way around.

The ferment of gospel joy needs the wineskin of new hearts (Ps. 119:32; Ezek. 36:26; 2 Cor. 6:13). We must be born again to be a new creation.

As we look to however many more days God will grant us, for ourselves as Christians and for our churches, let us commit to proclamation of the gospel, that it would settle deep into our bones, soaking into the marrow, enlarging our hearts that we might run in spreading the news that Christ is King, casting aside all that hinders us, including even religious, churchy things.

And when the gospel changes our attitude to depths of joy, it will change the latitude of our missional boundaries to widespread transformation. This is the joy inexpressible and full of glory (1 Pet. 1:8).

This is the world into which the parables are windows. We see in these little stories that God's big biblical story of redemption—the joyful restoration of the cosmos, the joyful expansion of the sovereignty of King Jesus, and the joyful redemption of sinful exiles—is coming true. It is coming true through and in and by Jesus.

Even so, come quickly, Lord Jesus!

# Conclusion

N. T. Wright has said that writing a book about the Bible is like building a sand castle at the base of the Matterhorn. True. This is my experience in writing this book about the parables. I have not sought to provide much academic commentary. That is for the scholars. I have not sought to plow new ground or offer new insights. You should be as skeptical of new ideas about the Bible as I am. I have only tried to show what the parables mean in as plain a way as I can and thereby glorify the Teller of the parables as well as I can.

French psychoanalyst Jacques Lacan explored the concept of the "irruption of the real," typically referring to the moment a traumatic event interrupts life as usual, stripping away the artifice and projection of our routines to bring us face-to-face with our stark mortality, the existence of suffering, and the depths of fears and feelings we normally ignore or subdue. 9/11 is often referred to as an irruption of the real. The Sandy Hook Elementary School murders in Newtown, Connecticut, were an irruption of the real. But a divorce or the death of a loved one can be an irruption of the real, too. I bring this point home at every funeral I preach. "Your life has been interrupted now; your attention is focused because of this loss," I say to the gathered grieving. "And now this is what God has to say to you about death and what happens next."

The parables in their own way are irruptions of the real. This despite the fact that they are fictions. The stories Jesus told nevertheless are insertions of powerful truth meant to shake people awake. They are smart bombs, full of explosive life to those who would embrace the power behind them. The way these stories upend life as we know it is spiritually discombobulating, but for those with the eyes to see and ears to hear, the parables give great comfort. They are snapshots of the blessed hope, visions of the now-dawning future. The way they turn life inside out shows us in fact how life was ill-fitting all along. The parables show us the glory of the Lord who was and is and is to come.

In this sense, then, these irruptions of the real are signs of eucatastrophe. The eucatastrophe, according to tale-teller J. R. R. Tolkien, is the moment "of the good catastrophe, the sudden joyous 'turn',"[1] the moment that "denies (in the face of much evidence, if you will) universal final defeat and in so far is *evangelium*, giving a fleeting glimpse of Joy, Joy beyond the walls of the world."[2] The eucatastrophe is the moment in a story when all heaven breaks loose. It is a beautiful unraveling. It is, to borrow from Tolkien's Samwise Gamgee, the moment when "everything sad comes untrue."[3] For Tolkien,

> The Gospels . . . contain many marvels—peculiarly artistic, beautiful, and moving: 'mythical' in their perfect, self-contained significance; and at the same time powerfully symbolic and allegorical; and among the marvels is the greatest and most complete conceivable eucatastrophe. The Birth of Christ is the eucatastrophe of the story of Man's history. The Resurrection is the eucatastrophe of the story of the Incarnation. The story begins and ends in joy.[4]

What a great description of the parables and their purpose: artistic, beautiful, and moving. Mythical but real. Fiction but truth. Powerfully symbolic and allegorical (in a sense), but revelations of

---

[1] J. R. R. Tolkien, "On Fairy-Stories," in *Essays Presented to Charles Williams*, ed. C. S. Lewis (Grand Rapids, MI: Eerdmans, 1973), 81.

[2] Ibid.

[3] See J. R. R. Tolkien, *The Return of the King* (New York: Ballantine, 1987), 283. Sam's actual words were, "Is everything sad going to come untrue?"

[4] Tolkien, "On Fairy-Stories," 83.

the very true, very literal kingdom of God. The parables highlight the keys to life and death; they are postcards from the world of eternal glory.

One way the parables show us this glory is by showing in "real life" scenarios how there is this in fact *realer* life to be had. The stories reveal the deeper reality that gives the Christian "more than conqueror" status and "never die" confidence. They reveal the everyday realer life by which missionaries like Romanian pastor Josef Tson operate. Many of us first heard of Tson thanks to David Platt's message "Divine Sovereignty: The Fuel of Death-defying Missions" delivered at the 2012 Together 4 the Gospel Conference.[5] In his sermon, Platt quoted from an autobiographical article by Tson in *To Every Tribe* magazine in which Tson recounts being interrogated by six men. He said to one of them,

> What is taking place here is not an encounter between you and me. . . . This is an encounter between my God and me. . . . My God is teaching me a lesson. I do not know what it is. Maybe he wants to teach me several lessons. I only know, sir, that you will do to me only what He wants you to do—and you will not go one inch further—because you are simply an instrument of my God.[6]

Tson added, "[I saw] those six pompous men as my Father's puppets!"[7]

Of another incident, he said,

> During an earlier interrogation at Ploiesti I had told an officer who threatened to kill me, "Sir, let me explain how I see this issue. Your supreme weapon is killing. My supreme weapon is dying. Here is how it works. You know that my sermons on tape have spread all over the country. If you kill me, those

[5] David Platt, "Divine Sovereignty: The Fuel of Death-defying Missions," Together 4 the Gospel Conference (Louisville, Kentucky, 2012), http://t4g.org/media/2012/05/divine-sovereignty-the-fuel-of-death-defying-missions-2/.

[6] Josef Tson, "Thank You for the Beating," *To Every Tribe* (Fall 2009), 4–5, http://www.toeverytribe.com/uploads/TETM-Fall09.pdf.

[7] Ibid., 5.

> sermons will be sprinkled with my blood. Every-one will know I died for my preaching. And everyone who has a tape will pick it up and say, 'I'd better listen again to what this man preached, because he really meant it: he sealed it with his life.' So, sir, my sermons will speak 10 times louder than before. I will actually rejoice in this supreme victory if you kill me."
>
> He sent me home.
>
> Another officer who was interrogating a pastor friend of mine told him, "We know that Mr. Tson would love to be a martyr, but we are not that foolish to fulfill his wish."
>
> I stopped to consider the meaning of that statement. I remembered how for many years, I had been afraid of dying. I had kept a low profile. Because I wanted badly to live, I had wasted my life in inactivity. But now that I had placed my life on the altar and decided I was ready to die for the gospel, they were telling me they would not kill me! I could go wherever I wanted in the country and preach whatever I wanted, knowing I was safe. As long as I tried to save my life, I was losing it. Now that I was willing to lose it, I found it.[8]

This testimony from the persecuted church is a real-life parable of the kingdom life showcased in the parables. These Spirit-powered stories Jesus told reveal the glory of the life to be had by those willing to join up with the Son on his mission to save the lost, make all things new, and deliver it all brimming with infinite joy to the Father in the age to come. The parables are postcards from the saving saboteur.

Let him who has the ears hear. There is a revolution afoot.

[8] Ibid., 8.

# General Index

# Scripture Index

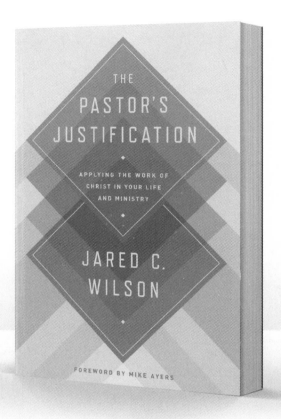